THE BEST KEPT SECRET TO PERMANENT WEIGHT LOSS

BARNET MELTZER, M.D.
JORDAN MELTZER

Published by Dr. Know • How Publications
1011 Camino Del Mar, Suite 234
Del Mar, CA 92014

Printed in the United States of America

ISBN: 978-0-9609040-4-4

The Best Kept Secret to Permanent Weight Loss

Acknowledgements

THE AUTHORS GRATEFULLY acknowledge the support of loved ones, friends, and patients who are in great measure responsible for the success of this book. Special thanks to Sky Meltzer, Brock Meltzer, Jessica Meltzer, Kristina Meltzer, Melanie Meltzer, Janice Johnson, and Marc Assaraf. Their contributions, inspiration, and support for this book will always be remembered.

CONTENTS

Part III: The Inner Strengths of Permanent Weight Loss

Introduction

LET me ask you a very important question. When it comes to losing weight, are you looking for short-term results or long-term results? That is, are you looking to lose your excess weight and not regain it? Great...then this book is for you. If you have previously tried to lose weight, you are probably familiar with the cycle of weight loss and weight gain. It goes something like this. You lose some weight—you may even maintain your new weight for a respectable amount of time—but eventually the weight has a way of making its way back. It's a frustrating, self-defeating cycle. For most people, losing weight is a challenge, yet keeping the weight off is even more difficult. I have good news for you. It doesn't have to be difficult and it doesn't have to be a struggle. I've written this book to demystify the weight-loss process. *The Best Kept Secret to Permanent Weight Loss* is your owner's manual to outsmart your weight gain and put an end to the cycle of weight loss and recurrent weight gain. ***The secret in this book will guide you to lose the weight you need to lose and keep it off, once and for all.***

It Can Be Done...You Can Do It

The purpose of this book is simple—to empower you with the tools to lose weight *permanently*, safely, and effectively. The emphasis on *permanent* weight loss is an important distinction I want to make. It is time you know the truth about the weight-loss industry. Unfortunately, most diets and weight-loss programs are not designed for long-term results. Whenever you see or hear of a diet or weight-loss program on the radio, the T.V., or the internet, they all make similar claims about losing weight. There is just one problem. They leave out that the weight loss they promise is ***temporary***. I see the repercussions of this all the time in my medical practice. Oftentimes, my patients are referred to me after several attempts—and sometimes lifelong attempts—to lose weight. Inevitably, one of the first questions they ask is "Dr. Meltzer, what is so different about this weight-loss plan that makes it a permanent weight-loss solution?" You may be wondering the same thing. Let me give you a firsthand account of what I tell my patients in their first visit.

You Have a Choice

Carrying excess weight is like being in a fifteen foot ditch. You can choose a weight-loss plan that helps you out of the ditch, or you can get caught in a cycle of losing and regaining your weight and dig yourself further in the ditch. You see, when it comes to losing weight, you have a choice. You can choose whether you are interested in losing weight for the short term, or if you are interested in long-term, permanent weight loss. If you are interested in losing weight for the short term, let me share with you something very interesting. It doesn't matter what you eat; just about every diet that has ever been invented works… *temporarily!* In fact, don't even bother picking up a diet book, because you can save some money and make up your own diet. It can be a cookie diet, an ice cream diet, a pretzel diet, a popcorn diet, an all-carbs diet, a no-carbs diet, and everything and anything in between. All you have to do is restrict your calorie intake, exercise a little bit, and you will undoubtedly lose some weight. That's right, if you are looking for a short-term solution, there are literally thousands of ways to lose weight, and they all work! They just don't work long term. They don't get you out of the ditch. Let me explain.

Prioritize Your Metabolism

So what is the difference between a short-term program and a permanent weight-loss plan? For short-term results, you can focus on calorie counting, better known as dieting. For long-term results, the emphasis needs to be on your metabolism—and the calorie and fat burning functions of your metabolism. You see, restricting calories, by its very nature, is unsustainable. Once you go back to eating normally, and even if you moderate what you eat, a slow or inefficient metabolism will inevitably cause you to gain back all of your weight and oftentimes more. To make matters worse, you will likely have done further damage to your metabolism and will be worse off than when you started. On the other hand, naturally accelerating your metabolism—so you can effectively burn through your meals and excess fat at an accelerated rate—is sustainable and leads to a lifetime of being fit and trim. ***What most people don't realize is they have the power to change their metabolism.*** Everyone can do it. That's right, everyone can change their metabolism.

That's essentially what I tell my patients. If you want a temporary weight-loss solution, you can focus on quantity of food intake like every other diet and weight-loss program out there, and unknowingly be digging yourself deeper in the ditch. If you want to lose weight permanently, the emphasis needs to be on your metabolism. Let me assure you that there is a science to naturally accelerating your metabolism. Over the past four decades, I have guided thousands of people of all ages, genders, and walks of life through this process. In this book, I'll give you the tools to transform your metabolism to achieve a naturally accelerated metabolic rate that burns through your meals and excess fat with ease, so you can achieve and maintain your ideal body weight. By the time you finish, not only will you understand what the underlying causes are of weight gain, obesity, and failed weight-loss attempts, but you will also be equipped with all of the knowledge, strategy, and support that you will ever need to achieve permanent weight loss.

Metabolic Fire is the Secret

To achieve permanent weight loss you are going to need Metabolic Fire. Yes, the best-kept secret to permanent weight loss is ***achieving*** and ***sustaining*** Metabolic Fire, the fire in your metabolism. You see, the fire in your metabolism burns food and body fat like the fire in a furnace burns wood. ***Therefore, I've coined the term "Metabolic Fire" to describe your body's ability to effectively burn carbohydrates and fats.*** It is a way of expressing a spirited metabolism. When you own Metabolic Fire, you have a healthy, wholesome metabolism that turns your nutritional fuel into energy instead of storing it as fat. It's simple really. The stronger your Metabolic Fire, the easier it is to burn through your meals, burn excess body fat, and achieve and maintain your ideal bodyweight. When you own Metabolic Fire, it's a simple matter to own permanent weight loss.

What I've realized is that, without an effective metabolism and without the necessary Metabolic Fire, it takes too much effort—in fact, it's a losing effort—to try to sustain any kind of weight-loss results. For thousands upon thousands, losing weight becomes a lifelong struggle of calorie counting and constant worrying about food intake. Even with the best attitude and strongest intention, losing weight and keeping it off can start to feel like a burdensome, uphill battle. In the end, without developing this Metabolic Fire, your weight-loss efforts become a source of frustration, a waste of your time, and more often than not, a waste of your money.

Let me share with you how you can achieve and sustain Metabolic Fire—and lose your excess weight for good.

The Three Pillars of Permanent Weight Loss

To achieve and sustain Metabolic Fire you are going to need to rely on the three pillars of permanent weight loss. Together, they build the bridge to permanent weight loss and your ideal weight.

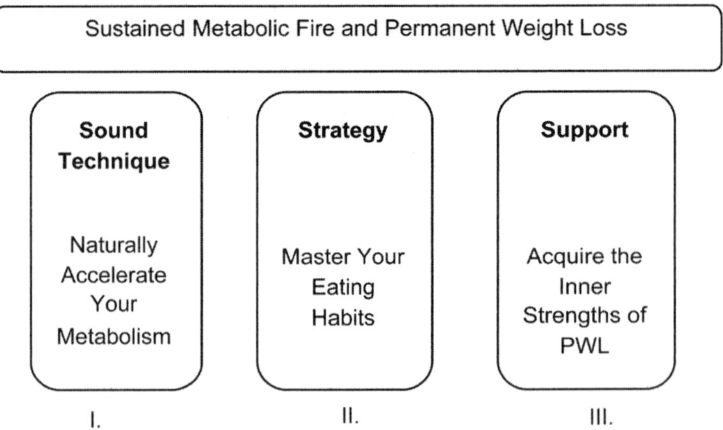

This program is unique. It is the only program that addresses how to naturally increase your metabolic rate while at the same time teaches you how to master your eating habits and acquire the inner strengths of permanent weight loss. In fact, these three pillars serve as the measuring stick for any permanent weight-loss (PWL) plan. Why is that? Because they *fully* address the two root causes of weight gain, obesity, and failed weight-loss attempts.

Root Causes of Weight Gain and Obesity:
• **Root Cause #1 - *Metabolic Dysfunction*** Metabolic dysfunction is a fancy way of describing a slow metabolism that has a tendency to store the food you eat as body fat. When you have a slow metabolism, managing your weight becomes a constant struggle of calorie counting and worrying about what you eat.
• **Root Cause #2 – *Emotional Overeating*** Emotional eating is the driving force behind overeating, cravings, food indulgences, poor food selection, and dysfunctional eating habits that undermine and derail most people's weight-loss efforts.

Together, the three pillars of permanent weight loss provide the sound technique, strategy, and support to overcome the root causes of weight gain and help you reach your weight-loss goals. Without these three pillars, you are merely trying to lose weight, not lose weight *permanently*.

Pillar I. Sound Technique: Learn How to Naturally Accelerate Your Metabolism

The first pillar to permanent weight loss is learning how to naturally accelerate your metabolism. The right technique keeps the fire burning. In other words, the nutritional plan and exercise program you follow need to be effective in the following areas:

- Accelerating your metabolism
- Shedding unwanted pounds
- Supporting your overall health and well-being

This may sound simple enough. In all of my time as a physician, however, I have not come across a single weight-loss program, except for ours, that satisfies all three criteria. The great majority of fad diets and weight-loss programs are geared toward short-term, unsustainable weight-loss results that compromise your metabolism and your health in the process.

Here's the good news. The technique I provide in this book works. It will work for you today, it will work for you tomorrow, and it will work for you years from now when you'll have a hard time remembering what it felt like to carry excess weight. This program will most certainly light your Metabolic Fire. By following our permanent weight-loss program, you will naturally accelerate your metabolism, burn your excess fat, look better, and feel better than you can imagine. All the while, this program will be promoting your long-term health, energy, and vitality. I have coached people of all ages and all backgrounds through this program and have watched them achieve their ideal weight, live their dreams, and change their lives forever. I am confident this program will do the same for you!

In part I, "How to Naturally Accelerate Your Metabolism," I will introduce you to this time-honored technique. This part of the book is divided into two distinct sections that you should be aware of. The first section, "LYF-Style Factors that Influence Your Metabolism," reviews the science behind why the program works to naturally accelerate your metabolism. The actual technique of your weight-loss plan comes in the second section, which we affectionately refer to throughout the book as the "Marching Orders." The Marching Orders takes into consideration all of the underlying information reviewed in "LYF-Style Factors that Influence Your Metabolism," and puts it together in an easy to follow, step-by-step weight-loss plan.

Pillar II. Strategy: Learn how to Master Your Eating Habits

What good is sound technique if you can't follow through on it? Not very good. This is particularly true when it comes to permanent weight loss. That's why you need a strategy. I came to this simple but important realization one day as I was sitting in my medical clinic in Del Mar, California. You see, despite knowing what to do, I observed that most of my patients had a difficult time being consistent with their eating habits. There were seemingly endless factors that, at one point or another, could derail their efforts and keep them from doing what they knew was best. Some were plagued with negative eating habits that were unconsciously learned in childhood and that took root through their adult life—such as using food as a reward system, for entertainment, or for emotional comfort. Others would become emotional overeaters or turn to food in the face of stress, emotional tension, anxiety, boredom, or bad moods. To top it off, the temptation and distraction of fast foods, junk foods, sweets, chocolate, cookies, ice cream, chips, crackers, and cheeses were sometimes too much for them to bear. It became clear to me that they needed help—they needed a strategy. They needed a system for overcoming negative eating habits that were deeply ingrained in their personal, social, and cultural upbringings.

In part II, "Master Your Eating Habits," I will take you through the strategies you can use to establish positive eating habits, so you can follow through on your permanent weight-loss plan. In this part of the book, you'll have the chance to become familiar with and size up your eating habits. Several quizzes and surveys will help you through this self-discovery process. You will then be introduced to the Golden Rules of Smart Eating. The Golden Rules will give you the strategies you need to eat well and to overcome the most common dysfunctional eating habits, which are notorious for undermining people's weight-loss goals.

Do you have a tendency to overeat? Do your cravings have a way of dictating your food selection? Do you find yourself indulging in food late at night or when you are lonely or bored? Not to worry. You can rely on the strategies outlined in "Master Your Eating Habits" to say good-bye to any self-destructive eating patterns that are holding you back from your slimmer, fitter, more confident self.

Pillar III. Support: Acquire the Inner Strengths of Permanent Weight Loss

Support is magical. With the right support in your life, it feels like you can accomplish anything. Support plays an integral role in permanent weight loss as well. The proper support will give your weight-loss plan lasting power. Through the ups and downs, the thick and the thin, you can rely on the right support to keep you on track. Support will give you the extra conviction you need to achieve and maintain your ideal weight.

Interestingly, when most people think of support, they think of social support—support from friends, loved ones, trainers, and coaches. This kind of support is important. However, that is not the kind of support that is ultimately going to get you the permanent results that you are looking for. So what kind of support could I be talking about? The type of support systems that you'll need to develop need to come from within—your own intrapersonal support systems. These support systems lie dormant within us all. They can come alive. It's just a matter of getting in touch with them and cultivating them. ***That's right—you are your most important support system!***

In part III, "The Inner Strengths of Permanent Weight Loss," we'll focus on developing your internal support systems, which will empower you to stick to the techniques and strategies outlined in parts I and II. We'll focus on developing the right belief systems that support self-empowering actions and self-enriching behaviors. We'll teach you how you can feed your mind, feed your heart, and feed your soul, so you won't be so preoccupied with filling yourself with food. We'll show you how to develop the essential inner strengths of Mind Power, Mood Power, and Soul Power. With these inner strengths on your side, you'll have the necessary support systems to overcome the restlessness, temptations, distractions, anxiety, and fatigue that have a way of antagonizing most people's weight-loss efforts.

Desire

Ok. So I said there were only three pillars to establishing and sustaining Metabolic Fire, and losing weight permanently. There is one more dimension that you need to know about. And it is an important one. The last component that you are going to need is something that I can't give you. I will do my best to inspire you throughout this process, but there is one final thing that you must bring to the table. It is your motivation. It is your intention. You have to want it. If you have a deep down desire to lose weight, then you and I can accomplish what we have set out to do—*achieve permanent weight loss!*

The Hole-in-the-Bucket Syndrome

If you have previously tried to lose weight and were unsuccessful, I don't want you to be discouraged. It's no secret that most diets and weight-loss programs fail. In fact, government studies have shown that 97 percent of diets and weight-loss programs fail to provide long-term results. Why is it that almost all of them are unsustainable? They are not focusing on the underlying causes of weight gain and obesity—metabolic dysfunction and emotional overeating. The weight-loss industry is suffering from what I like to call the hole-in-the-bucket syndrome. If you had a hole in a bucket, and you wanted to try to keep the bucket full of water, would it make more sense to try to continually pour more water into the bucket or fix the hole in the first place? Clearly, in the long run, it would take much less effort and be much more sustainable to repair the hole in the bucket.

The problem is, the weight-loss industry comes up with new ways every day of telling you how you can add more water to the bucket. Fad diets have people running around in a frenzy trying different ways to fill their buckets. This has resulted in a misleading and vicious cycle of weight loss, weight gain, and yo-yo dieting. How is it that no one is trying to fix the underlying problem and repair the hole in the bucket? The time has come to put an end to this cycle. The time has come to fix the hole in the bucket. The time has come to put an emphasis back on your metabolism and the three pillars of permanent weight loss.

Congratulations! You are about to embark on a journey. Committing to this process may be the best gift that you can ever give yourself. I hope you are excited. I have helped thousands of people through this process and I am excited for you.

How to Use This Book

FIRST off, I want to say congratulations! By reading this book, you are taking your first step toward losing weight and keeping it off for good. Our program is very results-oriented. To get the best results, it's well advised to take a gradual but consistent approach. Our weight-loss program is organized in three-month intervals. You can expect to lose fifteen to twenty-five pounds in the first six to ten weeks. Thereafter, you can expect to lose approximately two pounds a week or eight to ten pounds a month. It typically averages out to about twenty-five pounds of weight loss for every three months. In this manner, you will rejuvenate your metabolism and set yourself up for permanent results.

Therefore, expect to lose twenty-five pounds within the first three months. For every additional twenty-five pounds you are looking to lose, expect it to take an additional three months. For example, when you need to lose fifty pounds, expect it to take four to six months. If you are looking to lose seventy-five pounds, expect it to take seven to nine months. If you are looking to lose one hundred pounds, expect it to take ten to twelve months. The rate at which you lose the weight has to do with how closely you follow the program.

Keep in mind that there is a three-step process to permanent weight loss and establishing and sustaining Metabolic Fire. The process includes the following:

i. Naturally Accelerating Your Metabolism

ii. Mastering Your Eating Habits

iii. Acquiring the Inner Strengths of Permanent Weight Loss

These three pillars of permanent weight loss work together to teach you everything you need to know and everything you need to do to achieve and maintain your ideal weight. Let me tell you the best way to incorporate these key components to put your permanent weight-loss program into action.

The following table outlines what you would need to do for the first three months, assuming you were looking to lose twenty-five pounds. To achieve your goals, you will need a week-by-week nutritional program, weekly tactical strategies, and technical support. Here's how you do it.

Illustrative Three-Month Schedule for Twenty-five Pounds Weight Loss

Week	**Nutritional Program: What to Eat**	**Tactical Strategy and Technical Support: What to Do**
1	Power Cleansing • Read chapter 10	• How to Naturally Accelerate Your Metabolism – Read LYF-Style Factors 1–3
2	Nutritional Detox • Read chapter 11	• How to Naturally Accelerate Your Metabolism – Read LYF-Style Factors 4–7
3	Nutritional Detox	• Master Your Eating Habits – Read chapters 1–5
4	Nutritional Detox	• Master Your Eating Habits – Read chapter 6
5	Nutritional Detox	• Master Your Eating Habits – Read chapter 7
6	Nutritional Detox	• Master Your Eating Habits – Review chapters 6–7
7	Nutritional Detox	• Inner Strengths of Permanent Weight Loss – Read Introduction and Mind Power
8	Nutritional Detox	• Inner Strengths of Permanent Weight Loss – Review Mind Power
9	Nutritional Detox	• Inner Strengths of Permanent Weight Loss – Read Soul Power
10	Nutritional Detox	• Inner Strengths of Permanent Weight Loss – Review Soul Power

11	Nutritional Detox	• Inner Strengths of Permanent Weight Loss – Read Mood Power
12	Nutritional Detox	• Inner Strengths of Permanent Weight Loss – Review Mood Power
13	LYF Maintenance Plan • Read chapter 12	• How to Naturally Accelerate Your Metabolism – Read chapter 12, LYF Maintenance Plan

***Important Notes

1. If you reach your ideal weight before week 13, transition over to the LYF Maintenance Plan; however, continue studying the tactical strategies and technical support that correspond with each subsequent week.

2. If you have more than twenty-five pounds to lose, keep cycling the above schedule in consecutive three-month intervals for every additional twenty-five pounds you have to lose.

    a. It is well advised to go back to Power Cleansing for the first week of every three-month cycle.
    b. Also, upon a new three-month cycle, continue to review the tactical strategies and technical support corresponding with each given week to reaffirm your understanding and reassess your progress.

3. Once you reach your ideal weight, you can transition into the LYF Maintenance Plan.

    a. LYF Maintenance is described in detail in your Marching Orders in chapter 12.
    b. Keep in mind, when you reach the LYF Maintenance Plan, it is recommended that you cleanse for five days every quarter, at the time of the seasonal change. This cleansing will give you a chance to fine-tune your metabolism every three months.

Highlights of the First Three Months

Weeks 1–2

In weeks 1 and 2, you will go through one week of Power Cleansing and then transition to Nutritional Detox, as detailed in your Marching Orders. During this two-week period, I'd like you to read through "LYF-Style Factors that Influence Your Metabolism" so you can get a better understanding of why the program works. Pay particularly close attention to LYF-Style Factors #1 and #2, which will give you a strong working knowledge of your exercise plan and nutritional program. I have found that the better understanding my patients have of the underlying rationale for the weight-loss program, the more conviction they have in making the necessary changes to their eating, exercise, and living habits. You'll find that each chapter provides a one-page summary that highlights all of the major concepts and how they apply to your weight-loss plan.

Weeks 3–6

In addition to following your nutritional program as outlined in your Marching Orders, I want you to take these four weeks to study "Master Your Eating Habits." You will get a chance to size up your eating habits and become familiar with and identify your most harmful eating habits. In addition, you'll read about the Golden Rules of Smart Eating, which will give you the eating habit strategies you'll need to achieve permanent weight loss. Note well, it will be important for you to incorporate these pre-meal, mealtime, and post-meal strategies into your daily routine. You will also be introduced to the RIEXA technique, which will help you overcome your most vulnerable dysfunctional eating habits, such as overeating, cravings, and late-night food indulgences that can get in the way of your weight-loss goals.

Weeks 7–12

Continue to follow your nutritional program as outlined in your Marching Orders. In addition, take these next 6 weeks to learn about the Inner Strengths of Permanent Weight Loss and start cultivating your internal support systems. This final piece of the puzzle will solidify your permanent weight-loss plan.

You will need to rely on your mind power, soul power, and mood power to get long-term results. Allow yourself time for self-analysis and self-discovery. Be sure to practice the tangible action steps that accompany each chapter. In time, your inner strengths will be one of your greatest allies in helping you achieve and maintain your weight-loss goals.

ADDITIONAL RESOURCES AND SUPPORT

THIS book was intended to give you all of the information, tools, strategy, and support to lose your excess weight and keep it off for good. We do have additional resources, products, and services that we recommend for those interested in additional coaching, guidance, motivation, accountability, and support.

- **Additional Recipes and Online Support**—Be sure to check out our website for additional free resources, including recipes for Power Cleansing, Nutritional Detox, and LYF Maintenance.

  www.maketimeforwellness.com

- ***The Best Kept Secret to Permanent Weight Loss*** **(CD set)**—This CD set is designed to accompany the book. In addition to being motivational, the CDs will highlight the key principles of each chapter that you will need to focus on. If you purchased the book separately, make sure to check out our website for ordering information for the CDs.

  www.maketimeforwellness.com

- **Online Permanent Weight-Loss Program**—Our online weight-loss program is a great, cost effective way to get additional guidance and support for your weight-loss plan. Weekly video lessons will take you through a step-by-step process for naturally accelerating your metabolism, mastering your eating habits, and acquiring the inner strengths of permanent weight loss. If you are interested in more information regarding our online weight-loss program, please visit our website.

www.maketimeforwellness.com

- **Permanent Weight-Loss Coaching Services**—We offer a variety of weight-loss coaching services to provide you with personalized guidance, support, and accountability in working your way through our permanent weight-loss program. Make sure to check out our website for more information on our different weight-loss coaching programs.

  www.maketimeforwellness.com

- **Nutritional Supplementation / Super-Nutrients**—The super-nutrients we recommend as part of our weight-loss program can be found on our website as well.

  www.maketimeforwellness.com

Part I

How to Naturally Accelerate Your Metabolism for Permanent Weight Loss

SECTION I

LYF-Style Factors That Influence Your Metabolism

1

Introduction to the Light Your Fire "LYF" Permanent Weight-Loss Program

YOUR ability to burn body fat and keep it off has everything to do with your long-term results. This part of the book shows you how you can naturally accelerate your metabolism and increase your metabolic rate—a necessary and powerful step toward achieving permanent weight loss.

Before we start, let me assure you of something. Follow this program and you can lose your excess weight! You can outfox your genes. You can overcome your age. You can rejuvenate a sluggish metabolism. You can rally back from previous weight-loss failures. However, to do this you are going to need the right technique. I want this to be clear. You are going to need to know how to naturally accelerate your metabolism. Before we get into the details, however, let's take a look at the bigger picture of how weight gain and obesity are affecting our lives.

Weight Gain and Obesity Threaten Our Quality of Life

As a society, living with excess weight has become a way of life. Today, two out of three Americans are either overweight or obese. Why, even children are noticeably chubbier, and teenagers are more weight-conscious than ever. But it is more than just a social disorder. At the professional level, my fellow physicians and I have found out that weight gain and obesity are known predecessors to disease. In fact, weight gain and obesity are considered to be principal factors in the promotion of heart disease, cancer, diabetes, high blood pressure, and burn out. These chronic illnesses are undermining and threatening our quality of life.

Ninety-Seven Percent of Weight-Loss Programs Fail To Achieve Permanent Results

That isn't the end of it. Despite the media's obsession with weight loss and seemingly more information on health and nutrition than ever, there is a void of reliable resources to help people successfully lose weight. Sadly, the overwhelming majority of weight-loss programs are failures. Studies have shown that 97 percent of weight-loss programs fail to achieve permanent results. Fad diets have plagued the industry and have caused a state of confusion with each new diet craze contradicting the next. The low-carb frenzy that swept the nation boasted a low-carb, high-protein diet as the solution to weight loss. At the same time, other popular diets have sworn by low-fat or high-carbohydrate intake as the key ingredient to successful weight loss. As evidenced by recent studies, these diets have only one thing in common: they fail to achieve permanent weight loss and long-term health.

There is some good news amidst all of this and I am excited to share it with you. It does not have to be this way. There is an alternative. Permanent weight loss can be achieved—and so can a lifetime of better health, more energy, and greater vitality! I have helped thousands achieve their permanent weight-loss goals, and I am looking forward to sharing with you our LYF Permanent Weight-Loss Program. This lifelong plan is a simple, effective, and unique approach to weight control and permanent weight loss. I am confident that this dynamic and comprehensive LYF Program is more powerful and more successful than any other diet or weight-loss program you have ever seen or tried.

Let me explain why most weight-loss programs fail and why the LYF Plan is truly a *permanent* solution!

Why Most Weight-Loss Programs Fail

It is a scientific fact that, **when you burn more calories than you consume, you lose weight.** Let me repeat this. It is a scientific fact that when you *burn* more calories than you *consume*, you lose weight!

The vast majority of weight-loss programs center their attention DOWNSTREAM on the *consumption* of food calories instead of UPSTREAM on the *burning* process. Conventional dietetics focuses on the downstream. This kind of old school thinking teaches that the reduction of calories, commonly known as dieting, along with exercise results in effective weight loss. The emphasis on calorie counting and dieting is misleading. Diet after diet falls short of the mark, and history has proven that dieting and the overwhelming majority of weight-loss programs do not provide long-term results.

It is time for a new way of thinking. We all agree that the old weight-loss paradigm does NOT work. This has to change. We've all been waiting for a permanent weight-loss solution. Here's the answer. It is time to put your focus *upstream* on the *burning* process, better known as your metabolism or metabolic rate! The root cause of most people's weight gain is a slow metabolism that has a tendency to store fat instead of burning it. When you focus on accelerating your metabolism, you are looking for the answers upstream instead of downstream. This invites you to overcome the primary cause of your excess weight and take a permanent stand against weight gain.

Early on in my practice I learned that dieting, without changing the rate at which you burn through your meals, results in temporary weight loss followed by weight gain. The results are short-lived because no one can restrict consumption of calories forever, and a slow metabolism will eventually lead to the regaining of your weight. I hope that you are beginning to see the bigger picture. There is a fatal flaw in old school thinking. Dieting fails because the downstream focus ignores the most important factor in determining your weight loss success—the upstream burning process of your metabolism.

Accelerate Your Metabolism for Permanent Weight Loss

Your metabolism can be measured by your metabolic rate—the rate at which you burn fat and carbohydrates. In fact, it is your metabolic rate that determines whether you are slim and trim or overweight. When you know how to naturally accelerate your metabolism, your body will be geared to aggressively burn excess fat. You then will have created a powerful ally to help you achieve and sustain your weight-loss goals.

There are a number of nutritional, lifestyle, biological, and physiological influences on your metabolism. We will soon tell you everything you need to know on how to make these factors work to your advantage to accelerate your metabolism. For now, suffice it to say that, without fundamentally changing your underlying metabolism, you will have a very difficult time maintaining any kind of weight-loss results. Most diets and weight-loss programs fail to address your metabolism, which explains why they are destined to fail.

Your Metabolism Defined

I want to make sure that you understand what I am referring to when I talk about your metabolism. Let's get down to fundamentals. Your metabolism is essentially your body chemistry. Actually, the term metabolism literally means change. The word metabolism refers to all the biochemical changes in your body and all the metabolic interactions that take place when you transform food into energy. It involves many different sophisticated pathways and processes; it is not represented by a single organ or a single body part. Your metabolism is the summation of the interplay between vital organs, particularly your liver and pancreas; your glands; hormones; nervous system; digestion; and cellular enzyme systems. When you can support the superior function of these major metabolic players, as we'll show you how to do, you can naturally accelerate your metabolism and achieve your ideal weight.

Own an Efficient Metabolism

When you know how to naturally accelerate your metabolic rate, it leads to a healthy, wholesome, efficient metabolism. Your metabolic efficiency begins with your digestion. Digestive enzymes break down food into nutrients that can be absorbed and assimilated by the body and then metabolically converted into energy for human use. The best-case scenario is to eat wholesome, nutritious food that becomes biologically available to keep your body lean and energized. Yes, metabolic efficiency can be defined as a healthy metabolism that generates high energy levels and, at the same time, maintains superior weight control. This is important—take note. Metabolic efficiency generates high energy levels and activates the effective burning of fat.

The good news is metabolic efficiency is something that you can own. It was wired into your system from birth and it is just a matter of reprogramming it. The benefits of owning an efficient metabolism are twofold, as outlined in the chart below.

METABOLIC EFFICIENCY—PRIMARY BENEFITS	
1. Permanent Weight-Loss	Effectively utilize carbohydrates for immediate energy enabling your body to aggressively burn excess fat for longer-term energy
2. Endless Energy	Efficiently turn food into energy, nourish your body with vital nutrients, and neutralize and eliminate bodily toxins

Metabolic Dysfunction and Metabolic Burnout Lead to Weight Gain and Obesity

Whereas metabolic efficiency leads to permanent weight control, metabolic dysfunction is the principal cause of weight gain and obesity. Metabolic friction or burnout is defined by significant weight gain and fatigue. Metabolic burnout tends to creep up on the majority of people. In metabolic burnout, your bodily machinery slows down, causing you to gain weight. Oftentimes you are torn between eating more food to compensate for your lack of energy and depriving yourself for the fear of further weight gain. In any event, when you have developed metabolic dysfunction or metabolic burnout, the energy from the food you eat has a greater tendency to be stored as energy-rich compounds. You are well familiar with these compounds. They are better known as fats!

METABOLIC BURNOUT / METABOLIC DYSFUNCTION—PRIMARY SYMPTOMS	
1. Weight Gain and Obesity	Carbohydrates are more easily converted to fat in addition to dietary fat being converted to fat
2. Fatigue	Inefficiency in turning food into cellular energy and a buildup of bodily toxins lead to fatigue

Size Up Your Metabolic Burnout: Your BMI Counts

As doctors, we have ways to categorize and gain perspective on your degree of weight gain. Weight conditions can be classified by your Body Mass Index (BMI). Your BMI takes into consideration your weight relative to your height. For example, to say someone weighs 165 pounds does not tell the whole story. Being 5'3" and 165 pounds is a different case scenario than being six feet tall and weighing 165 pounds. In fact, your BMI is calculated by dividing your weight in kilograms by your height in meters (squared). Your BMI is commonly used to determine the degree of weight gain or obesity. Based on my experience, there are five known categories of weight management, as outlined in the following table.

BMI CATEGORY	BMI	DESCRIPTION
Metabolic Balance	19.0–24.9	• Healthy weight-to-height ratio
1st Degree Burnout	25.0–29.9	• Clinically overweight, typically by fifteen to thirty pounds
2nd Degree Burnout	30.0–34.9	• Clinically obese, typically thirty to sixty pounds overweight
3rd Degree Burnout	35.0–39.9	• Severe obesity, typically sixty to one hundred pounds overweight
Morbid Obesity	Greater than 40	• Morbid obesity, typically more than one hundred pounds overweight

BMI (kg/m^2)	19	20	21	22	23	24	25	26	27	28	29	30	35	40
Height (in.)	Weight (lb.)													
58	91	96	100	105	110	115	119	124	129	134	138	143	167	191
59	94	99	104	109	114	119	124	128	133	138	143	148	173	198
60	97	102	107	112	118	123	128	133	138	143	148	153	179	204
61	100	106	111	116	122	127	132	137	143	148	153	158	185	211
62	104	109	115	120	126	131	136	142	147	153	158	164	191	218
63	107	113	118	124	130	135	141	146	152	158	163	169	197	225
64	110	116	122	128	134	140	145	151	157	163	169	174	204	232
65	114	120	126	132	138	144	150	156	162	168	174	180	210	240
66	118	124	130	136	142	148	155	161	167	173	179	186	216	247
67	121	127	134	140	146	153	159	166	172	178	185	191	223	255
68	125	131	138	144	151	158	164	171	177	184	190	197	230	262
69	128	135	142	149	155	162	169	176	182	189	196	203	236	270
70	132	139	146	153	160	167	174	181	188	195	202	207	243	278
71	136	143	150	157	165	172	179	186	193	200	208	215	250	286
72	140	147	154	162	169	177	184	191	199	206	213	221	258	294
73	144	151	159	166	174	182	189	197	204	212	219	227	265	302
74	148	155	163	171	179	186	194	202	210	218	225	233	272	311
75	152	160	168	176	184	192	200	208	216	224	232	240	279	319
76	156	164	172	180	189	197	205	213	221	230	238	246	287	328

19.0-24.9	**Healthy Weight-to-Height Ratio**
25.0-29.9	**Clinically Overweight**
Above 30.0	**Clinically Obese**

Use the table above to identify your BMI. Once you have done so, take a look at what your weight would need to be to establish a healthy weight-to-height ratio. This will give you a general idea of your optimal weight to target as you begin your weight-loss efforts.

Take Charge of your Metabolism: The Light Your Fire "LYF" Permanent Weight-Loss Program

Our LYF Program will give you a powerful system for losing weight and keeping it off permanently. It gives you lifelong tools that will empower you to take charge of your metabolism. When you know how to fire up your metabolism, you can eat substantial amounts of food and still lose weight. I have had remarkable success stories, time and time again, with the LYF Plan. Your body gets fit; your mind gets tough; your stamina grows; your appearance glows; and you sustain your weight in a healthy range. Get ready to say good-bye to metabolic burnout, calorie counting, yo-yo dieting, and—most importantly—those extra pounds … for good!

As the name of the program implies, the key to the LYF Plan is *lighting your metabolic fire*. Let's take a look at what that means.

Metabolic Fire Is Everything

The LYF Program is designed to "Light Your Fire"—your Metabolic Fire. Just like fire burns wood, ***Metabolic Fire burns calories***. Metabolic Fire is the immunological and biochemical energy that burns food and burns up your fat. Metabolic Fire energizes you and regulates your weight. Yes, Metabolic Fire is the best-kept secret to permanent weight loss! You can safely say that those who struggle with excess weight lack the necessary Metabolic Fire.

Your Metabolism Is Like a Furnace

There is a simple way to understand how the LYF Program works. Your metabolism is a biochemical furnace. When you burn wood in your home furnace, it generates heat and warms up the room. When food enters your metabolic furnace, it is metabolized; and like the wood, the food generates heat. Your metabolism then converts this heat into energy to carry out bodily functions and to keep you energized. In other words, your metabolism is the fire within your system that regulates the burning of the food you have eaten. Your metabolism burns food just as the fire in a furnace burns woods. Keep this in mind. Wood is to the fire just as food is to your metabolism.

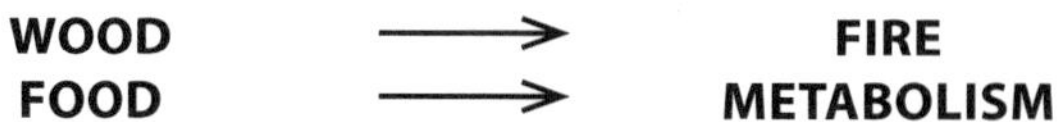

In building a fire, which is more important, the wood or the fire? Well, of course, they are both important. But with a strong fire, the wood burns well. It would not make any sense to focus only on the wood and not on the development of the fire. Similarly, when trying to lose weight permanently, it would not make any sense to focus only on quantity of food intake without taking into consideration your metabolism. The LYF Program is unique because it focuses on building the fire in your metabolism so you can effectively burn through your meals and excess body fat.

Metabolic Fire Can Govern Your Metabolism

Let's review the major benefits of Metabolic Fire. The stronger your Metabolic Fire, the easier it is to burn unwanted fat. Metabolic Fire is metabolic power. It results in a healthy, wholesome, and efficient metabolism. It is more than empowering. In fact, it gives you the power to take command of your weight. What is the purpose of owning Metabolic Fire? There are three main benefits. Metabolic Fire will do the following:

1. Provide you with endless energy.
2. Help you achieve permanent weight control.
3. Defend against obesity.

Yes, Metabolic Fire is key to achieving your ideal weight and defending against weight gain. When your body lacks substantial fire, your body chemistry shifts into metabolic sluggishness and weight gain is the rule.

How to Develop Metabolic Fire

The straightest, most direct path to cultivating Metabolic Fire is to learn how to create and construct an accelerated metabolic rate. I have discovered that sustaining an increased metabolic rate, in a natural and drugless fashion, is one of the secrets to a sizzling Metabolic Fire. How do you go about naturally accelerating your metabolism and lighting your Metabolic Fire? I can assure you that counting calories does not light your Metabolic Fire. Sizing up the woodpile is not what lights the fire.

So what does light your fire, you might ask? The following table summarizes the most important LYF-Style Factors that accelerate your metabolism, along with the biggest offenders of putting the fire out.

Metabolic Fire Is a Lifestyle!

METABOLIC FIRE **LYF-STYLE FACTORS THAT ACCELERATE YOUR METABOLISM**	**METABOLIC BURNOUT** **LYF-STYLE FACTORS THAT SLOW DOWN YOUR METABOLISM**
Exercise	Sedentary Living
Smart Foods: High-Fiber, Low Glycemic, High-Alkaline, etc.	Unintelligent "Dense" Foods: High-Fat, High Glycemic, High-Acid Proteins, etc.
Self-Regulated Carbohydrate Metabolism	Dysfunctional Carbohydrate Metabolism
Insulin Sensitivity	Insulin Resistance
Superior Liver Function	Liver Stress and Fatty Livers
Hormonal Balance	Chronic Stress / Hormonal Imbalance
Super-Nutrients	Anti-Nutrients
Positive Belief System	Depression
Antioxidants	Prescription Drugs

The key to accelerating your metabolism is the same as the key to starting a fire. There are three steps to get a fire going:

1. Ignite the fire.
2. Build the fire.
3. Sustain the fire.

In order to ignite a fire, you need tools and materials such as paper, matches, and twigs. To build the fire, you need some instruments such as a fire poker to stoke the fire, a good set of lungs to blow on the fire, and maybe even some kerosene to really get the fire going. Once the fire catches, you can then add some kindling wood and thin to medium-sized branches to give it some durability. Once the fire is established, you can move on. To sustain the fire, you can progressively add bigger and thicker pieces of wood. Eventually, you can put a big log on a roaring fire, and it will burn well.

It is imperative to start your Metabolic Fire in the same way. All of the tools that you need to ignite, build, and sustain your Metabolic Fire can be found in the preceding table under "LYF-Style Factors That Accelerate Your Metabolism." As it relates to food, you will be given a proven, three-step strategy to produce Metabolic Fire and naturally accelerate your metabolism.

The three main steps to the LYF Nutritional Program are below.

I. LYF Power Cleanse: Igniting Your Metabolic Fire	**Start with Paper and Twigs** This stage will be based on foods that are easiest for your body to metabolize and are most powerful in accelerating your metabolism and reversing metabolic dysfunction.
II. LYF Nutritional Detox Plan: Building Your Metabolic Fire	**Add Kindling and Medium Branches** This stage will add additional foods that support an increased metabolic rate and a healthy, sustained weight-loss effort.
III. LYF Maintenance Plan: Sustaining Your Metabolic Fire	**Add Thicker Logs** This stage is designed for maintaining your ideal weight and energy.

The LYF Nutritional Program is designed to effectively match up your metabolic furnace with the best, high-octane nutritional fuel. The driest and oldest wood makes for the best fires. The highest-quality nutritional fuel makes for the best Metabolic Fire. Poor to average nutritional fuel cannot sustain Metabolic Fire. We are going to start you with foods that:

- Burn quickly
- Stimulate the burning of fat
- Activate your metabolism
- Boost your metabolic rate

The LYF System is designed to teach you how to naturally accelerate your metabolism and boost your metabolic rate. Keep in mind that the foods that essentially slow down your metabolism are the forbidden foods of the plan. While we will not ask you to give anything up indefinitely, we do not want to put sand or water on the fire as we are building it up. Creating Metabolic Fire and naturally accelerating your metabolic rate is the most sensible path to being well and keeping your weight in a healthy range.

The LYF Program outlines for you, in detail, everything you need to know to accelerate your metabolic rate. I am confident that, by the time you finish reading this book, you will be able to ignite, build, and sustain your own efficient Metabolic Fire. This will enable you to lose any excess pounds and achieve your ideal body weight … permanently!

It is now time for us to learn how each LYF-Style Factor increases your metabolic rate. Remember—*YOU CANNOT PURCHASE METABOLIC FIRE … YOU HAVE TO EARN IT!*

2

LYF-Style Factor #1—Exercise

Exercise—Increasing Your Oxygen Consumption Increases Your Metabolic Rate

REGULAR exercise has a stimulating and beneficial effect on your metabolism and metabolic rate. Exercise not only increases the burning of calories and fat while you are working out, but it accelerates your metabolism for many hours well after you have worked out. I'm sure you have heard about the health benefits of regular exercise; they range from improved cardiovascular health to reducing stress. So why is exercise such an important tool in achieving your permanent weight-loss goals? Because regular exercise has four major benefits that can permanently accelerate your metabolism.

Exercise Accelerates Your Metabolism in Four Ways:
1. Increasing oxygen consumption increases your metabolic rate.
2. Sustained muscular exertion accelerates the burning of carbs and fat.
3. Building muscle mass accelerates your metabolism at rest and at play.
4. Regular exercise improves your carbohydrate metabolism.

Let's take a quick look at how these factors can permanently boost your metabolic rate.

1. **Increasing Oxygen Consumption Increases Your Metabolic Rate.**

   It is a scientific fact that increasing your oxygen consumption increases your metabolic rate. The best way to increase your oxygen consumption is through aerobic activity, which is why aerobic conditioning is so good for you. Aerobic conditioning consists of uninterrupted physical activities, such as jogging, swimming, and cycling.

2. **Sustained Muscular Exertion Accelerates the Burning of Carbs and Fat.**

   Sustained muscular exertion accelerates your metabolic rate. How so? Continuous exercise significantly increases your muscles' energy demands. This results in accelerated burning of glycogen, your body's immediate source of stored carbohydrates, and body fat. This elevated metabolic rate continues for some time after you have stopped exercising.

3. **Building Muscle Mass Accelerates Your Metabolism at Rest and at Play.**

   Strength training and regular exercise help build and sustain muscle mass. This is important because your muscle mass plays a significant role in accelerating your metabolism. Muscle tissue has a much more rapid metabolism than fat tissue. For example, a pound of muscle will burn between thirty and fifty calories a day to sustain itself compared to one to three calories a day for a pound of fat. Now here's the best part. By building and sustaining muscle mass, you automatically accelerate your metabolic rate throughout the day, regardless of whether you are exercising, working, sleeping, or at rest!

4. **Regular Exercise Improves Your Carbohydrate Metabolism.**

   The final major benefit of exercise has to do with its effect on carbohydrate metabolism. This is just a fancy way of describing how well your body burns carbohydrates. Your carbohydrate metabolism is covered in greater detail in LYF-Style Factor #3. For now, all you need to know is that regular exercise improves your body's ability to convert carbohydrates into energy instead of storing them as fat. Regular exercise will turn your body into a carb-burning machine!

Exercise: There Are Two Kinds

The kind of exercise that accelerates your metabolism can be broken down into two basic categories: (1) aerobic conditioning and (2) strength training. Both are important components to lighting your Metabolic Fire.

Aerobic Conditioning

Aerobic exercise requires sustained metabolic and muscular exertion. As previously discussed, aerobic conditioning will afford you the benefits of accelerated carbohydrate and fat burning both during and after your exercise. It also helps to improve your carbohydrate metabolism (your body's ability to burn carbohydrates) throughout the day.

Strength Training

Resistance training, such as lifting weights or doing pull-ups or push-ups, works to build muscle mass. Building muscle, as previously described, accelerates your metabolic rate when you are active and at rest, due to the significant calories and energy required to sustain muscle fibers. Similar to aerobic conditioning, strength training improves your carbohydrate metabolism as well.

Take Action: Move Your Feet!

Movement of all kinds is beneficial, so do not give up on a leisurely hike or some afternoon gardening. Simply keep in mind that the more vigorous and prolonged the activity, the bigger the impact on your metabolic rate. For example, a twenty-minute jog accelerates your metabolism considerably more than a brisk twenty-minute walk. The more demanding, the longer, the more biologically aggressive your workout—and the more often you exercise—the better it is for your Metabolic Fire. It is important, however, to build up your endurance slowly to avoid injury.

In order to initiate significant change to your metabolism and accelerate your metabolic rate, it is necessary to incorporate aerobic exercise into your daily routine. Keep in mind that it is critical to break a sweat. If you aren't breaking a sweat during your aerobic activity, make sure to increase the intensity of the exercise until you do. Furthermore, for best results, make sure to exercise in the morning before you eat breakfast. By exercising in the morning, you send the right message to your body from the get-go and can fully enjoy the metabolic benefits, such as improved burning of carbohydrates, for the entire day. Below are some general guidelines for incorporating aerobic conditioning and strength training into your daily and weekly routine.

LYF Exercise Guidelines

- Incorporate aerobic exercise into your daily routine.
- Make sure to break a sweat at least once and up to two times a day.
- Exercising in the morning will maximize the benefits to your metabolism.
- Incorporate strength / resistance training on a weekly basis (at home or your local gym).

BASIC PLAN

	Minimum Duration	Frequency
Aerobic Conditioning	• 30 minutes of brisk walking or • 20–25 minutes – Jogging / Running – Cycling – Swimming – Machine Workouts • Elliptical • Treadmill • Stationary bike • Stairmaster • Make sure to break a sweat!	• Once a day • Before breakfast for best results
Strength / Resistance Training	• 30 minutes***	• Once a week

*** Strength training can be divided up into ten minutes three times per week or fifteen minutes twice a week.

ADVANCED PLAN

<table>
<tr><th></th><th>Minimum Duration</th><th>Frequency</th></tr>
<tr><td>Aerobic Conditioning</td><td>• 30 minutes of brisk walking or
• 20–25 minutes
– Jogging / Running
– Cycling
– Swimming
– Machine Workouts
• Elliptical
• Treadmill
• Stationary bike
• Stairmaster
• Make sure to break a sweat!</td><td>• Twice a day
• Once before breakfast
• Once before dinner</td></tr>
<tr><td>Strength / Resistance Training</td><td>• 30 minutes</td><td>• 2–3 times a week</td></tr>
</table>

By following these guidelines above, you will make a significant difference in accelerating your metabolism.

LYF Summary: LYF-Style Factor #1—Exercise

"The Skinny" on Exercise—Here's What You Need to Know

- Exercise increases your metabolic rate, allowing you to burn extra calories while you are working out and while you are at rest!
  - Exercise increases the rate at which you burn carbs and fat during your workout.
  - Regular exercise increases your metabolic rate and helps burn calories throughout the day—even when you are not working out.
  - Exercise improves your carbohydrate metabolism, that is, your body's ability to burn carbohydrates instead of storing them as fat. Again, this persists throughout the day, not just while you are working out.
- Exercise Accelerates Your Metabolism in Four Ways:
  - Increasing oxygen consumption increases your metabolic rate.
  - Sustained muscular exertion accelerates the burning of carbs and fat.
  - Building muscle mass accelerates your metabolism at rest and at play.
  - Regular exercise improves your carbohydrate metabolism.

LYF Applications

- Be sure to follow your LYF exercise plan laid out on pages 46-47.
  - Be sure to incorporate aerobic exercise into your daily routine and strength training exercises into your weekly routine.
  - Aerobic conditioning is most effective if performed every day and is encouraged up to two times a day for the fastest results. Make sure to break a sweat!
  - Strength training to build muscle, maintain muscle, and accelerate your metabolic rate is recommended one to three times a week.

3

LYF-Style Factor #2—
Smart Food Selection

Smart Food Selection—Quality of Food Selection Effects Your Metabolic Rate

THE quality of your food has a decisive influence on your Metabolic Fire. Let me share with you a little secret. It turns out that the *type* and *quality* of food you eat is actually more important than the *quantity* of food you eat. This doesn't give you the license to overeat, but knowing what to eat makes all the difference in determining whether you are going to be fit or overweight. The truth is, not all food is good for your metabolism. Just as there are superior foods that naturally boost your metabolism, increase your metabolic rate, and stimulate the burning of fat, there are also harmful foods that slow down your metabolism and result in the storage of fat. In this chapter we'll teach you how to know the difference. If you don't catch every last detail, don't fret. Your LYF Nutritional Program takes all of this information into consideration and is all worked out for you step-by-step, detail-by-detail, morsel-by-morsel, in your Marching Orders.

Smart Foods

For now, this is what you'll need to know. We like to call the foods that naturally accelerate your metabolism "Smart Foods." Regulating your metabolism is an important benefit of eating Smart Foods, but this is just the beginning. You'll be happy to know that in addition to helping you lose weight permanently, Smart Foods promote long-term health, help prevent disease, and increase your energy and vitality!

Conventional Dietetics: The Traditional Approach to Food Selection

No wonder there is so much confusion about what are the best foods to eat. A food's nutritional value can be measured in many different ways, often leading to misconceptions and misunderstandings in what is good for you and what is not. From the perspective of traditional dietetics, nutritional fuel is typically measured in calories and is derived from foods that are classified as carbohydrates, fats, or proteins. So how do you decide which foods are good for weight loss and which foods are bad for your metabolism? The most traditional way of doing this, which most people are familiar with, is judging a food based on its protein, carbohydrate, and fat content.

Unfortunately, this methodology for food selection is misleading and does not work. You will soon find out that all carbohydrates are not the same. They may have equal caloric value at four calories/gram, but they do not have the same nutritional or metabolic value. For example, brown rice is better for you than white rice. Similarly, while all fats contain nine calories per gram, some unsaturated fats—like those found in nuts—are nutritious and metabolically stimulating. Alternatively, saturated fats, like those found in butter, can be destructive to your health and metabolism. All proteins also have equal caloric value at four calories per gram. You will soon discover, however, that high-fiber, alkaline proteins, such as beans, accelerate your metabolism while low-fiber, acidic protein, such as pork, can impair liver function and slow your metabolism.

Fats, Carbohydrates and Proteins Don't Tell the Whole Story

As discussed, most diets—and people for that matter—attempt to identify a food's nutritional value based on its carbohydrate, fat, or protein content. For example, foods can be considered high or low in carbohydrates, high or low in fat, or high or low in protein. Keep in mind, carbohydrates, fats, and proteins play an important role in your health, whether it is providing your body with energy or supporting the growth and maintenance of body tissues. For this reason, carbohydrates, fats, and protein must be taken into consideration in determining an effective nutritional plan. But there is more to it than meets the eye.

Let's test your nutritional IQ. I want you to tell me the answer to the following questions. If a food is high in protein, low in fat, and low in carbohydrates, does that make it an effective, healthy choice for weight loss? How about if the food is low in protein, low in fat, and high in carbohydrates—does that mean that it is good or bad for your metabolism? If you answered that there is too little information to draw an accurate conclusion, congratulations! You came to the right answer.

You see, there is a fundamental problem with only looking at a food's carbohydrate, fat, and protein content in trying to evaluate a food's nutritional or metabolic value. It does not take into consideration the *quality* of the food.

- Traditional dietetics ***ignores*** the significance of key vital nutrients that do not contribute to the caloric value of the food, but are crucial for determining the quality and the metabolic impact of the food.

Again, if you were to compare whole grain brown rice to refined white rice, there would be a similar carbohydrate, fat, and protein content. The whole grain brown rice, however, is much better for your health and metabolism. It gets even more interesting. Let's compare two completely different foods that share the commonalities of being high in protein and moderate in fat, such as a serving of Canadian bacon and a serving of tofu. These two foods have drastically different effects on your metabolism. The minerals, vitamins, antioxidants, fiber, and unsaturated fats in the serving of tofu would be much more stimulating to your metabolism than the Canadian bacon. The point is, knowing whether a food is high or low in carbohydrates, fats, or proteins will not lead you to appropriate food selection. This is why most diets and weight-loss programs are misguided when it comes to proper nutrition. This is one of the main reasons why diets fail. They do not answer to your metabolism. It is so important, I'm going to say it again. This is where conventional dieting falls short of the mark. You need to know this; it is non-negotiable. ***Focusing on***

the restriction of calories by moderating carbohydrates, fats, and proteins without identifying the right foods will not restore metabolic balance.

So how do you restore metabolic balance? To own the best metabolism, you need to find out which foods are endowed with key, metabolically stimulating nutrients, so you can determine the following:

- What are the good carbs and what are the bad carbs
- What are the good fats and what are the bad fats
- What are the good proteins and what are the bad proteins

Our guidelines for Smart Food selection will help you do exactly that.

Smart Foods to the Rescue

It takes smarts to get ahead. I have coined the term Smart Foods to describe the energizing, nutrient-rich foods that are the best sources of food for your metabolic furnace. We call them Smart Foods because it takes *smarts* to know what foods increase your metabolic rate. Smart Food selection will provide you with everything you need to know to distinguish between good and bad carbohydrates, fats, and proteins. With this knowledge, you will be able to make the appropriate food selections to accelerate your metabolism, burn fat, and achieve your ideal weight.

The long-term goal of the LYF Program and smart eating is to achieve metabolic balance. This inner metabolic harmony leads to outstanding health, endless energy, and permanent weight control. Wouldn't you prefer to be fit, trim, and physically appealing? Most of us do. Unfortunately, many common foods such as fast foods, junk foods, high fat foods, processed foods, sweetened foods, convenience foods, and comfort foods are not Smart Foods. They are a self-prescribed form of recreational eating. I have discovered that the nutritional pollution from poor food selections, coupled with self-destructive overeating habits, is enough to put out your Metabolic Fire. Poor food selection may very well sentence you to a life of undesirable weight gain, fatigue, and health problems.

Smart Foods Work

This is what you need to know. It is of the utmost importance that you ***select your food on the basis of its nutrient quality and its impact on your Metabolic Fire***. This is very smart. You see, it is the underlying nutrient content of a food that determines the food's quality and its impact on your metabolism. I want you to strongly consider making your food selections based on metabolic value. Why? Because it would smart to not know what foods are smart!

Choosing Smart Foods calls for selecting foods based on its ***nutrient quality*** instead of its ***caloric content***. I've said it before and I'll say it again. Not every calorie is created equally when it comes to promoting a healthy metabolism, energizing your body, and supporting long-term health. Not all food offers the same health benefits, and not all foods provide the same metabolic bounce or benefit per ounce. For example, an ounce of butter is high in calories but low in nutrient value. Alternatively, an ounce of vegetables is low in calories but loaded with nutrients. Which one do you think is the smarter food choice? The vegetables, of course!

So, let's take a closer look at how to identify the Smart Foods you want working for you. Selecting Smart Foods comes down to two simple concepts.

SMART FOODS

1. Smart Foods deliver a high concentration of life-giving nutrients relative to their caloric content.
    - Simply put, they are high-quality, nutrient-rich foods.
2. Smart Foods are free of common toxins, pollutants, and preservatives that interfere with your metabolism and long-term health.
    - You don't pay taxes for eating Smart Foods. They are clean foods and are not chemically altered.

Smart Foods Create Metabolic Power

I want to make sure you understand this important point. Choosing Smart Foods that are nutrient-rich and free of common toxins will shift your metabolism into high gear, activate your fire, and energize your body. Smart Foods are powerful because they keep your metabolic machinery running well by providing nutrients that sustain and protect your metabolism's major players. That is to say that Smart Foods deliver nutrients that promote superior organ function, nourish your master glands, and balance your hormones. Not only are they free of common nutritional pollutants, but Smart Foods also fight off toxins that can interfere with the inner workings of an efficient metabolism. In this manner, Smart Foods create metabolic power, feed your Metabolic Fire, and support an accelerated metabolic rate. This will enable you to permanently shed those unwanted pounds.

Smart Foods: A Call to Action

Thought precedes action. New thinking, new actions! It's time to take a new look at your relationship with food. I want you to listen very carefully. This new perspective could very well be the turning point in your life. I want you to know how to achieve permanent weight loss. I know how to do this. I have seen people from every walk of life achieve success. Never lose sight of what I am about to tell you.

Smart Food choices are about selecting food on the basis of quality, and more specifically, nutrient quality. These choices maximize the benefits you derive from your food choices while minimizing the risks to your body. How do you recognize Smart Foods? What are the criteria for determining Smart Foods from toxic foods that work against your best interest? This is where I come in. For four decades, I have been practicing preventive medicine and using clinical nutrition to better my patients' lives. I want to give you the proven and trustworthy guidelines that thousands of my patients have used to make the Smart Food choices required to achieve permanent weight loss. Below are the guidelines for selecting these Smart Foods. They will help you make the appropriate food selections to keep your Metabolic Fire burning well.

Nutritional Guidelines to Select Smart Foods

All of the nutritional guidelines that we are about to review are taken into consideration and fully integrated into your Marching Orders. Before we get to the Marching Orders, however, I want you to understand the philosophy of the nutritional program so you know why it is you are doing what you are doing.

This knowledge will strengthen your conviction in following through on your nutritional plan. Remember—the better the fuel, the better the fire.

NUTRITIONAL GUIDELINES FOR SMART FOODS	
Section I Macro Guidelines: The Big Picture	1. Select whole nutrient foods over refined and processed foods.
	2. Select fresh, living food nutrients over devitalized food.
	3. Select pure, natural food nutrients over chemically polluted foods.
Section II Micro Guidelines: The Nitty-Gritty	1. Select foods rich in phytonutrients: phytonutrient power.
	2. Select foods rich in antioxidants: antioxidant power.
	3. Select high-fiber foods over low-fiber foods.
	4. Select foods free of trans fats and low in saturated fats.
	5. Select alkaline food over acid-forming foods.
	6. Select low-glycemic foods over high-glycemic foods.

I find it interesting that by following the "Big Picture" guidelines, the micro guidelines generally fall into place. I think of the framework of the macro guidelines as the hardware and the inner workings of the "Nitty-Gritty" as the software. They are designed to work together. Let's start by taking a look at the big picture.

Macro Guidelines: Principle #1— Select Whole Food Nutrients

Whole, living foods deliver the highest concentration of vital, life-serving nutrients that have the ability to activate your metabolism. That is why it is so smart to eat whole foods. Whole foods—such as whole fruits and vegetables, whole grain breads, whole grain cereals, and whole grain rice—are naturally packed with vitamins, minerals, and enzymes. They are Smart Food choices for sustaining a healthy metabolism.

Unfortunately, the goal in the mass production and commercialization of food products is to extend shelf life and facilitate the processing of the food, not to keep the original nutrient content of the whole food intact. This processing of foods can often take what once was a nutrient-rich, Smart Food and turn it into empty calories. When you are trying to reestablish a healthy metabolism and lose weight, consuming empty calories is the worst-case scenario. What's the point of getting the empty calories without the nutritive value?

For example, in the refining process of a whole grain such as wheat, both the bran of the outer coat and the germ at its center are removed. This is not smart. This process depletes the wheat of more than twenty vital nutrients, including vitamins B and E and calcium. When four of the twenty nutrients are returned to the denatured carbohydrate, packagers label it "enriched." Why interfere with Mother Nature's brilliant handiwork to begin with? Refining damages many natural, beneficial, living nutrients and enzymes that enrich your metabolism.

To make matters worse, refined, empty calories actually impair your metabolism. For example, the removal of fiber in the refining process causes refined carbohydrates to be absorbed more quickly into the blood. This causes metabolic abnormalities that impede the burning of fat and lead to the accelerated storage of food you eat as body fat. (This topic is covered in detail in LYF-Style Factors 3–4.) Furthermore, instead of adding to your body's pool of vitamins, refined foods can deplete your body's vitamin reserves. For example, refined white bread and refined sugar require your body to borrow necessary B vitamins from your liver to metabolize the food. This makes the B vitamins unavailable for other metabolic processes.

In summary, whole, living foods are the metabolic food of choice. They are superior to refined and processed foods.

Refined foods are empty calories, which are:

1. Stripped of the nutrients that support long-term health and a healthy metabolism.
2. Processed differently and undesirably by the body.
    a. Can ultimately lead to the accelerated storage of food you eat as body fat.
    b. Can deplete your body's vitamin reserves.

Macro Guidelines: Principle #2—Select Fresh, Living Food Nutrients over Devitalized or Processed Foods

It is smart to eat fresh foods. They support an accelerated metabolic rate. When you select fresh, ripe foods, you can enjoy the benefit of eating food at the peak of its nutritive value, where all of the key nutrients are alive and intact. Fresh foods abound with life-enriching enzymes and performance-enhancing nutrients. I encourage all of my patients to eat a plentiful supply of fresh living foods.

Over the years, I have made an interesting observation with countless patients who have come to see me for conditions ranging from high blood pressure to asthma. When I put them on a live food nutritional plan, a remarkable change happens. Not only do they start getting healthier from the therapeutic values of live, fresh foods; but to the patients' pleasant surprise, they also begin to lose excess weight! What is happening? I have observed that fresh, living foods have a thermogenic effect and naturally accelerate your metabolism. Let me tell you why fresh fruits and vegetables promote a highly efficient metabolism. They nurture the liver, stimulate the thyroid glands, and help regulate and achieve hormonal balance. I see this happen time and time again. The net effect of these metabolic interactions is an accelerated metabolic rate. You see, fresh, living foods fire up your metabolism, generate Metabolic Fire, and enable you to burn fat more readily.

The overall health benefits of fresh, living food are extraordinary. Let me share with you another common scenario I see in my office. When a patient comes to me with a cold, flu, or upper respiratory infection, I typically prescribe fresh citrus juices. I have found that fresh-squeezed orange, grapefruit, and pineapple juice clean out the mucus and phlegm that build up in your inner ear, nose, and throat. I always stress the importance of fresh juices and do not prescribe orange juice from concentrate or reconstituted from a powder. Why is that? The therapeutic and nutritive value of the fresh juice is compromised when it goes through the devitalizing process of being turned into a powder. The orange juice from concentrate does not yield the same cleansing and healing benefits as fresh-squeezed juice, and it is no longer effective in treating these upper respiratory conditions.

The point is, there are health benefits—whether they are therapeutic or metabolically stimulating in nature—that are lost when a food is processed, preserved, devitalized, and no longer fresh and alive. Fresh peaches and apricots deliver more health benefits than preserved peaches and apricots. Fresh spinach is healthier than canned spinach. Fresh-squeezed orange juice is better for you than orange juice from concentrate. What I find particularly interesting, however, is that foods that have been processed, preserved, canned, or frozen, by and large, have retained an equivalent caloric content to the fresh alternatives. Fresh spinach and canned spinach, for example, have the same calories. Again, you get the same calories but have lost the original nutritive and therapeutic value. That is a poor strategy for achieving good health and your ideal weight. Hopefully my point is clear. Eating fresh, living foods delivers superior health and metabolic benefits to processed or devitalized foods.

Raw fruits, fresh vegetables, nuts, and seeds are the ultimate example of selecting fresh, living foods. Incorporating raw fruits, vegetables, nuts, and seeds into your diet through fruit salads, vegetable salads, and fresh fruit and vegetable juices will provide your body with the nutrients it needs to activate and sustain a healthy metabolism.

Macro Guidelines: Principle #3—Select Pure, Natural Foods over Chemically Polluted Foods

Pure, natural foods rejuvenate your metabolism. It is smart to select pure foods over foods entrenched with chemical toxins and nutritional pollutants. The more natural the food, the higher the nutritional value and the lower the health risk. What do I mean by pure foods? Pure foods are free of common toxins and preservatives involved in the growing, processing, storing, and preserving of foods. The SAD (Standard American Diet) diet is plagued with nutritional pollutants as well as chemically altered foods. These inflammatory toxins stress your health and can slow your metabolism.

Fast foods, junk foods, canned foods, prepackaged microwave meals, TV dinners, and delicatessen meats are all bad for your metabolism. They all commonly contain an assortment of chemical insecticides, chlorinated pesticides, artificial flavorings, additives, sodium nitrates and nitrites, monosodium glutamate (MSG), and colored gums and dyes. Toxic preservatives, chemical sprays, and injected hormones impair your Metabolic Fire and invite obesity and metabolic sluggishness. Further, polluted, drugged, contaminated foods weaken the immune system and increase the risk of cancer. Not exactly an appetizing thought, is it? Why chemically alter your food?

Select Organic Foods when Available

Keep this tip in mind. Select organically grown items whenever possible. Organic foods contain more vitamins and minerals, and don't contain the pesticides and additives typically found in conventionally grown foods.

Minerals and trace minerals are required for optimal health and metabolic function. Today, most soil is chemically treated to the point that magnesium and potassium levels are lower, and some trace minerals—such as selenium and vanadium—are eliminated. Organic foods are raised in soil rich with natural fertilizers, enabling them to retain the highest content of trace minerals. Organic foods are also grown without the use of chemical pesticides, thereby reducing your exposure to these harmful toxins.

Whole, organic, living food is the best nutrition for your metabolism. If organic food is not yet readily available where you live, don't worry about it. You can still achieve nutritional excellence with fresh, whole, and pure foods. They are far superior to the devitalized, refined, synthetic, or artificial alternatives.

Now that we've covered the macro guidelines, let's take a look at the specifics of the micro guidelines to see why they are so important in achieving your weight-loss goals and optimal health.

Micro Guidelines: Principle #1— Select Foods Rich in Phytonutrients

Conventional dietetics calculates calories as a measure of the amount of energy a particular food item can provide. But, as we've been highlighting, calories can be a most misleading index. Even though butter, for example, is very high in calories, eating a lot of it will not energize your body. On the contrary, it will have exactly the opposite effect. When you are looking for foods that energize the body, support superior metabolic function, and promote overall health, it is important to prioritize phytonutrient quality over caloric quantity. Fresh, whole, living food is rich and plentiful in phytonutrients. Phytonutrients are life-enriching elements that often make the difference between permanent weight loss and weight gain.

What exactly do I mean by phytonutrients? The word *phyto* is derived from the Greek prefix which means "from the plant." Phytonutrient, then, refers specifically to the health-promoting compounds found within edible plants in the plant kingdom.

- **Thousands of phytonutrients can be found in fresh vegetables, fruits, whole grains, and legumes.**

For example, genistein is a phytonutrient derived from soy, and tomatoes are rich in the phytonutrient lycopene. In fact, scientists have recently isolated more than five hundred health-providing phytonutrients in just one tomato! No wonder they are so good for you!

The study of phytonutrients is an emerging field, and it's anticipated that continued breakthroughs in the health benefits of phytonutrition are on the horizon. To date, scientific research has revealed that the benefits of these health-promoting compounds are based on their antioxidant and anti-inflammatory properties. Not only are phytonutrients important for your health, but they can also play an important role in helping you lose weight.

Phytonutrients provide antioxidant and anti-inflammatory properties that are important for your metabolism.

- Antioxidants and nutritive anti-inflammatories support the proper function of your organs, glands, hormones, cells, and tissues involved in creating superior metabolic processes and interactions.

My experience in treating thousands of patients with foods rich in phytonutrients not only supports these findings, but suggests much more.

Phytonutrient Power Increases Metabolic Power

It is clear to me that phytonutrients bring the body to life and pep up your metabolic rate. In fact, I have come to think of phytonutrients as sparkplugs to your metabolic machinery. I've witnessed countless patients improve their overall health and shed excess pounds with the simple emphasis of consuming phytonutrient-rich foods. Why is that? When it comes to permanent weight control, your metabolic pathways are heavily influenced by your food choices. I believe phytonutrient-rich foods activate, rejuvenate, and restore your digestive and cellular enzyme systems that are responsible for the regulation of your metabolism and neurotransmitters. Neurotransmitters are the messenger chemicals that enable nerves to communicate with other nerves, glands, and hormones. I have further come to realize that phytonutrients energize the daily workings of your liver and pancreas. They keep the crucial liver and pancreatic metabolic axis running smoothly and with seemingly effortless precision. In this manner, phytonutrients act as catalysts that naturally accelerate your metabolism and feed your Metabolic Fire.

Are you beginning to see that the source of a food's metabolic power goes far beyond its caloric value? A food's ability to stimulate the burning of fat can be measured by its phytonutrient content and its subtle interactions with nerves, hormones, and glands. Looking for the phytonutritive quality of each particular food item is an important criterion for making food selections that support permanent weight loss.

Phytonutrients "Phyt-off" Disease

I find it interesting that phytonutrients are the biologically active substances that give plants their unique flavors, colors, and therapeutic value. Even more remarkable is that the benefits of phytonutrient compounds that protect plants against their own plant diseases and environmental stresses can be transferred to humans as well. When the human body absorbs these phytonutrients, they can work in the same way that they work in plants, promoting overall health and preventing disease.

There is an expanding body of evidence supporting the belief that phytonutrients bestow medicinal and healing properties upon natural food. Fruits, vegetables, whole grains, legumes, nuts, and seeds are rich in phytochemicals that fight back and fight off heart disease, cancer, obesity, stroke, and premature aging. Phytonutrients are thought to reduce restrictive coronary artery disease. They have been found to block the oxidation of LDL cholesterol, preventing it from turning into artery-clogging plaque. And finally, they help protect your major organs, such as your liver and pancreas, from damaging free radicals. These therapeutic qualities have been attributed to the anti-inflammatory, antioxidant, and anti-cancerous properties of phytonutrients.

In forty years of practice, I have observed that foods rich in phytonutrients are effective in energizing the body, naturally stimulating master glands and invigorating organs and tissues.

In summary, I recommend foods rich in phytonutrients because they:

- Secure metabolic efficiency
- Fight off metabolic sluggishness
- Facilitate permanent weight loss
- Fight disease
- Promote overall health
- Increase energy

Micro Guidelines: Principle #2— Select Foods Rich in Antioxidants: Antioxidant Power

Antioxidants are a buzzword in today's culture. Everyone knows about them … but do they? If knowledge is power, then an understanding of smart nutrition leads to the stockpiling of nutrients that have antioxidant power. Antioxidants are important to your metabolism because they are the faculty nutrients in your Smart Food plan that defend your body against obesity. Antioxidants also safeguard your metabolic machinery by protecting your liver against liver stress and your pancreas from pancreatic burnout. Top sports coaches know that defense wins championships. In permanent weight loss, antioxidants are your nutritional defense that will help you win the battle of the bulge. How so? Antioxidants play a critical role in protecting the integrity of major organs and metabolic pathways. Eating foods with a high concentration of antioxidants is a sure way to build a strong defense and achieve your permanent weight-loss goals. It's simple, really. High antioxidant levels support permanent weight loss whereas low levels of antioxidants invite metabolic failure and excessive weight gain.

Nutritional Defense Counts

So what exactly does your body need to defend itself against? In the face of poor food choices, stress, environmental pollution, alcohol, caffeine, added sugar, and empty calories, your metabolism can get worn out and fall out of gear. In essence, your major organs, glands, and hormones responsible for maintaining a healthy metabolism can become less effective. Accelerated aging and disease can also negatively affect major functions of your metabolism. Your nutritional antioxidant power guards you against these kinds of metabolic assaults and injury.

Antioxidants Defend Against Damage from Free Radicals

The main benefit of antioxidants is that they inactivate and protect your body from free radicals. Why is that important? Metabolic stress can result from the damage and oxidation (rusting) caused by free radicals. Free radicals are bad for you. They damage vital tissues.

Where do free radicals come from? Some free radicals can be produced in the body through the normal wear and tear of metabolic and bodily functions. In small amounts, the body is equipped to handle these free radicals. However, poor food choices, nutritional toxins such as pesticides and herbicides, and environmental factors such as pollution, radiation, and cigarette smoke all contribute to the buildup of free radicals in your body. Free radicals are highly reactive substances that damage the body's vital cells and tissues at the cellular level. This free radical damage can interfere with metabolic efficiency and, ultimately, lead to target organ failure. In other words, free radicals can decay and impair liver, pancreatic, and cellular enzymatic functions. Furthermore, free radicals can cause an inflammatory reaction by your body. This can impair the functioning of major hormones responsible for converting food you eat into energy and lead to accelerated storage of food you eat as body fat.

Free Radicals	Antioxidants
• Sabotage your metabolism	• Protect and fortify your metabolism
• Accelerate weight gain	• Promote weight loss
• Accelerate aging and disease	• Slow aging and help prevent disease

The degree to which free radicals damage the body is determined by the amount of antioxidants on hand to fight back. If your diet is chock-full of antioxidants, the free radicals will be largely neutralized into harmless molecules. The good news is by selecting Smart Foods, you will have the antioxidants on hand to defend against the damaging effects of free radicals on your overall health and your metabolism.

Foods High in Antioxidants	Foods with Low (or Zero) Antioxidants
• Fresh fruit	• Dairy products
• Fresh vegetables	• Beef and pork
• Whole grains	• Refined carbohydrates
• Legumes and beans	• Fish
• Sprouts	• Chicken
• Nuts and seeds	• Refined white sugar

Micro Guidelines: Principle #3— Select High-Fiber Food Nutrients

Smart Foods are high-fiber foods. Select high-fiber over low-fiber foods. This one is a no-brainer. In the medical community, it's undisputed that a high-fiber diet is far superior to a low-fiber one. Fiber does more than regulate your intestinal tract and increase the efficiency of your digestive and waste disposal systems. High-fiber diets lower cholesterol and play an important role in establishing an accelerated metabolic rate and initiating the burning of fat. Fiber also improves the absorption rate of vital nutrients and binds to toxins, helping to eliminate them from your digestive tract. Furthermore, high-fiber foods have been shown to help prevent various cancers such as breast, colon, and rectum cancers.

As it relates to your metabolism, fiber plays a couple of interesting roles. High-fiber foods promote superior function of two of your most important organs responsible for your metabolism: your liver and your pancreas. As mentioned previously, fiber has the ability to bind to toxins in your digestive tract so that they can be eliminated from your body. Since everything absorbed in the intestine passes through the liver to be filtered and detoxified, this subjects your liver to less harmful toxins and reduces liver stress.

Fiber also has a positive effect on the pancreas. One of the major roles of the pancreas is to manage the absorption of blood sugar. High-fiber foods slow the absorption rate of carbohydrates into the bloodstream and prevent your blood sugar from spiking. This puts less stress on the pancreas and renders the hormones it secretes more effective in managing your blood sugar. We will get into the details of this in a later section, but the effectiveness of the pancreas and the hormones it secretes play a major role in your ability to burn calories versus storing them as body fat.

An additional benefit of fiber is that it increases satiety and a sense of fullness without adding any calories. Therefore, you can feel full after eating high-fiber foods without consuming a lot of calories.

In summary, high-fiber foods are essential for long-term health, a healthy metabolism, and an accelerated metabolic rate. Eating high-fiber meals can also naturally keep you from overeating because it can make the food you eat more filling without adding any calories. Make sure to include high-fiber foods in every meal. The only source of dietary fiber comes from foods in the plant kingdom, such as fruits, vegetables, whole grains, legumes, nuts, and seeds.

Micro Guidelines: Principle #4—Select Foods Low in Saturated Fats and Free of Trans Fats

Many people make the mistake of assuming that a food that is high in fat is bad for you while a food that is low in fat is good for you. There are foods that are moderate to high in fat that are good for you, such as avocados, nuts, and seeds. There are also foods low in fat—such as pretzels, refined white bread, or white rice—which are nutrient-deficient and are not so good for you. While your total dietary intake of fat should be moderated, in selecting Smart Foods, it is equally important to distinguish the *type* of fat you are consuming.

The primary distinction that you need to make is between saturated fats, unsaturated fats, and trans fats. In general, the fats that are bad for you, your metabolism, and your liver are those that are solid at room temperature. This includes saturated fats, which are most prominently found in animal products such as meat and dairy. This also includes trans fats, which are chemically altered or hydrogenated vegetable oils that prolong the shelf life of processed foods. Diets high in saturated and trans fats contribute to liver and pancreatic stress. We will cover this in detail in LYF-Style Factor #5.

The good fats are the unsaturated ones. These fats have been linked to various health benefits, such as improved arterial and brain function. Unsaturated fats can be classified as monounsaturated fats or polyunsaturated fats. Monounsaturated fats come in the form of omega-3 fatty acids and omega-6 fatty acids, and are found in foods such as avocados, nuts, flaxseeds, and olive oil. Polyunsaturated fats can be found in foods that contain vegetable oils and sesame oils.

GOOD FATS = UNSATURATED FATS	
Monounsaturated Fats	Avocados, nuts, flaxseeds, and olive oil
Polyunsaturated Fats	Vegetable oils and sesame oils

BAD FATS = SATURATED AND TRANS FATS	
Saturated Fats	Beef, pork, chicken, fish, and dairy
Trans Fats	Margarine, cookies, chips, and junk food

Micro Guidelines: Principle #5— Select Alkaline Foods over Acid-Forming Food

The issue of alkaline versus acidic foods will come up often when you're deciding which proteins work best in your Smart Food plan. What exactly do I mean by alkaline or acidic foods? A food's alkalinity or acidity is based on the ash or byproduct of the food once metabolized. Foods that leave a residue with a ph above 7.0 are considered alkaline, and foods that leave an ash with a ph below 7.0 are considered acidic. Interestingly, it is the mineral composition of the food that determines whether they are alkaline or acidic. For example, foods high in phosphorous or sulfur tend to be acidic whereas foods high in potassium and magnesium tend to be alkaline.

Smart Food is alkaline food. Blood, serum, and other vital fluids are all optimally alkaline, operating at a pH level of 7.4. Alkaline foods are kinder to your liver, kidneys, and pancreas than their acidic counterparts. They naturally maintain the appropriate ph in your bloodstream and tissues.

Alternatively, acidic foods have been associated with various health consequences. For example, osteoporosis is commonly associated with acidic foods. Calcium is leached from your bones to buffer the acidity, and ultimately the calcium is excreted in the urine. I find that patients who consume an overly acidic diet commonly suffer from metabolic burnout and obesity. I have also observed that excess acidity increases the risk of many chronic and degenerative diseases, such as atherosclerosis, multiple sclerosis, arthritis, liver and kidney disease, cancer, Alzheimer's, and Parkinson's disease.

So which foods promote an alkaline vs. acidic body chemistry? As mentioned previously, this often comes down to your protein choices. As a rule of thumb, plant proteins are generally alkaline whereas animal proteins are acid-forming.

Highly Alkaline Foods	Highly Acidic Foods
• Almonds	• Beef products
• Broccoli	• Chicken
• Carrots	• Fatty Fish (e.g., sardines)
• Papaya	• Organ Meats
• Potatoes	• Pork Protein
• Soybeans (e.g., tofu)	• Shellfish
• Sunflower Greens	• Egg Protein
• Green Leafy Vegetables	• Soft Drinks
• Watermelon	• Coffee
• Wheat Grass	• Dairy Products

Micro Guidelines: Principle #6—Select Low-Glycemic Foods over High-Glycemic Foods

We are now down to the last principle of Smart Food selection. You are close to being able to determine which carbohydrates, fats, and proteins are smart—and which are not so smart. There is just one more critical thing to know. And here it is. As you may recall, there are three stages to your LYF Program and to creating Metabolic Fire. Therefore, within the boundaries of Smart Foods, there are:

- The Smartest Foods for igniting the fire; that is, the Smartest Foods for Power Cleansing;
- The Smartest Foods for building the fire; that is, the Smartest Foods for Nutritional Detox; and
- The Smartest Foods for sustaining the fire; that is, the Smartest Foods for Nutritional Maintenance.

How do you determine which are the best foods for each stage of the LYF Plan? The Glycemic Index of these foods is our primary guide.

The Glycemic Index (G.I.) refers to the rate at which a food raises your blood sugar. Low G.I. foods are absorbed slowly into the blood and promote stable blood-sugar levels. Alternatively, high G.I. foods are absorbed quickly into the blood and can cause havoc. High G.I. foods spike blood sugar and trigger stress on the pancreas. Your pancreas, and the hormones it produces, serves an important role in regulating your blood sugar. Therefore, the G.I. of a food has a direct effect on the functioning of your pancreas.

Low G.I. foods, because of their slow absorption, are gentler on the pancreas and promote healthy pancreatic function. This is critical for accelerating your metabolism and getting your Metabolic Fire started. When you are in the process of restoring your metabolism, low G.I. foods defend against the accelerated conversion of carbohydrates you eat into body fat. ***As your Metabolic Fire heats up and you establish significant weight loss, you can gradually add medium G.I. foods to your Nutritional Detox and higher G.I. foods to your Maintenance Plan.***

LYF STAGE	ACCEPTABLE G. I. FOODS
LYF Cleansing	Low G.I. Foods
LYF Nutritional Detox	Low G.I. Foods and Some Medium G.I. Foods
LYF Maintenance	Low G.I. Foods, Medium G.I. Foods, and Some High G.I. Foods***

*** There are some nutrient-rich foods that happen to be high-glycemic, which will be added in the Maintenance stage.

The following table summarizes all of the "nitty-gritty" criteria that will enable you to identify good carbohydrates from bad carbohydrates, good proteins from bad proteins, and good fats from bad fats. In the following pages I've outlined which carbohydrates, proteins, and fats are the best for you based on each individual criterion. I will then delineate which foods are best based on all of the criteria combined.

Micro Guidelines to Smart Food Selection

Criteria	Smart Foods	"Dense" Foods
1. Phytonutrients	Rich in Phytonutrients	Phytonutrient-Deficient
2. Antioxidants	Rich in Antioxidants	Antioxidant-Deficient /High in Oxidants
3. Fiber	High in Fiber	Fiber-Deficient
4. Saturated Fat	Low in Saturated Fat	High in Saturated Fat
5. Alkalinity	Alkaline	Acidic
6. Gycemic Index	Low-Glycemic	High-Glycemic

Let's review which foods satisfy the criteria above to help you better understand your LYF Nutritional Program.

Micro Guidelines #1 and #2—Select Foods That Are Rich in Phytonutrients and Antioxidants

Choose foods rich in antioxidants and phytonutrients to promote superior pancreatic and liver function. These micronutrients nourish your organs for optimal metabolic function and neutralize toxins which contribute to liver and pancreatic stress. They also contain anti-inflammatory properties that promote overall health and an accelerated metabolic rate.

	Rich in Phytonutrients and Antioxidants	Deficient in Phytonutrients and Antioxidants

PROTEINS

Plant Proteins		
Beans	√	
Lentils	√	
Peas	√	
Tofu	√	
Soy Products	√	
Animal Proteins		
Beef and Pork		√
Chicken		√
Fish		√
Dairy Products		√

CARBOHYDRATES

Whole Carbohydrates		
Fruits	√	
Vegetables	√	

Whole Grains and Rice	√	
Potatoes	√	
Refined Carbohydrates		
Refined Bread		√
White Rice		√
Enriched Pasta		√

FATS

Plant Fats		
Nuts	√	
Seeds	√	
Avocados	√	
Animal Fats		
Beef and Pork		√
Chicken		√
Fish		√
Dairy Products		√

Micro Guideline #3—Select Foods That Are High in Fiber

Transitioning toward fiber-rich foods is essential for establishing metabolic efficiency and maintaining permanent weight loss and long-term health. Fiber promotes superior pancreatic function, which supports your body's ability to turn carbohydrates into energy instead of turning them into unwanted fat. Fiber-rich foods also promote superior liver function.

	Fiber Content	
	High	**Low**
Proteins		
Plant Proteins		
Beans	√	
Lentils	√	
Peas	√	
Tofu	√	
Soy Products	√	
Animal Proteins		
Beef and Pork		√
Chicken		√
Fish		√
Dairy Products		√
Carbohydrates		
Whole Carbohydrates		
Fruits	√	
Vegetables	√	
Whole Grains and Rice	√	
Potatoes	√	

Refined Carbohydrates		
Refined Bread		√
White Rice		√
Enriched Pasta		√

Fats

Plant Fats		
Nuts	√	
Seeds	√	
Avocados	√	
Animal Fats		
Beef and Pork		√
Chicken		√
Fish		√
Dairy Products		√

- Fiber is only found in plant-based foods.
- Animal products, such as meat and dairy products, are zero-fiber foods.

Micro Guideline #4—Select Foods That Are Low in Saturated Fats and Free of Trans Fats

In general, the fats that are bad for you include saturated fats, which are most prominently found in animal products such as meat and dairy, and trans fats, which are chemically altered or hydrogenated vegetable oils that prolong the shelf life of processed foods. Diets high in saturated and trans fats contribute to liver and pancreatic stress, as well as hardening of the arteries and heart disease.

	Significant Source of Saturated Fat?	
	Yes	**No**
Proteins		
Plant Proteins		
Beans		√
Lentils		√
Peas		√
Tofu		√
Soy Products		√
Animal Proteins		
Beef and Pork	√	
Chicken	√	
Fish	√	
Dairy Products	√	
Carbohydrates		
Whole Carbohydrates		
Fruits		√

Vegetables		√
Whole Grains and Rice		√
Potatoes		√
Refined Carbohydrates		
Refined Bread		√
White Rice		√
Enriched Pasta		√

Fats

Plant Fats		
Nuts		√
Seeds		√
Avocados		√
Animal Fats		
Beef and Pork	√	
Chicken	√	
Fish	√	
Dairy Products	√	

- Minimize saturated fat consumption and avoid trans fats to promote optimal liver and pancreatic function.

Micro Guideline #5—Select Foods That Are Alkaline Forming vs. Acid-Forming

Foods are classified as alkaline or acidic based on the byproduct (alkaline or acidic) that is produced once the food is metabolized. An alkaline diet supports superior liver function, a key to building and maintaining Metabolic Fire. Blood, serum, and other vital fluids are all optimally alkaline, operating at a pH level of 7.4. (A pH above 7.0 is alkaline, below 7.0 is acidic.) Excess acidity promotes stress on the liver, your most important organ as it relates to your metabolism.

	Alkaline	Acidic
Proteins		
Plant Proteins		
Beans	√	
Lentils	√	
Peas	√	
Tofu	√	
Soy Products	√	
Animal Proteins		
Beef and Pork		√
Chicken		√
Fish		√
Dairy Products		√
Carbohydrates		
Whole Carbohydrates		
Fruits	√	
Vegetables	√	

Whole Grains and Rice	√	
Potatoes	√	
Refined Carbohydrates		
Refined Bread		√
White Rice		√
Enriched Pasta		√

Fats

Plant Fats		
Nuts	√	
Seeds	√	
Avocados	√	
Animal Fats		
Beef and Pork		√
Chicken		√
Fish		√
Dairy Products		√

- Alkaline vs. acidic foods will come up often when deciding which proteins work best for weight loss.
- As a general rule of thumb, I have observed that plant proteins are better for your metabolism and promote an alkaline body chemistry whereas animal proteins (beef, pork, chicken, fish, and dairy products) are more acidic to your system.

Micro Guideline #6—Select Foods That Are Low-Glycemic

The Glycemic Index ("G.I.") refers to the rate at which a food raises your blood sugar. Foods with a high G.I. rapidly increase your blood sugar and eventually lead to stress on the pancreas. Choose low G.I. foods to promote proper pancreatic function and defend against the accelerated conversion of carbohydrates into body fat.

	GLYCEMIC INDEX		
	High	**Med**	**Low**
Proteins			
Plant Proteins			
Beans			√
Lentils			√
Peas			√
Tofu			√
Soy Products			√
Animal Proteins			
Beef and Pork			√
Chicken			√
Fish			√
Dairy Products			√
Carbohydrates			
Whole Carbohydrates			
Fruits		√	
Vegetables			√
Whole Grains and Rice		√	
Potatoes	√	√	

Refined Carbohydrates			
Refined Bread	√		
White Rice	√		
Enriched Pasta	√		

Fats

Plant Fats			
Nuts			√
Seeds			√
Avocados			√
Animal Fats			
Beef and Pork			√
Chicken			√
Fish			√
Dairy Products			√

- The biggest offenders of a high Glycemic Index are refined carbohydrates and added sugars (e.g., high-fructose corn syrup).
- Diets that only take into account the Glycemic Index can be misleading. There are many foods that have a low Glycemic Index but can cause liver stress and slow down your metabolism.
- The key is to identify foods that are low-glycemic that also qualify based on the rest of the food selection criteria for Smart Foods. Not to worry, we will do this for you at the end of this section!

With these guidelines in mind, it is time to get your fire started. The following table will show you how to get your fire going with the right kinds of Smart Foods. Alternatively, the foods that slow the burning of fat, add to your fat reserves, and have a way of putting out the fire will be avoided or at least restricted until you have reestablished a strong Metabolic Fire and an efficient metabolism.

	Glycemic Index			Fiber Content		Alkalinity		Saturated Fat	Rich in Antioxidants and Phytonutrients
	High	Med	Low	High	Low	Alkaline	Acidic		
Proteins									
Plant Proteins									
Beans			√	√		√			√
Lentils			√	√		√			√
Peas			√	√		√			√
Tofu			√	√		√			√
Soy Products			√	√		√			√
Animal Proteins									
Beef and Pork			√		√		√	√	
Chicken			√		√		√	√	
Fish			√		√		√	√	
Dairy Products			√		√		√	√	
Carbohydrates									
Whole Carbohydrates									
Fruits		√		√		√			√
Vegetables			√	√		√			√
Whole Grains and Rice		√		√		√			√
Potatoes	√	√		√		√			√
Refined Carbohydrates									
Refined Bread	√				√		√		
White Rice	√				√		√		
Enriched Pasta	√				√		√		

	Glycemic Index			Fiber Content		Alkalinity			Rich in Antioxidants
								Saturated	and
	High	Med	Low	High	Low	Alkaline	Acidic	Fat	Phytonutrients

Fats

Plant Fats									
Nuts			√	√		√			√
Seeds			√	√		√			√
Avocados			√	√		√			√
Animal Fats									
Beef and Pork			√		√		√	√	
Chicken			√		√		√	√	
Fish			√		√		√	√	
Dairy Products			√		√		√	√	

	These foods are the best carbohydrates, fats, and proteins for your nutritional plan. Some of these foods will be transitioned into different stages of your LYF Nutritional Program based on their glycemic index.

So What Are the Best Carbohydrates, Fats, and Proteins?

The previous chart highlights the best foods for your LYF Nutritional Program based on all of the micro guidelines to selecting Smart Food. By way of summary, the best carbohydrates, fats, and proteins for your metabolism are highlighted below.

What are the Best ...

Carbohydrates	• Vegetables
	• Fruit*
	• Whole Grains**
	  • Whole grain bread
	  • Whole grain rice
	  • Whole grain cereal
	  • Whole grain pasta
	• Potatoes (starchy vegetables)**

Fats	• Unsaturated plant fats
	  • Nuts
	  • Seeds
	  • Avocados

Proteins	• High-fiber, alkaline proteins
	  • Beans
	  • Lentils
	  • Peas
	  • Tofu
	  • Soy Products

* Fruit is a medium G.I. food and, therefore, is slowly phased into your LYF Nutritional Detox stage once you can handle medium G.I. foods better.

** Whole grains and starchy vegetables are medium G.I. foods that are introduced in your LYF Maintenance stage. These foods are good for maintaining weight but can slow down the weight-loss phase.

Putting it All Together

As demonstrated in the preceding tables, the most effective foods for weight loss are the ones that are low-glycemic, alkaline, high in fiber, and rich in phytonutrients and antioxidants. They are also the foods that are free from significant sources of saturated fat and free of trans fats altogether. There are a variety of smart, high-quality foods that satisfy all of these criteria.

The foods that satisfy all of these criteria are:

- **Vegetables, Legumes, Beans, Nuts, and Seeds.**

These above foods are the paper, twigs, kindling wood, and light-weight and medium-sized logs that create a foundation for igniting and building Metabolic Fire. You will soon experience how selecting these types of foods is far more powerful than calorie counting. These foods will also help you self-regulate your metabolism. As you progress through the three stages of (i) igniting your fire, (ii) building your fire, and (iii) maintaining and sustaining your fire, you can always rely on these foods to supercharge your metabolism.

As you reestablish a healthy metabolism and an accelerated metabolic rate, additional foods—such as fruit and whole grains—will be added as staples to your diet. Finally, you will have the option to add a variety of middleweight and heavyweight proteins once you approach your ideal weight and enter the LYF Maintenance stage.

What we have yet to discuss is the proportion in which these foods should be consumed and how to achieve a proper balance between carbohydrate, protein, and fat consumption. In your Marching Orders, we will outline detail-by-detail and week-by-week instructions based on each stage of the weight-loss program. For the long term, we will aim for a diet rich in whole, complex carbohydrates; high in whole, simple carbohydrates; low in fat; and moderate in protein.

LYF Summary: LYF-Style Factor #2—Smart Food Selection

"The Skinny" on Smart Food Selection—Here's What You Need to Know

- Certain foods accelerate your metabolism while other foods slow your metabolism.
- To own the best metabolism, you need to find out which foods are endowed with key, metabolically stimulating nutrients, so you can determine the good carbs, fats, and proteins from the bad ones.
- I've coined the term "Smart Foods" to describe the foods that are endowed with these metabolically stimulating nutrients.
- Smart Foods are characterized by the two following principles:
    - Smart Foods are high-quality, nutrient-rich foods. They deliver a high concentration of life-giving nutrients relative to their caloric content.
    - Smart Foods are free of common toxins, pollutants, and preservatives that can interfere with your metabolism and long-term health.

LYF Applications

- In your Marching Orders, your nutritional program will be described in detail, step-by-step. However, take note of the guidelines that underlie the LYF Nutritional Program
    - Take note of the nutritional guidelines for selecting Smart Foods on page 55.
    - Take note of the best carbs, the best proteins, and the best fats for your metabolism on page 84.

4

LYF-Style Factor #3—Your Carbohydrate Metabolism

Your Carbohydrate Metabolism—Self-Regulate Your Carbohydrate Metabolism First and Foremost to Increase Your Metabolic Rate

CARBOHYDRATES are a class of food substances and compounds that contain carbon, hydrogen, and oxygen (carbon-hydrates). Carbohydrates are everywhere. They will always be everywhere. You will inevitably find carbohydrates at parties, fine dining, special events, fast food restaurants, and in your cupboard and refrigerator. I have observed time and time again that dietary carbohydrates have a major impact on your metabolic rate. More specifically, your body's ability to metabolize carbohydrates efficiently can determine whether your body is active in storing fat or burning fat. Keep in mind, not all carbohydrates are the same. Specific dietary carbohydrates can accelerate your metabolism and build Metabolic Fire. Other carbohydrates can dampen Metabolic Fire. Adverse carbohydrate metabolism invariably shows up as weight gain. It is also turning out to be the precipitating cause of diabetes.

Not only has my personal experience in treating thousands of weight patients strongly suggested this correlation, but scientific research has proven it as well.

- **Your carbohydrate metabolism, or your body's ability to burn carbs, is crucial to your metabolic rate.**

In the simplest of terms, a healthy carbohydrate metabolism increases your metabolic rate. The LYF Program is designed to give you the tools and know-how to implement a wholesome, vibrant, and empowering carbohydrate metabolism. Learning how to self-regulate your carbohydrate metabolism is essential for achieving Metabolic Fire just as learning to play the scales is a prerequisite to becoming a concert pianist. First things first. Metabolic life begins with the scales of your carbohydrate metabolism.

It is very important to know that self-regulating your carbohydrate metabolism is one of the keys to having a powerful Metabolic Fire. What does it mean to self-regulate your carbohydrate metabolism? It means that you have the ability, through Smart Food selection and sound lifestyle choices, to create and self-manage an efficient carbohydrate metabolism. That is, you can influence how well your body burns carbohydrates.

An efficient carbohydrate metabolism provides a seemingly effortless conversion of dietary carbohydrates into energy and facilitates aggressive burning of excess fat. Alternatively, an inefficient carbohydrate metabolism results in a slower, less effective transformation of dietary carbohydrates into energy for your body—resulting in a conversion of carbohydrates into body fat. A strong, sound carbohydrate metabolism always leads to Metabolic Fire, and the subsequent benefits of Metabolic Fire:

- An effective carbohydrate metabolism leads to Metabolic Fire.

Benefits of Metabolic Fire include the following:

- Provides energy to your body
- Stimulates the efficient burning of fat
- Defends against obesity

An efficient carbohydrate metabolism takes a crucial biochemical stand against obesity by protecting against the conversion of carbohydrate fuel into fat—a dangerous process that plagues the overweight.

Efficient Carbohydrate Metabolism	Inefficient Carbohydrate Metabolism
Efficient Conversion of Carbs into Energy	Inefficient Conversion of Carbs into Energy
↓	↓
Burn Carbohydrates for Energy	Storage of Carbohydrates as Fat
↓	↓
Increased Metabolic Rate	Decreased Metabolic Rate
↓	↓
Metabolic Fire Burns through Fat Reserves	Fat Reserves Accumulate
↓	↓
Weight Loss and Energy	Weight Gain and Fatigue

Proper Carbohydrate Metabolism Results in Proper Fat and Protein Metabolism

There is one more crucial piece of this biochemical puzzle that you need to be aware of. You just found out that effective regulation of your overall metabolism begins with an efficient carbohydrate metabolism. Here's what else you need to know. ***By self-regulating your carbohydrate metabolism, you automatically set into motion the proper regulation of your fat and protein metabolism!*** It reminds me of an old political adage from my college days referring to the presidential election: "As New Hampshire goes, so goes the nation." Similarly, as your carbohydrate metabolism goes, so goes your fat and protein metabolism. When your carbohydrate metabolism is working well, your body burns fat instead of storing fat. Alternatively, a poor carbohydrate metabolism leads to the accelerated storage of both dietary carbohydrates and dietary fat as body fat!

Carbohydrates Spare Proteins

When your carbohydrate metabolism is on track, not only do you benefit from efficient fat metabolism, but you promote proper protein metabolism as well. With a healthy carbohydrate metabolism, dietary proteins are largely shunted into the vital process of protein synthesis and are spared from being used as fuel. Can you begin to see the value of a well-oiled, well-lubricated, carbohydrate-governed metabolic machinery? When it is working for you, your carbohydrate metabolism ensures you have enough fuel to be energized, that you are ready to burn fat at a moment's notice, and sees to it that protein can do its thing silently and smoothly. Way to go! When your carbohydrate metabolism is working efficiently, it is truly an amazing process!

Your Carbohydrate Metabolism Is Your Thermostat

Yes, your carbohydrate metabolism, like a thermostat, is a device that turns the heating and the cooling of your Metabolic Fire on and off. So how is it that you can self-regulate your metabolic thermostat to achieve permanent weight loss? The secret lies in regulating your blood-sugar level. Before we get into the details of how you can self-regulate your blood sugar, let's take a biochemical crash course in the metabolic conversion of carbohydrates to blood sugar.

The Normal Carbohydrate Metabolic Cycle

Dietary carbohydrates are broken down by enzymes in the small intestine. The principal end product of carbohydrate digestion is glucose. The small intestine has a vast array of capillaries (the villi) that absorb the glucose into your blood. The glucose in your bloodstream is commonly known as your blood-sugar level. Your blood sugar is an essential source of bodily fuel, and your fuel line is measured by your blood glucose level. The normal and healthy fasting level of blood glucose is in the 70 mg to 85 mg/100 ml range. Readings higher than 100 mg suggest high blood sugars, and readings below 65 mg to 70 mg are considered low blood sugars. The purpose of regulating your carbohydrate metabolism is to stabilize your blood-sugar level.

Every time you eat a meal your blood sugar rises. How does your body handle this and bring the glucose level back to normal? When your blood glucose rises there are bodily mechanisms in place that transfer glucose from the blood into cells and tissues to be converted into energy or stored as fat. Alternatively, if your blood sugar drops too low, there are mechanisms in place that release stored glucose into the blood to maintain glucose homeostasis and equilibrium. This in turn sustains proper bodily and organ function. The idea is to effectively stabilize blood sugar to a normal level of 70 mg to 85 mg.

Let's summarize what we've discovered:

The LYF Program exposes a poorly known secret of the nutrition industry.

- The secret to permanent, steady weight control is a self-regulating carbohydrate metabolism.
- The primary goal in regulating your carbohydrate metabolism is stabilizing your blood-sugar level.

Now let's take a look at what impacts blood-sugar levels and how you can start taking steps toward self-regulating an efficient carbohydrate metabolism.

Factors Determining Blood-Sugar Levels

The blood-sugar level at any given time is determined by the difference between the amount of glucose entering the bloodstream and the amount leaving it at that moment. There are four principal factors that interplay to determine your blood sugar.

The Four Principle Factors that Influence Blood Sugar
1. Dietary intake of carbohydrates
2. The rate at which carbohydrates are absorbed in the bloodstream (Glycemic Index)
3. Insulin sensitivity
4. The glocostatic activity of the liver

Factor #1—Dietary Intake of Carbohydrates

Dietary carbohydrates are your body's preferred immediate energy source because they are the primary source of glucose for your body. In general, the carbohydrates you consume are primarily responsible for the dietary effects on your blood-sugar level. In extreme situations—such as in starvation or if you are on a low-carbohydrate diet, both of which we do not advise—the body can convert protein into glucose as well. Avoiding or limiting carbohydrate consumption is not a long-term solution for weight loss or for your health.

It is a must for you to dial into the Light Carbs that lubricate your metabolism and ignite your Metabolic Fire. Eating the Light Carbs is eating the right carbs. Alternatively, eating bad carbs have a disruptive effect on your blood-sugar levels. The important thing to keep in mind is choosing carbohydrates with a slow rate of absorption into the blood.

Factor #2—The Rate at which Carbohydrates Are Absorbed into the Bloodstream (better known as the Glycemic Index)

As you know, not all carbohydrates are the same. The fact is that all carbohydrates have not been created equally. Different carbohydrates behave differently in your body. Different carbohydrates affect your metabolism differently—some good and some not so good. In other words, each carbohydrate has its own distinct characteristics and distinct impact on your blood sugar.

The Glycemic Index (G.I.) is a system devised to rank the quality of carbohydrates according to each food's individualized impact on your blood glucose or blood-sugar level. Carbohydrates can have a low G.I. (Light Carbs), a medium G.I., or a high G.I. For example, romaine lettuce and tomatoes rank very low on the G.I., whereas sweets, sodas, baked goods, and refined breads all rank high on the G.I.

Low-glycemic carbohydrates are preferred because they are gentle on your system and produce smaller fluctuations in your blood-sugar level. In other words, wholesome, low-glycemic foods contribute to a steady blood-sugar level. This is conducive to utilizing blood sugar for immediate energy as opposed to storing elevated blood sugar as fat. As we get into more detail on the importance of a stabilized blood sugar, you will better understand how wholesome, low-glycemic foods increase your metabolic rate.

Carbohydrates ... The Good

Good carbohydrates for your weight-loss plan and for your health come in two forms. Those carbohydrates that are good for losing weight and those carbohydrates that are good for maintaining your weight.

As a general rule of thumb, vegetables are very low on the G.I. and are the best source of good carbohydrates for losing weight. Good carbohydrates can also come in the form of legumes, such as beans, lentils, peas, and soy products. Nuts and seeds rank low on the G.I. as well, yet are a less significant source of carbohydrates. Together, vegetables, legumes, nuts, and seeds represent the best source of carbohydrates for losing weight.

Medium-glycemic foods—such as fruits, corn, whole grain breads, whole grain cereals, and whole grain rice—are also good sources of carbohydrates. These foods, however, work better for maintaining your weight rather than losing your weight. As it pertains to your overall health, these carbohydrates are full of life-giving nutrients and are truly Smart Foods.

Carbohydrates ... The Bad and the Ugly

Finally, the carbohydrates to avoid that wreak havoc on your carbohydrate metabolism and your health, are refined carbohydrates and added sugars. Refined carbohydrates include white bread, refined pasta, enriched flour, and white rice. You can identify a refined carbohydrate by looking for these common descriptions in the food label: enriched, bleached, unbleached, semolina, durum, and rice flour. Added sugars can be prominently found in sodas, sweets, and baked goods. Foods high in sucrose or high-fructose corn syrup must be avoided. Unfortunately the great majority of breads and pastas in the supermarket are refined or enriched products, and many commercialized foods are loaded with added sugars. It's no wonder why Americans continue to struggle with their weight.

The Good Carbs		The Bad and the Ugly Carbs
Low-Glycemic "Light Carbs"	**Medium-Glycemic Carbs**	**High-Glycemic Carbs**
Vegetables	Fruit	Refined Carbohydrates
Beans and Legumes	Corn	Refined Bread
Nuts	Whole Grain Bread	Refined Pasta
Seeds	Whole Grain Pasta	Refined Cereals
	Whole Grain Rice	White Rice
	Whole Grain Cereal	Added Sugar

It's important to keep in mind that, just because a food is low-glycemic, it is not necessarily good for you and your metabolism. While low-glycemic foods are a must for getting your Metabolic Fire off to the right start, ***it is paramount to keep in mind that foods must be low-glycemic and good for your liver to be most effective in increasing your metabolic rate.*** This is one of the glaring problems and a drastic oversimplification of most of the low-carb diets that have been popular in recent years. While they rightly promote the consumption of low-glycemic foods, they don't take into consideration the impact many of the foods they suggest have on the most important organ of your metabolism: your liver. For example, many low-carb diets overemphasize meat, eggs, and dairy, which can be harmful to your liver and your overall health. Low-glycemic foods that are also good for your liver call for an alkaline liver chemistry. For example, vegetables, beans, legumes, nuts, and seeds are both low-glycemic and promote an alkaline liver chemistry. Working together, alkaline, low-glycemic foods construct the backbone and foundation to the LYF Program.

We will spend some more time on the importance of the liver in LYF-Style Factor #5. But first, let's take a closer look at how insulin plays a major role in regulating your blood sugar and influencing your carbohydrate metabolism and metabolic rate.

Factor #3—Your Insulin Sensitivity: The Rate of Entry of Glucose into Cells, Muscles and Organs

We've discussed how important the pancreas is in regulating your metabolism. When you talk about the pancreas, you automatically think of insulin. The pancreas secretes insulin, a major hormone in regulating your metabolism. Your sensitivity to insulin is a major factor in determining your blood-sugar level. Insulin facilitates the entry of blood-sugar molecules into muscle cells, organ cells, and fat cells by an action on the cell membrane. *Therefore, insulin sensitivity defines a cell's responsiveness to insulin.* Every time you eat a meal, your blood sugar rises. How does your body handle this and bring the glucose level back to normal?

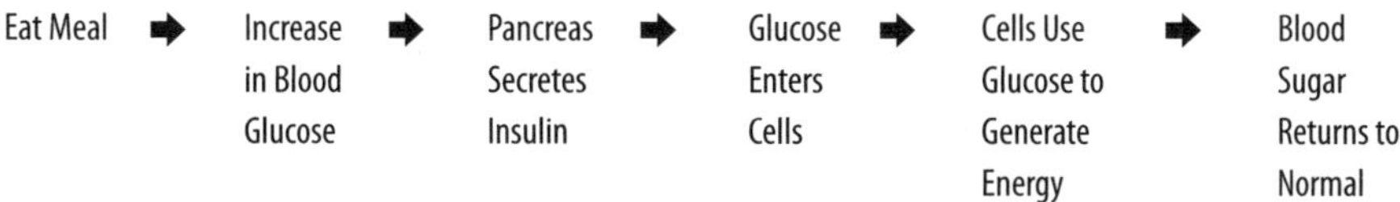

As you can see in the above diagram, in a person with a healthy metabolism, the pancreas releases insulin into the bloodstream, which enables muscle, fat, and organ tissues in the body to absorb the glucose and convert it into energy. As the cells in the tissues absorb the glucose, blood glucose levels return back to normal.

The Pancreas Acts Like a Thermometer

The pancreas acts like a thermometer in its ability to measure small amounts of change in your blood-sugar level. When the temperature rises, that is to say, after eating or drinking, there is a rise in blood sugar. The pancreas detects this and is stimulated to secrete the protein-based hormone insulin. Insulin, a messenger hormone, is secreted by the pancreas into the bloodstream and works to regulate your blood sugar.

The pancreas, therefore, in adjusting your insulin levels, has an important glandular function. The pancreas defends the stability of your fuel lines and the constancy of your blood-glucose level. Healthy insulin function maintains an even flow of glucose into the cells. Once insulin is taken up by the tissues, it can then exert its actions. Keep in mind the theme of insulin sensitivity. The more sensitive your cells are to insulin functions, the easier glucose is absorbed by your cells and the steadier the blood fuel and blood-sugar levels are.

Your Insulin Sensitivity Is Crucial to Permanent Weight Loss. Why?

- Your insulin sensitivity allows your body to make healthy adjustments to changes in your blood-sugar level.
- When your blood sugar can be stabilized and sustained at its normal range over long periods of time, you will have laid the groundwork for a healthy carbohydrate metabolism and an accelerated metabolic rate.
- An accelerated metabolic rate ignites the burning of fat.

Insulin Sensitivity Invites Glucose Tolerance

Insulin sensitivity defines and invites glucose tolerance. Glucose tolerance is a concept that means your body handles carbohydrates well and, in turn, burns fat. As a result of glucose tolerance, you have the following:

➡ Effective, healthy carbohydrate metabolism to fuel and energize your body

➡ Steady, even flowing blood-sugar levels

➡ Accelerated burning of fat reserves

➡ Successful weight loss

The end result is called glucose tolerance, and the net effect is that you lose weight.

Factor #4—Your Liver Glucostat

The liver is perhaps the most important organ when it comes to your metabolism. As such, the liver plays a vital role in permanent weight loss. (More detail on the factors that influence and support superior liver function is included under LYF-Style Factor #5. For now, the focus is on how your liver plays a critical role in managing blood-sugar levels.)

The Glucostatic Activity of the Liver

Did you know that the liver has the ability to release glucose into the bloodstream to increase your fuel and blood-sugar levels? In fact, Claude Bernard, a prominent physician in the 1800s, described the liver as an organ that secretes glucose. Your liver is a key player in regulating your glucose levels and your fuel lines. The liver has the ability to both (i) absorb glucose when your blood sugar is high, storing it as glycogen for later use, and (ii) release glucose into the bloodstream to meet energy demands when your blood glucose levels drop. That is why the liver is called a glucostat. The glucostatic function of the liver is to maintain a healthy, steady, and constant circulation of blood sugar. This even flow of blood sugar is crucial to self-regulate your carbohydrate metabolism, accelerate your metabolic rate, and sustain your Metabolic Fire.

The blood-sugar stabilizing function of the liver is not automatic. Glucose uptake and glucose discharge are mediated by the action of insulin and numerous other circulating hormones. Insulin is the key hormone. In fact, insulin has to work synergistically with the liver to achieve the desired insulin sensitivity and glucose tolerance previously discussed. When insulin and your liver work hand in hand, side by side, your blood sugar can be steady and stable. When your insulin levels and your liver are out of synch, blood-sugar instability is the rule. Therefore, the relationship between your liver function and the insulin functions of your pancreas is pivotal in determining your metabolic rate.

Due to the significance of your carbohydrate metabolism in achieving an accelerated metabolic rate, a summary of the key features of a healthy carbohydrate metabolism is in order, as follows:

1. Your carbohydrate metabolism is the thermostat to your metabolic furnace; that is to say, your carbohydrate metabolism can either heat up or cool down your Metabolic Fire.
2. To sustain a strong, healthy carbohydrate metabolism, you need to be able to effectively stabilize your blood sugar.
3. The most important factors for stabilizing your blood sugar are:
   - Eating Light Carbs (low-glycemic carbohydrates)
   - Developing insulin sensitivity
   - Proper glucostatic activity of the liver

LYF Summary: LYF-Style Factor #3—Your Carbohydrate Metabolism

"The Skinny" on Your Carbohydrate Metabolism—Here's What You Need to Know

- Your carbohydrate metabolism is a fancy way of referring to your body's ability to burn carbs as opposed to storing them as fat.
- A proper carbohydrate metabolism also sets in motion the proper fat and protein metabolism.
  - When you have an effective carbohydrate metabolism, not only do you burn carbs well, but your body is also better at burning excess fat.
  - Alternatively, a poor carbohydrate metabolism results in accelerated storage of dietary carbs and fat as body fat.
  - With a healthy carbohydrate metabolism, dietary proteins can be used for vital protein synthesis and are spared from being used as fuel.
- To sustain a strong, healthy carbohydrate metabolism, you need to be able to effectively stabilize your blood sugar. The most important factors for stabilizing blood sugar are:
  - Eating Light Carbs (low-glycemic carbs)
  - Developing insulin sensitivity
  - Proper glucostatic activity of the liver

LYF Applications

- Here are the two most significant things you can do to establish an effective carbohydrate metabolism:
  - Incorporate the right, Light Carbs into your diet (not to worry, we do this for you in your LYF Nutritional Program).
    - Light Carbs, or low-glycemic carbs, are easiest on your blood-sugar levels and can help reestablish a healthy carbohydrate metabolism by promoting insulin sensitivity and proper glucostatic activity of the liver.

- Take note of the Light Carbs on page 94.

– Exercise regularly.
  - Exercising regularly improves your insulin sensitivity and, therefore, improves your carbohydrate metabolism.

5

LYF-Style Factor #4—Insulin resistance

Insulin Resistance—One of the Biggest Impediments to Weight Loss

WHEREAS insulin sensitivity promotes a healthy metabolism, insulin resistance works against you. Insulin resistance is associated with a sluggish and slowed down metabolic rate and leads to weight gain and obesity. In fact, insulin resistance has been scientifically shown to be a major impediment to effective weight loss.

Insulin resistance (IR) is a metabolic condition where your blood sugar is out of balance. With IR, your insulin function is off; and the insulin cannot do its usual job of getting blood sugar into your body's cells for energy use and storage. Keep in mind that, after eating, insulin signals the body's insulin-sensitive tissues to absorb glucose and lower blood glucose to a normal level. In an insulin-resistant person, normal levels of insulin do not trigger glucose absorption by muscle, fat, and other tissues. To compensate for this, the pancreas in an insulin-resistant individual releases much more insulin in an effort to trigger these cells to adequately absorb glucose.

Insulin Sensitivity	Insulin Resistance
Eat a meal. ↓ Blood sugar rises. ↓ Insulin released into bloodstream. ↓ Blood sugar stabilizes.	Eat a meal. ↓ Blood sugar rises. ↓ Insulin released into bloodstream. ↓ Blood sugar remains high. ↓ More insulin released into bloodstream. ↓ Eventually, blood sugar stabilizes.

With higher insulin levels, you would expect to have low blood sugar. However, ***with IR, you wind up having elevated blood sugars and elevated insulin levels at the same time.*** So how does IR impact your metabolism and your weight-loss efforts?

Insulin Resistance Increases the Conversion of Carbohydrates into Body Fat

The end result of IR is twofold:

- Your body is less efficient in converting your dietary fuel into energy.
- Chronically elevated glucose and insulin levels accelerate the conversion of blood glucose into body fat.

In essence, your body has a difficult time utilizing dietary carbohydrates for cellular energy and, therefore, accelerates the storage of dietary carbohydrates (in the form of blood glucose) as body fat. Let me make this very clear.

IR triggers a dysfunctional carbohydrate metabolism and leads to weight gain and obesity.

Insulin Resistance Increases the Conversion of Dietary Fat to Body Fat

To make matters worse, insulin resistance increases the conversion of dietary fat to body fat. As insulin levels increase in your blood, your body increases the secretion of a particular enzyme, lipoprotein lipase, which increases the uptake of fat from the blood into fat cells. Furthermore, elevated insulin levels decrease the activity of hormone-sensitive lipase, an enzyme responsible for breaking down body fat to be burned and used as energy.

In summary, the metabolic friction known as insulin resistance creates the following complications:

- It accelerates the storage of carbohydrates as body fat.
- It accelerates the storage of dietary fat as body fat.
- It inhibits the breaking down and burning of fat reserves.

The net effect is that IR programs your metabolism to store fat instead of burning body fat.

Insulin Resistance

↓

Accelerated Conversion of Carbohydrates into Body Fat

↓

Accelerated Conversion of Dietary Fat into Body Fat

↓

Slows the Breakdown and Burning of Fat

↓

Slows Your Metabolism

Now let's go a little deeper.

Insulin Resistance Impairs the Liver's Glucostatic Function

In addition to accelerating the conversion of carbohydrates and dietary fat to body fat, IR impairs the liver's glucostatic function. This results in the liver discharging glucose into the bloodstream and elevating blood-glucose levels even further. Excess blood sugar is converted into fat, and you gain weight.

Just as body tissues and cells can be either insulin-sensitive or insulin-resistant, so can your liver. When your liver is sensitive to insulin, insulin works effectively in inhibiting the liver from discharging glucose into the blood. This would make good sense since there would be no need for the liver to release glucose into the blood if blood sugar is high and insulin is effectively working to lower it. However, when insulin sensitivity is lost and insulin resistance develops, liver function and the glucostatic function of the liver can become impaired. This ultimately damages your body's ability to stabilize blood sugar, which compromises your carbohydrate metabolism and leads to further weight gain and the storage of fat.

Insulin Resistance vs. Insulin Sensitivity

Now that we have covered the benefits of insulin sensitivity and the negative effects of insulin resistance on your metabolism, let's take a look at a side-by-side metabolic comparison.

	Insulin Sensitivity	**Insulin Resistance**
Muscle Metabolism	Increases the uptake of glucose by muscles, leading to the efficient conversion of carbohydrates into cellular energy	Decreases the rate of entry of glucose into muscle cells, leading to the inefficient conversion of carbohydrates into cellular energy and the accelerated conversion of carbohydrates into body fat
Fat Metabolism	Favorably influences fat metabolism and the burning of excess fat	Adversely affects fat metabolism and leads to the accelerated storage of dietary fat as body fat, along with abnormalities of triglycerides and cholesterol in the blood
Liver Metabolism	Promotes proper glucostatic function of the liver, which is critical to a healthy carbohydrate metabolism and accelerated metabolic rate	Impairs glucostatic function of the liver and leads to unstable blood sugar and accelerated conversion of dietary fuel into body fat
Carbohydrate Metabolism	Promotes a healthy carbohydrate metabolism and an accelerated metabolic rate	Impairs carbohydrate metabolism and leads to a slower metabolic rate, weight gain, and obesity

Many experts consider IR to originate with the overconsumption of bad carbohydrates.

This includes added sugars and high-fructose corn syrup found in soft drinks, breakfast cereals, sweets, desserts, cookies, and baked goods. Other harmful carbohydrates include high-glycemic, refined carbohydrates, such as such as white rice, refined bread products, refined cereals, and refined macaroni and pasta products. The rapid breakdown of these carbohydrates into blood sugar causes a spike in insulin levels and can eventually burn out the pancreas and decrease the effectiveness of insulin. That is why eating Light Carbs is so important in reestablishing a healthy metabolism. When low-glycemic foods are eaten, blood-sugar levels are sustained at normal levels over long periods of time. This puts less stress on the pancreas, allows for insulin to be released at a slower and more constant rate, and renders the insulin more effective.

Health Consequences of IR

In addition to impairing your metabolism and leading to weight gain and obesity, there are a number of adverse health consequences associated with IR. Let's start with diabetes.

IR and Diabetes

IR is another way of describing impaired glucose tolerance. Over time, the constellation of abnormalities associated with IR progresses from high blood sugars, elevated insulin levels, and impaired glucose tolerance to the pre-diabetic condition called "metabolic syndrome." This syndrome is accompanied by high blood pressure, elevated blood triglycerides, and other blood lipid abnormalities such as increased bad cholesterol (LDL) and decreased good cholesterol (HDL). Ongoing metabolic abnormalities converts pre-diabetic "metabolic syndrome" into full-blown diabetes. This is hazardous to your health because diabetes is associated with atherosclerosis or hardening of the arteries, high blood pressure, heart failure, kidney failure, and, in some cases, blindness.

There are two major components to high blood-sugar levels seen in type II diabetes.

Component #1

There is a reduction in the entry of glucose into the cells. In the absence of effective insulin function, the entry of glucose into heart muscle, skeletal muscle, fat tissue, and other tissues declines. As a result, there is extracellular (i.e., outside the cells) glucose excess and intracellular (i.e., inside the cells) glucose deficiency. This diabetic state has been coined "starvation in the midst of plenty".

Component #2

The second—and potentially the principal cause of elevated blood sugars in type II diabetes—is the derangement of the glucostatic function of the liver.

In simpler terms, the liver contributes to elevated blood sugar by releasing glucose into the blood even though blood-sugar levels are already elevated.

Indeed, the liver plays a crucial role in carbohydrate metabolism. The delicate synergistic mechanism between your diet, blood sugar, your insulin function, and your liver function is key to achieving an effective carbohydrate metabolism, creating Metabolic Fire, and losing weight. Alternatively, IR causes dysfunction between your liver and your insulin and is a root cause of metabolic burnout and weight gain.

Other Health Consequences of IR

Other consequences of IR are well documented. IR is often associated with the following:

- **A hyper-coagulable state**, resulting in increased risk for blood clots and stroke.
- **Increased C-reactive protein (CRP)**, a marker of inflammation and increased coronary risk.
- **Increased inflammatory cytokine levels**, associated with higher levels of inflammation.
- **Depressed levels of antioxidants**, such as vitamin E and lycopene, which are important nutrients that protect you from cellular damage and aging.
- **Increased glycation of proteins**. This means that the body, in an attempt to manage excess glucose levels, starts attaching glucose molecules to protein. Glycated proteins have been implicated in many age-related and stress-related chronic diseases, such as type II diabetes; cardiovascular disease; Alzheimer's disease; cancer; and sensory losses, such as deafness and blindness. Glycation of proteins interferes with molecular and cellular functioning throughout the body; at times, they release highly oxidizing free radical byproducts, such as hydrogen peroxide. All in all, IR and the glycation of protein are hazardous to your health.
- **Visceral adiposity,** a high degree of fatty tissue underneath the abdominal muscle wall. This condition is distinct from subcutaneous adiposity or fat between the skin and the muscle wall. Visceral adiposity

is associated with hypertension, hyperglycemia, and dyslipidemia. The blood fat abnormalities include elevated triglycerides, increased small dense LDL particles, and decreased HDL cholesterol levels.

LYF Summary: LYF-Style Factor #4—Insulin Resistance

"The Skinny" on Insulin Resistance—Here's What You Need to Know

- Insulin functions to facilitate the entry of your blood sugar into muscle tissues, fat tissues, and organ tissues to be used for energy or stored.
- In an insulin-resistant person, normal levels of insulin do not trigger glucose absorption by muscle, fat, and other tissues.
- To compensate for this, the pancreas in an insulin-resistant individual releases much more insulin in an effort to trigger these cells to adequately absorb glucose.
- Insulin resistance creates the following complications:
    - Accelerates the storage of carbohydrates as body fat;
    - Accelerates the storage of dietary fat as body fat; and
    - Inhibits the breakdown and burning of fat reserves.
- Insulin resistance develops as a result of eating the wrong foods and living a sedentary lifestyle.

LYF Applications

- To defend against insulin resistance and promote insulin sensitivity, be sure to do the following:
    - Stick to your Smart Foods. Smart Foods promote insulin sensitivity and defend against insulin resistance.
    - Eat the right Light Carbs and avoid high-glycemic carbs.
        - Take note of the Light Carbs vs. the high-glycemic carbs detailed on page 94.
    - Incorporate exercise into your daily routine. This renders insulin more sensitive and combats insulin resistance.
- All of the factors above are incorporated into your LYF Nutritional Program and LYF Exercise Program.

6

LYF-Style Factor #5—Superior Liver Function

Superior Liver Function: Your Liver Is the Key to Your Metabolism

THE liver is a most fascinating organ. It is named after life itself and being alive—the "live-r." In the previous section, we touched on the critical role the liver plays in stabilizing your blood sugar and achieving a healthy, proficient carbohydrate metabolism. Stabilizing blood sugar, however, is just one function of the multifaceted liver.

Of all the organs in the body, the liver has the distinction of being the governor of your metabolism. It is centrally involved in all of your metabolic processes and is the most important organ regulating your metabolism. The liver's complex metabolic functions include regulating carbohydrate, fat, and protein metabolism. Furthermore, everything that you digest and that is absorbed through your small intestine is emptied into the portal vein, which must first pass through the liver before being distributed to the body. Therefore, everything you eat and drink must answer to your liver.

The good news is your liver is blessed with natural intelligence. You see, your liver has astute powers of discrimination. It knows what's good for you and what's not good for you. In fact, your liver is a biochemical genius that converts the dietary nutrients you consume into a usable form that can be identified by and utilized by the body. Furthermore, your liver is an important filter. It is responsible for filtering and neutralizing toxins, as well as detoxifying (inactivating) chemical pollutants and drugs that are consumed and absorbed by the body. When we defined an efficient metabolism in an earlier section, we described it as a process that efficiently turns food into energy, nourishes your body with nutrients, and neutralizes and eliminates bodily toxins. Your liver plays a crucial role in all of these metabolic processes.

SUMMARY OF LIVER FUNCTION	
1. Regulates nutrient and vitamin metabolism	Converts nutrients and vitamins into a form that can be utilized by the body
2. Detoxification of Toxins, Steroids and other Hormones	Neutralizes toxins and inactivates steroids and hormones for elimination from body
3. Stabilizes Blood Sugar through Glucostatic Function	Storage of glucose when blood sugar is high and the release of glucose when energy is needed and blood sugar is low
4. Formation and Secretion of Bile	Bile is essential for fat metabolism
5. Manufacturing of Plasma and Blood Proteins	Synthesizes vital plasma and blood proteins
6. Promotes Immune Functions	Liver function is vital to your immune function

Given all of the liver's metabolic responsibilities, it should come as no surprise that superior "live-r" function is critical to creating Metabolic Fire and losing weight. Alternatively, liver stress can contribute to metabolic burnout and weight gain. Superior liver function can be achieved by (i) feeding your liver the right nutrients and (ii) minimizing liver stress by avoiding liver-toxic foods.

Liver Stress Contributes to Insulin Resistance and Weight Gain

The most direct path to metabolic burnout is to overstress your liver. When your liver is overtaxed and its time is taken up neutralizing and inactivating toxins, it burdens the liver. In fact, it compromises the liver's ability to govern all of the remaining intricacies of your metabolism. To make matters worse, in the process of combating toxins, the liver can produce inflammatory substances that inhibit the absorption of glucose into cells and contribute to insulin resistance. An overworked liver that is also contributing to insulin resistance is a recipe for disaster—metabolic dysfunction and weight gain. Let's take a look at how liver stress can negatively impact your metabolism. Remember, liver stress has everything to do with what you choose to eat and drink.

Bad Fats Stress Your Liver

Did you ever stop to think that the types of fats you consume have a significant impact on your liver function and your metabolism? In general, the fats that are bad for you and your liver are those that are solid at room temperature. This includes saturated fats, which are most prominently found in animal products such as meat and dairy, and trans fats, which are chemically altered or hydrogenated vegetable oils that prolong the shelf life of processed foods. Trans fats can be found in a variety of junk foods, cookies, baked goods, chips, and margarine.

Did you know that, in the process of metabolizing and neutralizing bad fats, such as saturated and trans fats, the liver produces inflammatory chemicals such as NF-kappa B? These inflammatory chemicals interfere with the transport of glucose to your cells, ultimately contributing to insulin resistance. To worsen matters, these inflammatory chemicals also contribute to the oxidation and accelerated aging of your cells, as well as the rusting and premature aging of your body. It doesn't take a rocket scientist to see the pattern.

Saturated and Trans Fats Consumption

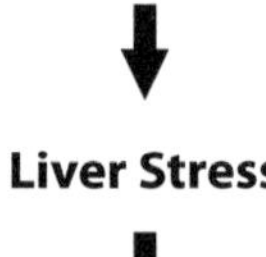

Liver Stress

Insulin Resistance, Weight Gain, Metabolic Dysfunction, and Accelerated Aging

The more saturated and trans fats you consume, the more stress you put on your liver and the more you contribute to insulin resistance, weight gain, metabolic dysfunction, and the accelerated aging of your cells!

Acidic Foods Stress Your Liver

In addition, foods that create an acidic byproduct, or post-metabolic acid residue, further contribute to liver stress. In general, animal proteins and animal fats create an acidic byproduct whereas plant proteins and plant-based foods create an alkaline byproduct. Acid toxins in the body drain the liver. The liver needs to conjugate and detoxify these toxins in order to convert them into harmless molecules. This takes work. It is also interesting that acid toxins and acid proteins antagonize insulin by increasing the fractions of albumin and beta-lipoproteins in the plasma that interfere with the smooth sailing associated with insulin sensitivity.

Keep in mind that alcohol, caffeine, refined sugars, refined carbohydrates, soft drinks, emotional stress, depression, and certain prescription drugs also contribute to liver stress.

How to Create Superior Liver Function

Avoiding the toxins that contribute to liver stress is only the beginning. It is not the whole story. Knowing what food and drink nourish the liver and support optimal liver function is an important component to your metabolic know-how. Let's take a look at the preferred ways to support optimal liver function.

Whereas acid toxins produce liver stress, an alkaline body chemistry enriches the liver's metabolic and glucostatic functions. For example, leafy, chlorophyll-rich vegetables have an alkaline effect on the liver. You see, blood, serum and other vital fluids are all optimally alkaline, operating at a pH level of 7.4 (a pH of 7 is neutral; above is alkaline, below is acidic). Therefore, selecting alkaline foods supports optimal liver function and minimizes liver stress.

Another way to promote superior liver function is through a high-fiber diet, which cleanses the intestinal tract and subjects the liver to fewer toxins. Lastly, eating antioxidant-rich foods that contain anti-inflammatory properties can prompt the liver to release substances, such as PPARs, that promote insulin sensitivity and support weight loss.

Keys to the "Live-r"

In summary, foods that are alkaline forming, high in fiber, phytonutrient dense, rich in antioxidants, and that contain anti-inflammatory dimensions promote superior liver function. Put more simply, these characteristics are prominently found in fruits, vegetables, nuts, whole grains, and legumes. Superior liver function results in the efficient burning of carbohydrates for energy and triggers and ignites the burning of unwanted pounds.

The Relationship between the Pancreas and the Liver

We've talked about the importance of the liver, the pancreas, and pancreatic insulin in regulating your metabolism. To take it one step further, I find it interesting that there is an undeniable interplay between your liver and your pancreas. The synergy between the two can make or break your metabolism. Physiology will tell you this is true. How so? Let's review. The pancreas secretes insulin into the bloodstream and sends its first message to the liver. In fact, insulin is secreted directly into the portal vein, which is the major blood supply to the liver. As such, the liver cells receive the highest concentration of insulin of any organ or tissue in the body. In other words, insulin must communicate with, and pass through the liver before it can exert its action on the rest of the body. Hopefully you are beginning to see the dynamic connection between the pancreas and the liver. Pancreatic insulin, in its purest form, must first answer to the liver.

Putting it All Together

Let's tie it all together with your eating habits. The key to owning an efficient metabolism boils down to the relationship between your food selection, your pancreas, insulin, and your liver. As discussed in a previous section, low-glycemic foods are necessary to restore proper pancreatic and insulin function. When you couple low-glycemic foods with foods that are liver-friendly, you create a powerful combination for achieving and maintaining your ideal body weight. As you can see in the following chart, there are a variety of low-glycemic foods—especially the saturated animal fats—which are not best for you liver. The point is, low-glycemic is not enough. That is why you need foods that are low-glycemic as well as alkaline, high in fiber, rich in phytonutrients and antioxidants, low in saturated fats, and free of trans fats. You can rely on these types of foods to construct the backbone and foundation to your LYF Program.

Liver Function	**GLYCEMIC INDEX** Low →		High
Superior Liver Function ↓	Vegetables Beans and Legumes Nuts and Seeds	Fruit Whole Grain Bread Whole Grain Cereal Whole Grain Pasta Whole Grain Rice	Baked Potato
Liver Stress	Dairy Products Fish Chicken Beef Pork		Refined Carbohydrates Refined Bread Refined Cereal Refined Pasta White Rice Added Sugar Alcohol

LYF SUMMARY: LYF-STYLE FACTOR #5—SUPERIOR LIVER FUNCTION

"The Skinny" on Superior Liver Function—Here's What You Need to Know

- Of all the organs in the body, the liver has the distinction of being the governor of your metabolism.
- The liver is centrally involved in all of your metabolic processes and is the most important organ regulating your metabolism.
- Liver stress compromises your liver's ability to govern your metabolism and contributes to insulin resistance and weight gain.
- The foods that cause liver stress, and therefore can slow your metabolism, include the following:
  - Trans fats—hydrogenated vegetable oils commonly found in junk foods, baked goods, chips, and margarine.
  - Saturated fats—bad fats most commonly found in meat and dairy products.
  - Highly acidic foods—foods that leave an acidic byproduct, such as animal proteins, antagonize the liver.
- Foods that promote superior liver function include the following:
  - Alkaline foods—foods that leave an alkaline byproduct, such as vegetables and plant proteins, promote superior liver function.
  - Foods rich in antioxidants, phytonutrients, and anti-inflammatory properties—such as those found in fruits and vegetables—promote superior liver function.
  - High-fiber foods—such as fruits, vegetables, whole grains, beans, legumes, nuts, and seeds—promote superior liver function.
- Foods that are both good for your liver and good for your pancreas are the best for your metabolism.

LYF Applications

- Smart Foods are designed to promote superior liver function and combat liver stress.
- Therefore, stick to your Smart Foods and LYF Nutritional Program.
- Check out the chart on page 116 to see the foods that are best for both your liver and your pancreas and, therefore, the best for your metabolism and losing weight permanently.

7

LYF-Style Factor #6—Chronic Stress & Your Hormones

Chronic Stress and Your Hormones—The Relationship between Chronic Stress, Your Hormones, and Weight Gain

IN the very first part of the twenty-first century, you could say that both stress and weight gain have become a way of life. Is it possible that there is a connection? Yes there is! In fact, there is a crucial connection between stress, your nerves, your hormones, and your metabolism. This neuro-physiologic relationship links prolonged or chronic stress to a decreased metabolic rate. Ultimately, prolonged emotional, mental, or social stress leads to insulin resistance along with other metabolic abnormalities that translate into unwanted pounds. Does knowing that stress can cause weight gain stress you out?

Not to worry, we have it covered. Stress management is part of your LYF Program. At the end of this section, we show you the take-charge steps you can implement to effectively manage stress instead of letting stress manage you. But first, let's take a closer look at the chemistry behind how stress, your nerves, your hormones, and your metabolism are all interrelated. It is most fascinating.

You see, the stress response is biochemically mediated by your nervous system (both voluntary and involuntary) and your hormones. When a stressor or stressful situation stimulates your nerves and nervous system, your body processes the information and releases hormones to equip your mind and body to handle the type of stress you are experiencing. These hormones, in turn, have a direct impact on your cellular metabolism and metabolic rate. In this way, stress has a direct and meaningful impact on your metabolism.

Stressor / Stressful Event ➡ Stimulates Nervous System ➡ Hormones Released to Prepare Your Mind and Body to Handle Stressor ➡ Hormones Affect Your Metabolism

Acute Stress and Chronic Stress Affect Your Metabolism Differently

It is important to note that there are two types of stress, each with a different impact on your body and metabolism. The first kind of stress is acute stress, a life-threatening type of stress, which signals to your body to prepare for a fight-or-flight scenario. Acute stress actually triggers hormones that speed up your heart rate, quicken your breathing, and rev up your metabolism. These hormones enable you to run faster, jump higher, and think faster. Note well the distinction between acute and chronic stress. Acute stress is of sudden onset, is typically episodic, and is non-sustaining. Acute stress is not the predominant type of stress experienced on a daily basis.

The second type of stress, which is the kind that is most prevalent and epidemic in our society, is the prolonged variety of chronic emotional, mental, or social stress. Whereas our ancestors may have experienced chronic stress in response to famine or starvation, we experience prolonged stress from things such as our jobs, finances, responsibilities, and relationships. In response to this type of mental and emotional strain, the body has a very different reaction relative to acute stress. Hormones released under chronic stress lead to a series of events that slow down the metabolism and can lead to weight gain. Eventually, prolonged stress alters your hormonal balance, taxes your nerves, antagonizes the sensitivity of your tissues to insulin, and disrupts several metabolic functions. ***Put more simply, chronic stress is bad for your nerves, it is bad for your hormones, it slows down your metabolic rate and ultimately leads to weight gain.***

Your Hormones, Insulin Resistance, and Your Metabolism

As we've established, the stress response is regulated primarily by the interplay between your nerves and your hormones. ***As it relates to weight gain, one of the most critical metabolic consequences of chronic stress is the promotion of insulin resistance.*** Let's follow the stress response and see how insulin resistance can develop. We'll start by taking a more detailed physiological look at the inner workings of stress, your hormones, and your metabolism.

To do this, you'll need to know the impact of stress on the following two systems. It turns out that these two systems regulate your body's hormonal function.

1. The "HPTA", or the Hypothalamus-Pituitary-Thyroid-Adrenal Axis
2. Sympatho-Adrenal System

Note well that the adrenal glands play a pivotal role in both regulatory systems (HPTA and Sympatho–Adrenal System). The bottom line is that stress increases the output of adrenal hormones. Adrenal health is crucial to your metabolism. A review of anatomy will tell you that the adrenal gland is structurally divided into two main sections: the adrenal medulla and the adrenal cortex.

- The adrenal medulla is responsible for producing catecholamine hormones, namely, epinephrine and norepinephrine.
- The adrenal cortex is responsible for producing steroids such as glucocorticoids, commonly referred to as cortisol.

Elevated levels of adrenal hormones, such as catecholamines and cortisol, are the rule in chronic stress. Increased levels of epinephrine and cortisol impair and antagonize insulin function, thereby decreasing insulin sensitivity and contributing to insulin resistance.

Stress and Your Adrenal Glands

So exactly how does prolonged stress elevate adrenal hormones? Take a look at the diagram below, which details a stress response through the body's two main self-regulatory systems for managing stress. Take note that the end result is higher cortisol levels and weight gain.

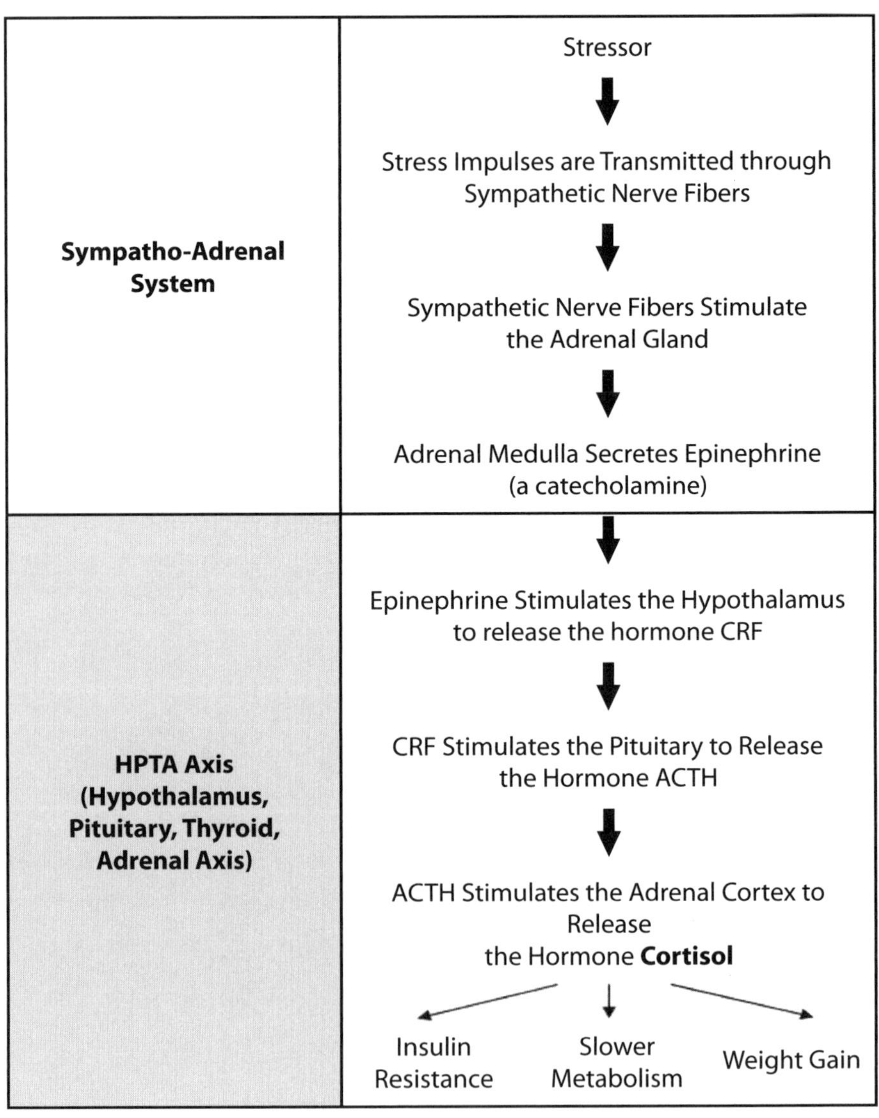

Let me walk you through the preceding chart. I want to start with the Sympatho-Adrenal System and then follow the Hypothalamus-Pituitary-Thyroid-Adrenal Axis (HPTA). First, stress impulses are transmitted through sympathetic nerve fibers and stimulate the adrenal medulla to secrete the catecholamine epinephrine. Epinephrine then stimulates the **h**ypothalamus to release a hormone called corticotrophin-releasing factor (CRF), which stimulates the **p**ituitary to release a hormone called adrenocorticotrophic hormone (ACTH), which stimulates the **a**drenal cortex to release cortisol—the final messengers of the HPTA axis.

This chain of events illustrates how stress can interfere with your PWL plan. Blood-cortisol levels are increased rapidly and actually peak thirty to sixty minutes after the onset of the stress. Elevated blood-cortisol levels are an obstacle to permanent weight loss. As you are learning, the chronic production of cortisol can negatively affect your metabolism and lead to weight gain.

Effects of Cortisol on Insulin and the Metabolism

Excessive and prolonged accumulation of catecholamines and cortisol can initiate a destructive chain of metabolic events that lead to metabolic dysfunction and insulin resistance. Cortisol directly contributes to insulin resistance by interfering with the transport of glucose into your cells. However, cortisol indirectly promotes insulin resistance as well through its disruptive impact on the glucostatic function of the liver. Under normal circumstances, glucose reserves are stored in the liver as glycogen. This is why you carb-load, for example, prior to running a marathon or racing in a triathlon. However, cortisol encourages the liver to stop storing glucose from the blood as glycogen. Instead, it activates the liver to break down glycogen, releasing glucose into the bloodstream. Cortisol also tells the liver to convert protein to glucose, which plays havoc on your blood sugar and raises your blood-glucose levels further. All in all, this can have an antagonizing effect on insulin, impair carbohydrate metabolism, and derail any attempts of permanent weight loss.

Another effect of chronic stress and elevated cortisol levels is the suppression of Insulin-Like Growth Factor (IGF-1). It has been shown that reduced levels of IGF-1 impair glucose and carbohydrate metabolism, ultimately contributing to insulin resistance and dyslipidemia, an abnormality in fat metabolism.

Cortisol Increases Visceral Fat

Cortisol not only impacts your metabolism through the promotion of insulin resistance, but it can also accelerate the storage of visceral belly fat. Visceral fat is located next to your organs, as opposed to subcutaneous fat which is located between your skin and muscle. The omentum is a storage area of visceral fat that hangs down from the stomach organ; it is perhaps the most hazardous and nefarious type of visceral fat as it relates to weight gain. You see, when your body has elevated levels of cortisol, your omentum has the ability to absorb and clear some of this cortisol from the bloodstream. The net effect is that the absorption of cortisol steroids accelerates the rate at which the omentum stores fat.

In summary, chronic stress negatively impacts your metabolism and can stifle weight-loss efforts.

- Chronic stress elevates the production of cortisol.
- Cortisol directly contributes to IR by interfering with the transport of glucose into your cells.
- Cortisol indirectly contributes to IR by:
  - Disrupting the glucostatic function of the liver.
  - Suppressing IGF-1.
- Cortisol accelerates the rate at which you store visceral belly fat.

Stress, Your Thyroid, and Your Metabolism

The stress response outlined above not only impacts the nervous system, the **h**ypothalamus, the **p**ituitary and the **a**drenal glands. Chronic stress—mediated through the hypothalamus, pituitary, **t**hyroid, adrenal axis (HPTA axis)—also leads to burn out of your **t**hyroid gland. Having an active thyroid gland actually increases your metabolic rate. On the other hand, decreased thyroid function slows your metabolism. The thyroid is exquisitely sensitive to anxiety, fears, buried anger, nervousness, and worry. All too often I have observed that patients with underactive thyroid function have this type of stress-related emotional profile. The point is, chronic stress wears out the thyroid and slows down your metabolic rate.

The Thyroid Is Your Metabolic Captain

The thyroid gland plays an important role in cellular metabolism and is thought of as the metabolic captain of your body. How did it earn such a title? The thyroid gland secretes an iodine-rich hormone called thyroxine, which is tailored to increase the oxygen consumption in most of the cells and tissues in your body. This calorigenic impact of thyroxine increases the rate at which you burn calories. That's not all. The presence of thyroid hormones increases the production of hormone-sensitive lipase, which accelerates the breakdown and burning of body fat. All in all, healthy thyroid function helps sustain an optimal metabolic rate to burn fat, protein, and carbohydrates efficiently.

Stress is known to interfere with thyroid function and promote weight gain. It is believed that stress causes a vasoconstriction, or a decrease in the blood supply to the thyroid. Further, as noted previously, chronic stress induces elevated cortisol levels, which negatively impact the thyroid. You see, cortisol increases the excretion of iodine into the urine, thereby making less iodine available to the thyroid gland to synthesize thyroid hormones. When iodine uptake is decreased in the thyroid gland, fewer thyroid hormones are produced, which can result in an underactive thyroid. This decreased thyroid function is detrimental to the proper rate of cellular metabolism. Everything slows down and you gain weight. Clinically, people diagnosed with hypothyroidism, or a low, underactive thyroid function, suffer from lethargy, mental and physical sluggishness, and weight gain. As a further note, prescription drugs, most commonly those used to treat type II diabetes, estrogens, and prednisone or other steroids, inhibit iodine uptake and can worsen an already stressed thyroid gland.

In summary, chronic, recurrent emotional stress and mental strain lead to a destructive cascade of metabolic and inflammatory changes that trigger the development of IR and weight gain!

- Chronic stress results in the elevation of cortisol and epinephrine, the reduction in IGF-1, and the disruption of the glucostatic function of the liver, all of which contribute to insulin resistance, the accelerated storage of fat, and weight gain.
- Cortisol can also accelerate the rate at which you store visceral belly fat.
- Chronic stress and elevated cortisol levels can weaken the thyroid gland and decrease the production of thyroxine, an integral hormone that regulates carbohydrate, fat, and protein metabolism through the accelerated burning of calories.

Now you can see why Metabolic Fire is a lifestyle and not just a diet. You'll have to learn how to effectively manage your stress levels.

Effective Stress Management Feeds Metabolic Fire

Here is the good news. Your metabolism can be protected by a dynamic, comprehensive and effective stress management program. In your tool kit, you can find the following resources for self-regulating stress levels. The table below highlights the essential techniques you can incorporate into your everyday life.

STRESS MANAGEMENT PROGRAM	
Exercise	• Exercise calms the mind and body and relieves any built-up stress. • Follow your LYF Exercise Program, as described in LYF-Style Factor #1, and it will go a long way in managing your stress.
Nutritional Balance	• The right nutrition will build up your body's resistance to stress. • Follow the LYF Nutritional Program, and you will be feeding your body what it needs to conquer stress.

Meditation	• Meditation is a powerful relaxation technique that is calming to the mind, body, heart, and soul. • We'll cover basic meditation techniques in "Master Your Eating Habits" as well as "The Inner Strengths of Permanent Weight Loss."
Mind-Body Disciplines	• Activities that integrate the mind and the body are very effective in counteracting stress. • Yoga, tai-chi, and kung fu are all good examples of mind-body disciplines.
Creative Relaxation	• Creative self-expression rechannels your energy into relaxed productivity. • Creativity is healing therapy for your mind and your nerves. • Playing a musical instrument, painting, and writing are all good examples of creative self-expression that can be incorporated into your daily routine.
Self-Nurturing Activities	• Spend your free time doing the things you really love to do. • Have fun and share laughter with friends and loved ones.

LYF Summary: LYF-Style Factor #6—Stress and Your Hormones

"The Skinny" on Stress and Your Hormones—Here's What You Need to Know

- There is an important relationship between chronic stress, your hormones, and weight gain.
- Chronic stress elevates the production of hormones, such as cortisol, which negatively impact your metabolism and promote weight gain.
    - Chronic stress elevates the production of cortisol.
    - Cortisol directly and indirectly contributes to insulin resistance, and therefore weight gain.
    - Cortisol accelerates the rate at which you store visceral belly fat.
- The thyroid gland and the hormones it produces (thyroxine) play an integral role in regulating carbohydrate, fat, and protein metabolism through the accelerated burning of calories.
- Chronic stress and elevated cortisol levels can weaken the thyroid gland and decrease production of thyroxine, thereby contributing to weight gain.

LYF Applications

- By following your LYF Nutritional Program and LYF Exercise Program, you will go a long way in combating the negative effects of chronic stress on your metabolism.
- Check out additional stress management techniques you can incorporate into your daily life on pages 126-127.

8

LYF-Style Factor #7—Nutritional Supplementation

Nutritional Supplementation: How to Use Super-Nutrients to Accelerate Your Metabolism

ARE nutritional supplements really necessary? I believe they are. Knowing what nutrient-rich foods are the best to boost and regulate your metabolism is important, but not enough. Nutritional supplementation is an integral component to achieving permanent weight loss. You see, it is up to each one of us to supply our bodies with what we need to metabolically thrive. The soil depletion and the commercialization and processing of our food sources have left us with a need for supplementing a healthy diet. In other words, supplementation is not optional for the best metabolic machinery—it is a must!

Let's quickly review why certain nutrients are so important to your metabolism. First off, you need to be certain that you have all the nutrient players from vitamin A to zinc in your metabolic pool. The governing intelligence of your metabolic furnace can then select what it needs, from the available metabolic pool, to act and create the most efficient and dynamic Metabolic Fire. Keep in mind that a diet rich in essential nutrients, vitamins, minerals, amino acids, fatty acids, antioxidants, and phytonutrients is critical for sustaining an accelerated metabolic rate. It is absolutely necessary to have a wholesome, comprehensive, balanced supply of these nutritive cofactors in your nutritional program to feed your Metabolic Fire.

Super-Nutrients Are the Supplementation of Choice

The supplementation program of choice for the LYF Plan is invested in super-nutrients. What exactly are super-nutrients? Super-nutrients are specialized, high-energy, nutrient-rich supplements and whole food sources that can fire up and increase your metabolic flame. For example, spirulina, a high-energy, nutrient-rich blue-green algae, is considered to be a super-nutrient. The recommended super-nutrients in your LYF program can be used to serve two main functions.

- Super-nutrients can aid in accelerating your metabolic rate.
- Super-nutrients can be used as liquid, high-energy, low-calorie, nutrient-rich alternatives to snacks between meals. You'll come to know this better as one of your options for liquid nutrition to curb your appetite between meals.

When used properly, supplementation with super-nutrients delivers lasting benefits. Super-nutrients provide your body with the highest degree of nutritional excellence. They accelerate your metabolic rate and help you avoid unnecessary eating between meals.

Super-Nutrients Are the Catalyst to Your LYF Plan

In LYF-Style Factor #2, we discussed in detail the importance of the nutrient and micronutrient makeup of foods in determining what are the Smartest Foods that accelerate your metabolism. In this section, you will learn how to build upon the foundation of Smart Foods by using super-nutrients as a metabolic catalyst to lose weight.

Super-nutrients have an immediate effect. They have kindling power—they brighten, enrich, and sustain Metabolic Fire. They make sure the fire breathes well and gets the necessary oxygen to keep the fire alive and burning. They naturally stoke the fire much like a blower, bellows, or a steady drip of oil or wax would help keep the fire strong and keep it from going out. Super-nutrient power translates to metabolic power.

By now, you know that Smart Foods are rich in essential nutrients that support a healthy metabolism. Super-nutrients are essentially Super-Smart Foods. Why is that? Super-nutrients have the following:

- Higher concentrations of powerful phytonutrients and antioxidants found in Smart Foods.
- Higher concentrations of specialized nutrients, such as chromium, which have distinctive beneficial actions on the workings of your metabolism.

Keep in mind, however, that without the foundation of Smart Foods, super-nutrients are not as effective. Working synergistically together with Smart Foods, however, super-nutrients can act as the necessary catalysts that take your metabolism to a higher gear.

Let's take a`look at the most vital nutrients that must be present in your supplementation program. We will then recommend the super-nutrients that are rich in these nutritive factors.

- **Phytonutrients**

  Phytonutrients are naturally occurring enzymes and life-giving nutrients found in fruits and vegetables that bring the body to life, naturally stimulate master glands, invigorate organs and tissues, revitalize nerves, and recharge brain batteries. Phytonutrients support proper liver function. In addition, phytonutrients have anti-inflammatory properties that protect against insulin resistance and promote insulin sensitivity.

- **Antioxidants**

  Antioxidants protect against the rusting and aging of the body's cells by neutralizing harmful substances such as free radicals that cause cellular damage. Commonly known antioxidants include vitamin C, vitamin E, and beta-carotene (which is converted to vitamin A in the body). Antioxidants support proper liver function and have anti-inflammatory properties that protect against insulin resistance and promote insulin sensitivity.

- **B-Vitamins**

  The all important B vitamins are critical cofactors to the enzyme systems in the Krebs cycle. The Krebs cycle, or the citric acid cycle, in the mitochondria of your cells, is the crucial intracellular metabolic pathway involved in the chemical conversion of carbohydrates and fats into a form of usable energy. Therefore, B vitamins are critical for supporting a healthy metabolism.

- **Chromium**

  Chromium is an important trace mineral for weight loss because it promotes insulin sensitivity and defends against insulin resistance. Biochemically, chromium has an affinity for insulin and renders insulin more effective. Therefore, chromium plays an important role in self-regulating your carbohydrate metabolism. The FDA agrees that chromium may be of benefit in reducing the risk of insulin resistance and, possibly, of type II diabetes. Interestingly, the adequate daily dietary intake for chromium is 50 to 200 micrograms, but most diets contain less than 60 percent of this intake!

- **Potassium**

  Potassium has a very important relationship to insulin. Insulin causes potassium to enter the cells, just as it causes your blood glucose to enter the cell. Potassium and insulin work hand in hand. Healthy potassium levels have been shown to contribute to an effective carbohydrate metabolism. In addition, potassium has an alkalinizing effect on your liver and blood chemistry, which supports a healthy metabolism.

  Alternatively, potassium depletion decreases glucose tolerance and impairs your carbohydrate metabolism. Potassium-depleted patients are prone to a diabetic metabolism. Certain diuretics, such as the thiazides, that are commonly used to treat high blood pressure and heart disease, increase potassium excretion in the urine. As physicians, we know that potassium-depleted patients are prone to an impaired carbohydrate metabolism and a worsened diabetic state.

- **Zinc**

  Insulin is known to have an affinity for zinc. Zinc plays a critical role in the synthesis, storage, and secretion of insulin.

Recommended Super-Nutrients

Let's take a look at the recommended super-nutrients and how their powerful nutrient makeup can act as a catalyst to shedding excess weight.

Super-Nutrient #1: Spirulina ... Why Re-Vita!

Spirulina, a blue-green microscopic algae, is one of nature's super-foods and most potent proteins. Spirulina has a rich history. It is believed to have been a food source for the Aztecs in sixteenth-century Mexico. Its harvesting from Lake Texcoco is legendary, as described by Spanish explorers and soldiers of Hernando Cortez. Spirulina was found in abundance at this lake by French researchers in the 1960s. The first large-scale spirulina production plant was established there in the early 1970s.

Spirulina occurs naturally in tropical and subtropical lakes that are saturated in minerals and have a highly alkaline pH. In fact, spirulina thrives in such alkaline waters that no other plants can live there! The high concentration of minerals and alkalinity of the water in which it is grown are transferred into cell structure of the spirulina. Spirulina is referred to as a "super-green" because of its high chlorophyll content. Chlorophyll's molecular structure closely resembles that of hemoglobin, the oxygen-carrying protein found in red blood cells. Chlorophyll has cleansing and purification benefits on the cells and tissues. So why is spirulina so good for your metabolism? Let's review.

Important Nutrients	Good Source?	Notes
Phytonutrients	✔	• Spirulina is phytonutrient-rich, containing phytonutrients such as chlorophyll-a, xanthophylls, and diatoxanthin. • These phytonutrients are important in stabilizing liver function and defending against liver toxicity. • It contains anti-inflammatory properties that defend against IR and promote IS.
Antioxidants	✔	• Spirulina is a concentrated source of anti-oxidants, including beta-carotene, vitamin C, vitamin E, and selenium. • It defends against the rusting and aging of your cells. • It promotes superior liver function. • It contains anti-inflammatory properties that defend against IR and promote IS.
B Vitamins	✔	• Spirulina offers the complete B vitamin complex, including the most plentiful source of B-12 in the plant kingdom. • B vitamins play a critical role in cellular metabolism.
Chromium	✔	• Spirulina is a good source of chromium. • Re-Vita, the form of spirulina we recommend, contains 60 mcg per serving. • Chromium improves insulin sensitivity and overall carbohydrate metabolism and defends against insulin resistance.
Potassium	✔	• Spirulina is a known source of potassium, a key mineral in supporting a healthy carbohydrate metabolism. • Potassium also contributes to an alkaline blood chemistry and supports superior liver function.

Zinc	✔	• Spirulina is a rich source of zinc.

Additional Benefits

- **Alkaline Protein**

  Spirulina qualitatively contains unusually high amounts of protein, between 55 percent and 77 percent by dry weight depending upon the source. Spirulina is a complete protein, containing all essential amino acids. It is also a super-alkaline protein which is a sparkplug to liver metabolism. When liver metabolism is healthy, superior weight control is the rule.

- **Essential Fatty Acids**

  Spirulina is a rich source of essential fatty acids, which have been noted for their anti-inflammatory properties, along with many other health-promoting benefits.

- **Natural Appetite Suppressant**

  It is important to note that spirulina is a natural appetite suppressant.

How to Incorporate Spirulina into Your LYF Plan ... Choose Re-Vita!

The harvesting and processing method is critical to the quality of spirulina. In the extraction procedure, it is best that the temperature does not exceed 88 degrees. This method of processing spirulina at lower temperatures preserves and keeps intact all of its nutrients. At higher temperatures, spirulina is devitalized, and many of the nutrients become denatured. For this reason, I strongly recommend Re-Vita, a liquid-based spirulina supplement that retains all of the enzymes and nutrients of the live, whole food.

In general, we recommend adding one tablespoon of Re-Vita to a fresh-squeezed juice (preferably a lower-glycemic juice such as grapefruit juice) in the morning. Re-Vita can also be used as a pick-me-up in between meals. It is a healthy, high-energy, low-calorie alternative to snacks. Check your Marching Orders for further application of Re-Vita.

Super-Nutrient #2: Brewer's Yeast

Brewer's yeast (in the active form) can be used to make beer but is also a nutrient-rich byproduct of brewing that can be used as a nutritional supplement. As a supplement, brewer's yeast consists of the dried, inactive, pulverized cells of *Saccharomyces cerevisiae*, a type of fungus.

Brewer's yeast, the preferred form of nutritional yeast, is known for its high concentration of B vitamins, trace minerals, and essential amino acids. Brewer's yeast is a powerful cleanser of the liver and promotes healthy pancreatic function. This makes brewer's yeast an important super-nutrient for your metabolism and overall health. Let's take a closer look at the combination of nutrients that makes this super-nutrient so effective.

Important Nutrients	**Good Source?**	**Notes**
Chromium	✔	• Brewer's yeast is considered to contain a superior form of chromium, both in terms of quantity and bio-availability. • High-quality brewer's yeast powder or flakes contain as much as 60 mcg of chromium per tablespoon. • Chromium improves insulin sensitivity and overall carbohydrate metabolism and defends against insulin resistance.
B Vitamins	✔	• Due to an unusually high concentration of B vitamins, brewer's yeast is rapidly metabolized by the body. • The dense supply of B vitamins functions to increase cellular metabolism and, likewise, increase the conversion of carbohydrates and fats into usable energy.

Additional Benefits

- **Protein / Amino Acids**

  Brewer's yeast is a rich source of complete protein, containing all essential amino acids. It is also naturally low in fat and sodium.

How to Incorporate Brewer's Yeast into Your LYF Plan

Brewer's yeast should not be confused with other forms of yeast like baker's yeast, other nutritional yeasts, or torula yeast. While other forms of nutritional yeast may be equally rich in B vitamins, they can be low in chromium. Therefore, other forms of nutritional yeast are not as effective as brewer's yeast in aiding weight loss.

In general, we recommend mixing one to two tablespoons of brewer's yeast with a fresh-squeezed fruit juice (preferably a lower-glycemic fruit juice such as grapefruit juice). When using brewer's yeast, start with one to two teaspoons daily because it may cause gas in some individuals. As you tolerate it, gradually increase your dose to one to two tablespoons, in the morning and the evening, at least twice daily. Check your Marching Orders for further application of brewer's yeast.

Important Notes on Brewer's Yeast

- As discussed, brewer's yeast contains a highly biologically active form of chromium. Therefore, supplementation with brewer's yeast could potentially enhance the effects of drugs for diabetes and possibly lead to hypoglycemia. People with diabetes taking insulin or other blood-sugar-lowering agents should not supplement with brewer's yeast (or chromium) without a doctor's supervision.

- Side effects have not been reported from the use of brewer's yeast although allergies to it exist in some people.

- Brewer's yeast is not related to *Candida albicans* fungus, which causes yeast infection.

Super-Nutrient #3: Mangosteen ... Why VEMMA!

Mangosteen is a nutrient-rich, tropical fruit that grows in the wild forests of Malaysia and Thailand and has been heralded as the "Queen of Fruits." It has been used for centuries by Asian health practitioners for its health benefits. Its unique concentration of phytonutrients and antioxidants makes it a powerful super-nutrient and one of nature's super-fruits. Let's take a closer look at the nutrient makeup of mangosteen.

Important Nutrients	Good Source?	Notes
Phytonutrients	✔	• Mangosteen is the ultimate in phytonutrition. The Mangosteen rind may be the single greatest supply of phytonutrients, such as xanthones, found in any fruit. • These phytonutrients support superior liver and pancreatic function and have anti-inflammatory properties that protect against IR.
Antioxidants	✔	• Mangosteen is the world's most potent source of xanthones, a rich source of antioxidants. • It defends against the rusting and aging of your cells. • It promotes superior liver function. • It contains anti-inflammatory properties that defend against IR and promote IS.

How to Incorporate Mangosteen into Your LYF Plan

I recommend taking mangosteen in the form of the liquid supplement VEMMA. Mangosteen is the most active ingredient in VEMMA, an all purpose, liquid supplement that stands for **V**itamins, **E**ssential Trace **M**inerals, **M**angosteen, and **A**loe Vera. As the name suggests, in addition to the health benefits of mangosteen, VEMMA is a quality source of all-purpose vitamins, essential minerals, and trace minerals.

In general, I recommend taking one ounce of mangosteen, in the form of VEMMA every day. Check your Marching Orders for further application of VEMMA.

Super-Nutrients: Honorable Mention

For the sake of completeness, I have included a quick discussion on additional super-nutrients known for their benefits on the metabolism and aiding in weight loss. It is important to note that people with diabetes who take insulin or other blood-sugar-lowering agents should consult with a doctor before incorporating any of these super-nutrients into their supplementation program.

Gymnema Sylvestre

Gymnema sylvestre is an herb of Southeast Asian origin. It is native to the tropical forests of southern and central India, where it has been used as a naturopathic treatment for diabetes for nearly two thousand years. Gymnema sylvestre is also a well-known and highly respected ayurvedic remedy that is also known as the "sugar killer." It gets its reputation because it is said to remove the taste for sweet foods. The major biologically active constituents of gymnema sylvestre are the gymnemic acids. These organic compounds have an array of anti-diabetic, anti-sweetener, and anti-inflammatory activities.

Gymnema Sylvestre and IR

Gymnema sylvestre has been shown to help in the maintenance of healthy blood-glucose levels. The herb has been known to increase insulin sensitivity, fight off insulin resistance, lower blood sugar, and exert a blood-sugar stabilizing effect. The following are some possible mechanisms by which gymnema sylvestre does this:

1. It increases the secretion of insulin.
2. It increases the utilization of glucose. It has been shown to increase the activities of enzymes responsible for effective utilization of glucose by insulin-dependent pathways. This metabolic process causes an increase in insulin efficiency.

3. It has been linked to pancreatic rejuvenation because it is said to promote regeneration of pancreatic islet cells, where insulin is manufactured.
4. It causes inhibition of glucose absorption from the intestine, resulting in a lower blood-sugar level.

Gymnema Sylvestre and Sugar Cravings

Gymnema sylvestre reduces the taste of sugar when it is placed in the mouth. Therefore, it is sometimes used to fight sugar cravings. This effect, however, is short-lived, lasting a mere fifteen to twenty minutes. Interestingly, the gymnemic acids in gymnema sylvestre have a very similar atomic structure to that of glucose molecules. Some postulate that these gymnemic molecules fill the receptor locations on the taste buds. This prevents the activation of the taste buds by the sugar molecules present in food, thereby curbing the sugar craving.

Ginko Biloba

Ginkgo Biloba dates back about 200 million years. It is highly prized for its therapeutic medicinal role in traditional Chinese medicine. For weight loss, ginkgo has been shown to support healthy blood-glucose levels and insulin sensitivity. It is also a natural antioxidant that protects against oxidative cell damage from free radicals and inflammatory chemicals that contribute to IR.

Gingko biloba is also known to thin the blood and improve blood flow to most tissues and organs. This helps prevent blood clots that can lead to a number of cardiovascular, renal, respiratory, and central nervous system disorders.

Galega Officinalis

Galega officinalis (G.O.) is an herb commonly known as goat's rue, French lilac, Italian fitch, or professor-weed. It is native to the Middle East, but it has been popularized in Europe, Western Asia, and Western Pakistan.

G.O. was traditionally used in medieval Europe to help support pancreatic health, encourage healthy insulin levels, and relieve symptoms of diabetes. Recent clinical trials and studies have also suggested that this potent herb can help the body in maintaining a balanced glucose level in the bloodstream.

Upon analysis, it turns out that G.O. contains guanidine, a substance that decreases blood sugar by decreasing insulin resistance. This has evolved into some practical advantages for traditional medical doctors. Glucophage and metformin are commonly prescribed drugs for diabetics. I find it interesting that they are chemical derivatives from this biguanide class of guanidine.

Other Notable Herbs

Banaba	• Documented for its ability to lower blood sugar and act as a glucose transport in the blood stream. • Known by some as botanical insulin.
Bitter Melon	• Noted for its ability to improve glucose tolerance. • Bitter Melon is recommended by the Department of Health in the Philippines as one of the best herbal medicines for diabetes management.
Cinnamon	• USDA research indicates that cinnamon reduces the amount of insulin necessary for glucose metabolism. • Furthermore, cinnamon has been shown to stimulate glucose uptake and glycogen synthesis to similar levels as insulin.
Ginseng	• Ginseng has been documented to help regulate blood-sugar levels and improve insulin sensitivity.

These featured super-nutrients work together with Smart Foods to get the job done. Now it's time for the rubber to meet the road. What exactly do I want you to eat to:

- Ignite your fire.
- Build your fire.
- Sustain your fire.

Read along and you shall find…

LYF Summary: LYF-Style Factor #7—Nutritional Supplementation

"The Skinny" on Nutritional Supplementation—Here's What You Need to Know

- Nutritional supplementation is not optional for the best metabolic machinery; it is a must.
- The supplementation program of choice for your LYF Plan is invested in super-nutrients.
- Smart Foods are foods rich in essential nutrients that support a healthy metabolism.
- Super-nutrients are essentially Super-Smart Foods:
  - Super-nutrients have higher concentrations of powerful phytonutrients and antioxidants found in Smart Foods.
  - Super-nutrients have higher concentrations of specialized nutrients, such as chromium, that have distinctive beneficial actions on the workings of your metabolism.
- Working synergistically together with Smart Foods, super-nutrients can act as the necessary catalysts that take your metabolism to a higher gear.

LYF Applications

- Your Marching Orders will detail exactly how to incorporate super-nutrients into your nutritional program.

SECTION II

The Marching Orders

9

INTRODUCTION TO YOUR MARCHING ORDERS

NOW for the fun part of the program. Welcome to section II, the action steps affectionately known as your Marching Orders for your LYF Permanent Weight-loss Plan. The time has come to light your Metabolic Fire and accelerate your metabolic rate! Section I has been devoted to reviewing all of the major factors that influence your metabolism. In section I, you get to know what to do. In section II, you get to do what you know. Here you get to apply all of the knowledge underlying "How to Naturally Accelerate Your Metabolism." The idea is to favorably influence all of the LYF-Style Factors that increase your metabolic rate. The goal is simple. Lose your excess weight and keep it off forever. At the very core, however, this permanent weight-loss process is part of something bigger. It follows a time-honored process of nutritional healing.

Let me explain this process. To begin with, I am certain that you realize a healthy metabolism is the key to Metabolic Fire and an accelerated metabolic rate. Therefore, to achieve permanent weight loss, you must first repair and restore your metabolism and save it from the jaws of metabolic dysfunction. This metabolic dysfunction, or a wounded metabolism, is the leading cause of obesity. At the end of the day, it is absolutely imperative to revitalize, refresh, and rejuvenate your metabolism to get long-term results. A wounded metabolism calls for nutritional healing. The purpose of nutritional healing is to transform your metabolism from dysfunction, or a wounded state, to a healthy, whole, healed state.

In surgery, postoperative wound healing after an appendectomy or hysterectomy is a process. So is nutritional healing. You would not expect someone to lift weights at the gym a few days after they have gotten out of surgery for a hernia repair. They will have to wait for the wound to heal for strenuous exertion. Similarly, it is essential to avoid certain foods while your metabolism is healing. Better said, specific foods and dietary patterns promote wound healing. Other foods and dietary patterns interfere with and delay your metabolic healing. I have studied these patterns over the past four decades. What needs to be healed? Your metabolism does. That means your organs, glands, metabolic pathways, blood chemistry, and hormonal imbalances all need to be restored to good running order. By following the nutritional process outlined in this section, you will have a full wind at your back in reaching and sustaining your ideal body weight.

There are three important steps in nutritional healing that work to keep you fit and slim and looking good. The three steps in the process are:

1. LYF Power Cleansing
2. LYF Nutritional Detox
3. LYF Maintenance Plan

STAGE	DESCRIPTION	DURATION
Stage 1: LYF Power Cleansing	Ignite Your Metabolic Fire	Five to Seven Days
Stage 2: LYF Nutritional Detox	Build Your Metabolic Fire	Until You Reach Your Desired Weight
Stage 3: LYF Maintenance Plan	Sustain Your Metabolic Fire	The Rest of Your Life

Stage 1, the LYF Power Cleansing, is the first step to rejuvenating your metabolism. This stage is designed for the first five to seven days. You are well advised to start your program with the best foods that can get your fire started. Power Cleansing calls for the specific foods that are easiest for your body to metabolize. These foods are the paper and twigs to starting your Metabolic Fire. This weeklong process will purify your liver, pancreas, kidneys, lymph system, bloodstream, and other organs, and initiate the burning of fat. Although results may vary, most people usually lose in the range of five to seven pounds during this initial stage of Power Cleansing.

Stage 2, the LYF Nutritional Detox, is designed to build upon the Metabolic Fire ignited in the Power Cleansing stage. It is the nutritional program of choice for achieving your desired weight. Whether you are looking to lose 35 pounds or 135 pounds, you are well advised to stay in the Nutritional Detox stage until all of the excess weight is lost. In other words, the more weight you need to lose to reach your ideal body weight, the longer the Nutritional Detox will be for you. This stage adds a variety of additional good carbs and proteins and supports a healthy, sustained weight-loss effort. Weight-loss results are individualized, but you can expect to lose on average two pounds per week, or eight to ten pounds per month, over the duration of this period.

Stage 3, the LYF Maintenance Plan, begins once you have achieved your ideal body weight. This stage introduces a comprehensive system of food selection designed to last for the rest of your life! Additional foods, that is to say, medium to heavy logs, will be added in LYF Maintenance that will help you sustain your Metabolic Fire and maintain your ideal body weight.

Before you start on the LYF Program, here are a few things to keep in mind:

- The closer you follow the prescribed nutritional plan, the better your results will be.

- Once you have achieved your ideal body weight, you will transition into the LYF Maintenance Plan, which is designed to be a system of food selection for the rest of your life. If you ever stray from the LYF Maintenance Plan and need to reestablish your ideal body weight, you can either transition into the Nutritional Detox stage until you reestablish your ideal body weight or start with a week of Power Cleansing followed by Nutritional Detox if you need to take more aggressive action.

Now it is time to get the fire started. Get ready to transform your metabolism and start losing weight with Power Cleansing.

10

STAGE I—LYF POWER CLEANSING

PURIFY YOUR ORGANS AND TRANSFORM YOUR METABOLISM

POWER Cleansing is the first step to restoring your metabolism and lighting your Metabolic Fire. Nutritional Cleansing is a time-honored pearl for initiating the nutritional healing process. It is a crucial step that lays the foundation for permanent weight loss. When you are Power Cleansing, you will feed your body with alkaline, high-enzyme, nutrient-rich, whole, living foods that will support your metabolic machinery. You will be asked to avoid commonly eaten foods that introduce unwanted toxins to your system and can result in organ stress and metabolic dysfunction. Power Cleansing works from the inside out. I like to tell my patients that Power Cleansing is like having the oil changed in your car. A clean engine works the best. Power Cleansing purifies all of the key players of your metabolism: your liver, pancreas, digestive organs, blood stream, kidneys, bile, and bodily fluids. This purification process transforms your metabolism into unparalleled running order and removes the metabolic friction that can stand in the way of weight loss. In effect, Power Cleansing ignites your Metabolic Fire, leads to an accelerated metabolic rate, and results in significant burning of unwanted fat.

As previously discussed, it is recommended to spend from five to seven days in the Power Cleansing stage to get your program started. This will give you enough time to favorably activate your metabolic rate.

Power Cleansing Foods Must Meet and Satisfy All of the Following Criteria:

- High-Fiber
- Low-Glycemic
- High-Alkaline
- Rich in Antioxidants
- Rich in Phytonutrients
- Low in Saturated Fat / No Trans Fat

As discussed in LYF-Style Factor #2, the most effective foods for permanent weight loss are the ones that are high in fiber, high-alkaline, low-glycemic, and rich in phytonutrients and antioxidants. Note well that these foods must also be free from significant sources of saturated fats and free of trans fats altogether. So what are the foods that satisfy all of these criteria? Vegetables, legumes, beans, nuts, and seeds are the foundation to your cleansing process. They are the paper and twigs in the food chain that ignite your metabolic rate. In addition, we include specific super-nutrients such as liquid spirulina and brewer's yeast into the Power Cleansing stage to support healthy, accelerated weight loss.

Now let's take a look at detailed instructions for Power Cleansing. Follow the plan to the letter for the best results.

A Typical Day in the Life of Power Cleansing

Morning (7:00–8:00 AM)	• Grapefruit Juice with 1 tablespoon Re-Vita
Late Morning Snack (~10:30 AM)	• Grapefruit Juice with 1 ½ tablespoons brewer's yeast
Afternoon (12:30–2:00 PM)	• Garden-Green Chlorophyll Salad with herbal dressing, and – 1–2 teaspoons unsalted sunflower seeds – 5–6 garbanzo beans • Guacamole dip with veggies
Afternoon Snack (~3:30 PM)	• Grapefruit Juice with 1 tablespoon Re-Vita *and* 1 ½ tablespoons brewer's yeast
Night (5:30–7:00 PM)	• Spice-of-Life Spinach Salad w/ herbal dressing • Bowl of lentil vegetable soup • Steamed broccoli

Recommended Nutritional Supplementation

- Re-Vita, as described above
- Brewer's Yeast, as described above
- Chromium, 200 mcg, 2 times/day
  - 200 mcg with breakfast
  - 200 mcg with dinner

Exercise

- Refer to your LYF Exercise Plan in LYF-Style Factor #2
  - Aerobic exercise in morning before breakfast
  - Additional workout before dinner (for advanced exercise plan)

Guidelines for Power Cleansing: What's In, What's Out

The foods recommended are very specific and have dynamic cleansing actions.

What's In		
Vegetables	***Yes!***	Very low-glycemic vegetables are the backbone to Power Cleansing. Most of the vegetables in Power Cleansing are eaten raw, fresh, and whole, which captures the vegetables at the height of their nutrient, phytonutrient, and antioxidant value. This ensures maximum cleansing and nutritional properties.
Legumes	***Yes!***	Lentils and peas are high-alkaline, high-fiber, low-glycemic proteins that are free from saturated fat and promote proper liver, pancreatic, and insulin function. Garbanzo beans are also high quality proteins that are recommended in your salads.
Nuts and Seeds	***Yes!***	Almond butter and sunflower seeds are the right kind of unsaturated fats and alkaline proteins for effective Power Cleansing.
Sprouts	***Yes!***	Living sprouts, especially sunflower greens, add to your Metabolic Fire. Sprouts are whole, living foods. They energize your digestive system and support an accelerated metabolic rate.

These foods should be avoided during the Power Cleansing stage.

What's Out		
Whole Grains	***No!***	Whole grains are a medium-glycemic food that can slow down weight-loss efforts if you have not sufficiently accelerated your metabolism. Keep in mind, however, that whole grains are good choices for maintaining your weight once your excess weight has been lost. Whole grains are healthy foods that are a good source of fiber and nutrients and are usually low in fat. For this reason, whole grains will be incorporated as staples in stage 3, the LYF Maintenance Plan.
Fruit	***No!***	Other than grapefruit juice used with supernutrients, fruit consumption should be avoided in this phase. Fruit is a medium-glycemic food and therefore needs to be restricted until insulin sensitivity is reestablished. Don't lose sight that fruits are full of nutrients and antioxidants. Additional fruit consumption will be introduced in Phase 2, Nutritional Detox, once certain weight-loss goals have been met.
Dairy Products	***No!***	It is best to avoid dairy products in the Power Cleansing stage. Dairy products are a significant source of saturated fat, contribute to an acidic (vs. alkaline) body chemistry, and are a zero-fiber food. Dairy products can contribute to liver stress, slow down your metabolism, and stunt weight-loss efforts. Therefore, dairy products should be avoided until your reach your LYF Maintenance Plan.
Animal Protein	***No!***	It is best to avoid animal protein in the Power Cleansing stage. Animal protein, such as beef, pork, chicken, and fish, are significant sources of saturated fat, contribute to an acidic (vs. alkaline) body chemistry, and are a zero-fiber food. These heavier proteins are optional, particularly fish and rennet-free dairy, once you reach your LYF Maintenance Plan.

Blueprint for Power Cleansing: Your Complete Nutritional Options

Meal	Description
Breakfast	• 8 ounces fresh-squeezed grapefruit juice with 1 tablespoon Re-Vita
Late Morning Snack (~10:30)	• 8 ounces fresh-squeezed grapefruit juice with 1 ½ tablespoons brewer's yeast
Lunch	• Leafy Green, Phytonutrient-Rich, Low-Glycemic, Chlorophyll Salad* with herbal dressing, and – 1–2 teaspoons unsalted sunflower seeds – 5–6 garbanzo beans • In addition to salad, choose one of the following options – One 6-inch celery stalk with 1–2 tablespoons of almond butter, ***or*** – Guacamole dip with veggies • ½ avocado mixed with fresh salsa to create guacamole dip** • Use broccoli, celery, or cucumbers to dip in guacamole
Afternoon Snack (~3:30)	• 8 ounces fresh-squeezed grapefruit juice with 1 tablespoon Re-Vita and 1 ½ tablespoons brewer's yeast
Dinner	• Leafy Green, Phytonutrient-Rich, Low-Glycemic, Chlorophyll Salad* with herbal dressing, and – 1–2 teaspoons unsalted sunflower seeds – 5–6 garbanzo beans • 1 steamed vegetable – Broccoli, zucchini, asparagus, artichoke, spinach, ***or*** mushrooms • In addition, choose one of the following options – 1 bowl of lentil vegetable soup***, or – 1 bowl of split pea vegetable soup***

* For variations of the Leafy Green, Low-Glycemic, Phytonutrient-Rich, Chlorophyll Salad, see table 10.1 at the end of the chapter.

** This is a basic guacamole option. For an additional recipe, see recipes at end of chapter.

*** See end of chapter for recipes and preferred store-bought options.

Table 10.1: Recommended Leafy Green Salads

Leafy Green, Phytonutrient-Rich, Low-Glycemic, Chlorophyll Salad Combinations*		
1.	Sprouted Garden-Fresh Salad	romaine lettuce, tomato, sprouts, parsley, red onion, and red cabbage
2.	Garden-Green Chlorophyll Salad	romaine lettuce, spinach, Swiss chard, parsley, sprouts, tomato
3.	Spice-of-Life Spinach Salad	spinach leaves, romaine lettuce, sprouts, tomato, red onion, celery
4.	Mexican Cabbage Salad	red cabbage, green cabbage, red onion or green onion, romaine lettuce ,tomato
5.	Avocado-Tomato Grande Salad **	avocado, tomato, romaine lettuce, sprouts, cucumber, spinach
6.	Radiant Radish Salad	radishes, red onion, romaine lettuce, sprouts, tomato, parsley
7.	Raw Mushroom Salad	mushrooms, romaine lettuce, sprouts, tomato, cucumber, celery
8.	Cauliflower Salad	cauliflower, celery, mushrooms ,romaine lettuce, sprouts, tomato
9.	Garden Pea Salad	Chinese snow peas, green peas, green/ red bell pepper, romaine lettuce, sprouts, tomato
10.	Mustard Greens Salad	mustard greens, beet greens, dandelion greens, sprouts, tomato
11.	Super Sprouts Salad	mung bean sprouts, alfalfa sprouts, sunflower seed sprouts, romaine lettuce, tomato
12.	Cucumber Tomato Salad	cucumber, red onion, romaine lettuce, sprouts, tomato
13.	Basic Avocado Salad**	avocado, red onion, romaine lettuce, sprouts, tomato

* Carrots and beets can be added to any salad in Nutritional Detox and Maintenance stages.

** Avocado-based salads should not be combined with guacamole option in the Power Cleansing stage.

Power Cleansing: Basic Recipes

One of the great things about Power Cleansing is that it doesn't require a lot of cooking or food preparation. For the food that does need preparation, I've included recipes below. Where applicable, I have also noted preferred brands that you can buy at the supermarket.

Luscious Lentil Soup*

Ingredients:

- 1 cup dry lentils
- 2 bay leaves
- 1 carrot, sliced
- 2 cloves garlic, pressed
- 3 tomatoes, blended with scant water
- 1 red onion, chopped
- 1 stalk celery, chopped
- 1 vegetable bouillon cube

Seasonings of choice (optional): dill, ginger, cumin, cayenne, basil, (¼ teaspoon each)

Cooking Instructions:
Rinse lentils. Soak lentils and bay leaves in 3 cups water, in a covered pot, for at least one hour. Then, simmer for 30 minutes with pot partially covered. Add balance of ingredients and simmer until lentils and vegetables are tender. If necessary, add additional water for desired consistency. Makes approximately 4 servings.

* Amy's Lentil and Lentil Vegetable soups are good organic options for store-bought soups. For those with blood pressure concerns, choose *light in sodium* options when available.

Spicy Split Pea Soup*

Ingredients:

1 cup split peas
2 bay leaves
1 clove garlic, pressed
1 red onion, chopped
1 tablespoon chopped parsley
1–2 sliced carrots
1–2 stalks celery, chopped
5 mushrooms, sliced
1 ½ vegetable bouillon cubes

Seasonings of choice (optional): 1 teaspoon dill; ½–1 teaspoon curry, jalapeño, or green chili

Cooking Instructions:
Bring 4 cups water to a boil in covered pot. Rinse split peas. Add split peas and bay leaves to boiling water. Turn down heat and simmer for 30 minutes with pot partially covered. Add balance of ingredients and simmer 15 minutes longer or until peas are done. To make a creamy soup, you can put part or all of the soup in the blender and then return to pot. Makes approximately 4 servings.

* Amy's organic Split Pea soup is a good store-bought option. For those with blood pressure concerns, choose *light in sodium* option when available.

Wholly Guacamole*

Ingredients (for 1 serving):

½ avocado
Juice from ¼ lemon
¼ clove garlic, pressed
1 teaspoon cilantro, chopped
Chopped red onion (as desired)

Seasonings of choice (all optional): Spike seasoning (just a dash); red cayenne pepper (just a dash); 1 tablespoon fresh salsa; chopped, fresh, green chilies with seeds removed (as desired)

Cooking Instructions:
Squeeze lemon juice over the avocado and mash with a fork. Mix in other ingredients, as desired.

* Note: Make sure that store-bought guacamole or restaurant-made guacamole does not include any sour cream or mayonnaise.

Dr. Meltzer's Potassium-Rich Vegetable Broth

Make sure not to snack between meals. You may, however, drink the following vegetable broth as desired.

Ingredients:

1 cup zucchini	1 medium carrot
½ cup broccoli	1 medium potato
½ cup string beans	1 stalk celery
1 tablespoon parsley	1 medium beet

Cooking Instructions:
Add the above vegetables to 4 cups of boiling water and let simmer for 20 minutes. Discard vegetables and drink the broth. Season with garlic, onion, cayenne, and kelp.

11

Stage II—LYF Nutritional Detox

Achieve Your Ideal Body Weight through Nutritional Detoxification

IF you are looking to lose more than fifteen pounds, most of your weight will be lost during the Nutritional Detox stage. The Nutritional Detox shares similarities with Power Cleansing in that it clears out liver toxins and supports superior liver function, improves pancreatic and insulin function, has an alkalinizing effect on bodily fluids, cleans up the bloodstream, and promotes insulin sensitivity. Nutritional Detox feeds the ongoing cleansing and purification of organs, bodily fluids, cells, and tissues. With time and consistency, this builds a strong Metabolic Fire and leads to the accelerated burning of excess fat.

Nutritional Detox builds upon the fundamental foods established in Power Cleansing. This includes foods that are phytonutrient-dense, high in fiber, highly alkaline, and low-glycemic. They are also the foods that are free from significant sources of saturated fat and free of trans fats altogether. Here's what's new. What sets the Nutritional Detox apart from Power Cleansing is the addition of a variety of plant-based vegetable proteins, the addition of some starchy vegetables, and the addition of fruit once you have reestablished insulin sensitivity. The Nutritional Detox is a more robust diet that enables healthy and effective weight loss over a sustained period of time. The added foods in this stage represent the kindling wood in your diet that will get your body ready for bigger logs such as thicker carbohydrates and denser proteins.

The bottom line is that the Nutritional Detox stage will enable you to achieve your desired body weight in a healthy and effective manner and will shift your body into a more efficient, metabolically balanced state. Let's take a look at what is on the menu for this phase.

A Typical Day in the Life of Nutritional Detox

Morning (7:00–8:00 AM)	• Grapefruit juice with 1 tablespoon Re-Vita • One 6-inch celery stalk with 1–2 tablespoons of almond butter
Late Morning Snack (~10:30 AM)	• Grapefruit juice with 1 ½ tablespoons brewer's yeast
Afternoon (12:30–2:00 PM)	• Garden-Green Chlorophyll Salad with herbal dressing, and – 1–2 teaspoon unsalted sunflower seeds – 5–6 garbanzo beans • Hummus taco with warm corn tortilla
Afternoon Snack (~3:30 PM)	• Grapefruit juice with 1 tablespoon Re-Vita *and* 1 ½ tablespoons brewer's yeast
Night (5:30–7:00 PM)	• 6–8 ounces of carrot celery juice • Sprouted Garden-Fresh Salad with herbal dressing • Steamed broccoli • Scrambled tofu with sautéed mushrooms

Nutritional Supplementation

- Re-Vita, as described above
- Brewer's Yeast, as described above
- Chromium, 200 mcg, 2 times/day
    - 200 mcg with breakfast
    - 200 mcg with dinner

Exercise

- Refer to your LYF Exercise Plan in LYF-Style Factor #2
    - Aerobic exercise in morning before breakfast
    - Additional workout before dinner (for advanced exercise plan)

Guidelines for Nutritional Detox: What's In, What's Out

The foods recommended for Nutritional Detox are the following:

What's In		
Vegetables	***Yes!***	Very low-glycemic vegetables are a staple to the Nutritional Detox phase. Additional vegetables, such as carrots and beats, can be added to salads in this stage. Additionally, carrot juice is recommended for dinner three times per week given its alkalinizing effect on your body and the liver.
Legumes	***Yes!***	Additional legumes are added in this phase to meet up with longer-term protein requirements. Additional proteins include tofu, soy products, tempeh, veggie burgers, pinto beans, black beans, garbanzo beans, and red kidney beans.
Nuts and Seeds	***Yes!***	Additional nuts and seeds are added in this stage, including walnuts, cashews, non-hydrogenated peanut butter, and other nut butters. These are the good unsaturated fats that will keep your metabolism in good running order.
Sprouts	***Yes!***	Living sprouts, especially sunflower greens, add to your Metabolic Fire. Sprouts are whole, living foods. They energize your digestive system and support an accelerated metabolic rate.
Addendum		
Corn Tortillas	***Yes!***	Corn tortillas are added in this stage to complement certain lunch and dinner options.

Fruit	***Yes!***	Aside from grapefruit juice used with super-nutrients, fruit must be avoided for the first three weeks to reestablish sufficient insulin sensitivity. After three weeks, fruit can be added as soon as the following weight-loss goals have been achieved. • If you begin the program thirty pounds or more overweight, fruit can be added once you are within twenty-five pounds of your ideal weight. • If you begin the program thirty pounds or less overweight, fruit can be added once you are within fifteen pounds of your ideal weight.

The foods that should be avoided during the Nutritional Detox stage are the following:

What's Out		
Whole Grains	***No!***	Whole grains such as whole grain bread, whole grain cereals, and whole grain rice are to be avoided until stage 3, the LYF Maintenance Plan. As we've discussed, whole grains are healthy foods but are better options for maintaining your weight.
Dairy Products	***No!***	It is best to avoid dairy products in the Nutritional Detox stage. Dairy products are a significant source of saturated fat, contribute to an acidic (vs. alkaline) body chemistry, and are a zero-fiber food. Dairy products can contribute to liver stress, slow down your metabolism, and stunt weight-loss efforts. Therefore, dairy products should be avoided until your reach your LYF Maintenance Plan.
Animal Protein	***No!***	It is best to avoid animal protein in the Nutritional Detox stage. Animal protein, such as beef, pork, chicken, and fish, are significant sources of saturated fat, contribute to an acidic (vs. alkaline) body chemistry, and are a zero-fiber food. These heavier proteins are optional, particularly fish and rennet-free dairy, once you reach your LYF Maintenance Plan.

Blueprint for Nutritional Detox: Your Complete Nutritional Options

Meal	Description
Breakfast	• 8 ounces fresh-squeezed grapefruit or orange juice with 1 tablespoon Re-Vita • One 6-inch celery stalk with 1–2 tablespoons of almond butter ***

*** Celery and almond butter is optional. If you prefer a lighter breakfast, stick with the juice and Re-Vita.

Late Morning Snack (~10:30 AM)	• 8 ounces fresh-squeezed grapefruit or orange juice with 1 ½ tablespoons brewer's yeast

Lunch	• Leafy Green, Phytonutrient-Rich, Low-Glycemic, Chlorophyll Salad*, with – 2 teaspoons unsalted sunflower seeds – 5–6 garbanzo beans • In addition to salad, choose one of the following options from Group A or Group B.
Group A—Taco Combinations	
• Add fresh salsa to flavor any of the following options	
Option 1	• Guacamole taco with warm corn tortilla – ½ avocado mixed with fresh salsa to create guacamole dip** – 1–2 corn tortillas
Option 2	• Hummus taco with warm corn tortilla – Hummus*** and fresh salsa – 1–2 corn tortillas
Option 3	• Tempeh taco with warm corn tortilla – Tempeh spread*** – 1–2 corn tortillas

Option 4	• Tofu taco with warm corn tortilla – Egg-free Tofu Salad or Tofu Cottage Salad*** – 1–2 corn tortillas
Group B—Veggie Dips	
• Broccoli, celery, or cucumbers with your choice of vegetable protein spread***	
Option 1	• Guacamole dip with veggies – ½ avocado mixed with fresh salsa to create guacamole dip** – Use broccoli, celery, or cucumbers to dip in guacamole·
Option 2	• Hummus dip with veggies – Hummus and fresh salsa – Use broccoli, celery, or cucumbers to dip in hummus.
Option 3	• Tempeh salad with veggies – Tempeh spread – Use broccoli, celery, or cucumbers to dip in tempeh.
Option 4	• Tofu salad with veggies – Egg-free Tofu Salad or Tofu Cottage Salad – Use broccoli, celery, or cucumbers to dip in tofu spread.
Option 5	• Lentil dip with veggies – Lentil walnut pate – Use broccoli, celery, or cucumbers to dip in lentil spread.
Option 6	• 2 celery sticks with 1–2 tablespoons almond butter

* For variations of the Leafy Green, Phytonutrient-Rich, Low-Glycemic, Chlorophyll Salad, see table 10.1 in Power Cleansing.

** For additional guacamole recipe, reference Power Cleansing recipes.

*** Most of these spreads can be found at the health food section of your local supermarket or health food store.

Afternoon Snack (~3:30 PM)	• 8 ounces fresh-squeezed grapefruit juice with 1 tablespoon Re-Vita and 1 ½ tablespoons brewer's yeast

Dinner	• 6–8 ounces of carrot-celery juice (2 parts carrot: 1 part celery), 3x/week • Leafy Green, Phytonutrient-Rich, Low-Glycemic, Chlorophyll Salad* with herbal dressing, and – 2 teaspoons unsalted sunflower seeds (or 4–7 walnuts) – 5–6 garbanzo beans or red kidney beans • 1 steamed vegetable – Broccoli, zucchini, asparagus, artichoke, spinach, or mushrooms • In addition, choose one of the following dinner options from groups A–F
Group A—Soup Exchanges	
• Any vegetable soup combined with a plant protein (beans, lentils, legumes, tofu, etc.)	
Option 1	• Lentil Vegetable or Split Pea Vegetable soup**
Option 2	• Black Bean Vegetable soup
Option 3	• Mixed Bean Vegetable soup (Lima Bean, White Navy Bean, etc.)***
Option 4	• Pasta free, Vegan Minestrone Soup
Option 5	• Thai Peanut Soup
Option 6	• Tortilla Soup: Tomato Soup with Avocado and a Corn Tortilla
Group B—Tofu Exchanges	
• Any tofu dish combined with veggies or a corn tortilla	
Option 1	• Scrambled tofu with mushroom and onions***

Option 2	• Tofu chop suey with cabbage and mung bean sprouts***
Option 3	• Tofu enchilada with corn tortilla, veggies, and salsa or enchilada sauce
Group C—Mexican Foods	
• Your choice of Mexican food dishes that include beans, vegetables, and a corn tortilla. (Be sure to avoid rice, flour tortillas, and cheese.)	
Option 1	• Refried vegetarian beans and salsa in a warm corn tortilla
Option 2	• Vegetarian enchilada with beans and veggies in a warm corn tortilla
Group D—Veggie Burgers	
• Any choice of veggie burger (no bun). Use Dijon mustard or salsa to flavor.	
Option 1	• Tofu Burger or Soy Burger***
Option 2	• Tempeh Burger
Option 3	• Soy-Based Garden Burgers****
Option 4	• Falafel Burger
Group E—Tempeh Exchanges	
• Any tempeh dish mixed with vegetables or a corn tortilla	
Option 1	• Tempeh tacos with shitake mushrooms
Option 2	• Tempeh enchiladas with shitake mushrooms
Group F—Lentil Exchanges	
Any lentil dish with vegetables	
Option 1	• Lentil-mushroom-vegetable casserole
Option 2	• Lentil burger with sautéed mushrooms

* For variations of the Leafy Green, Phytonutrient-Rich, Low-Glycemic, Chlorophyll Salad, see table 10.1 in Power Cleansing.

** Refer to Power Cleansing recipes.

*** Refer to Nutritional Detox recipes.

**** For example, vegan Boca burger.

Nutritional Detox: Basic Recipes

To get you started, I have included recipes on some of the nuts and bolts of your Nutritional Detox program. Since breakfast and lunch options require minimal preparation, the following recipes will focus on dinner options. Where applicable, I have also noted preferred brands that you can buy at the supermarket. In addition, make sure to use our website as a resource for additional recipes—www.maketimeforwellness.com.

Soup Exchanges— Recipes

- Lentil Vegetable Soup—refer back to Power Cleansing recipes.
- Split Pea Soup—refer back to Power Cleansing recipes.

Lima Bean—Mixed Vegetable Soup*

Ingredients:

1 ½ cups dried lima beans
1 ½ cups celery, chopped
1 ½ cups carrots, chopped
1 ½ cups onions, chopped
2 bay leaves
½ cup green pepper, finely chopped
1 ½ cups green beans, cut into 2-inch peaces
1–2 tomatoes, chopped into small chunks
6 cups water
1 ½ vegetable bouillon cubes

Seasonings of choice (optional): ½ teaspoon black pepper, 2 tablespoons apple cider vinegar, ½ teaspoon kelp, basil

Cooking Instructions:
Rinse beans. Then, soak the beans in covered pot overnight or for several hours in 6 cups water. Simmer beans with bay leaves for 45 minutes. Then, add remaining ingredients (except for tomato) and simmer for an additional 15 minutes or until vegetables and beans are tender. Add tomato at end. For creamy consistency, blend ½ of soup content in blender and return to soup pot to reheat. Makes approximately 6 servings.

* Amy's Black Bean Vegetable soup is a good organic option for store-bought bean soups.

Tofu Exchanges— Recipes

Scrambled Tofu

Ingredients:

3 tablespoons olive oil
1 onion, diced
5 cloves garlic, crushed
2 cups firm tofu, drained and cubed
12 mushrooms

Seasonings of choice (optional): 1 tablespoon fresh ginger (grated), Spike or Bragg Liquid Aminos (to taste)

Cooking Instructions:
In a large skillet, heat oil. Sauté onion and garlic until golden brown, medium heat. Add tofu. Cover and steam in own juices, stirring often. Uncover, let brown, add mushrooms and seasonings. Cover and cook briefly. Uncover and cook until golden brown. Other vegetables may be included for vegetable chow mein.

Tofu Chop Suey

Ingredients:

1 celery stalk, chopped
1 large onion, chopped
1 tablespoon olive oil
1 cup mushrooms, chopped
1 cup mung bean sprouts
1 cup Chinese cabbage
1 cup tofu, drained and cubed
1 teaspoon minced ginger (optional)
Broccoli, snow peas, or sesame seeds (other optional additions)

Seasonings of choice: Bragg Liquid Aminos (2 tablespoons)

Cooking Instructions:
Sauté onion and celery in skillet until tender. Add mushrooms, sprouts, cabbage and Bragg seasoning. Toss and sauté for 3–5 minutes. Add tofu, stirring periodically until heated.

Veggie Burgers

- Preferred store-bought tofu burger is Wildwood Organics Tofu Veggie Burger

Soy Burger

Ingredients:

1 cup dry whole soybeans
¾ cup sesame meal (sesame seeds grounded in blender or food processor)
½ cup sunflower meal (sunflower seeds grounded in blender or food processor)
3 green onions, finely chopped
2 tablespoons olive oil
1 tablespoon agar agar, dissolved in $^{2}/_{3}$ cup water
½ small green pepper, finely chopped
2 cups mushrooms, chopped
1 stalk celery, finely chopped
2 bay leaves
1 teaspoon sea salt

Cooking Instructions:

Soak soybeans overnight in covered pot. Drain and rinse soybeans. Then, add 4 cups of water and bay leaves and simmer soybeans in partially covered pot. When the soybeans are tender and you can mash them with a fork on the side of the pot, they are done (approximately 4 hours). Yields 3 cups cooked beans. Remove bay leaves, drain, and mash with a potato masher while soy beans are still warm. Add agar agar mixture and stir evenly into soybean mixture. Then, add:

- 1 teaspoon salt
- Sesame meal
- Sunflower meal
- Onion
- Mushrooms
- Celery

Mix well and form into patties. Heat 2 tablespoons olive oil in skillet. Place patties on skillet and brown on both sides. When brown, place on baking dish at 350 degrees for 20-30 minutes. Makes six patties.

Golden Rules for LYF Nutritional Detox

Before we transition to the LYF Maintenance phase, lets' review the *Golden Rules* for following Nutritional Detox.

****Eat at prescribed times.

****Have leafy green salads with lunch and dinner.

****Select one lunch exchange and one dinner exchange each day.

****Vary your meal plan for balance and fun

****Avoid the forbidden foods at all costs.

****Avoid snacking and nibbling.

****Rely on Liquid Nutrition when you want something between meals.

- Drink the potassium broth, as referenced in Power Cleansing recipes.
- Make a cup of warm, herbal tea.
- Have a glass of grapefruit juice with Re-Vita and / or brewer's yeast.

****Work out every day—keep your attitude fired up, warm, bright, and light.

****Go back to your cleansing diet one day/week—five days every three months.

****Be certain to get six to eight glasses of pure water a day.

****Season your food with herbs.

12

Stage III—LYF Maintenance Plan

Take Charge Maintenance Plan: How to Keep Fit and Maintain Your Weight

CONGRATULATIONS! You have successfully completed the LYF Power Cleansing and Nutritional Detox. I can only imagine how good you must feel. I have to say, witnessing thousands of patients reach their weight-loss goals has been one of the most rewarding aspects of my years as a physician. As you well know, however, there is more to it than just that. Keeping the excess weight off is what counts. This is where your LYF Maintenance Plan comes into play. The take-charge Maintenance Plan is based on eating your way to superior weight and waist management. The purpose of LYF Maintenance is to sustain a nutritional program and supportive lifestyle that will maintain your ideal weight and prevent weight gain. LYF Maintenance empowers you with everlasting, long-lasting Metabolic Fire. The focus is to maintain and sustain this metabolic power to stay fit, toned, and healthy for the rest of your life. In essence, the Maintenance Plan maintains permanent weight control.

LYF Maintenance further builds upon the Smart Food foundation that makes up the Power Cleansing and Nutritional Detox stages. In addition to the whole, fresh, living food and complete protein ever present in the Power

Cleansing and Nutritional Detox plans, Maintenance includes the addition of three distinct food groups.

LYF MAINTENANCE ADDS THE FOLLOWING FOOD:
• Complex Carbohydrates***—Whole grain breads, whole grain pastas, whole grain cereals, and starchy vegetables such as potatoes are added.
• Fruit***—A wider assortment of fruit is added.
• Expanded Protein Choices—Additional protein options are included. You can choose from a Vegan, Vegetarian, or Modified Plant-Based protein plan.
*** By now you have established sufficient insulin sensitivity to effectively handle the medium-glycemic carbohydrates found in fruits, whole grains, and starchy vegetables.

The essence of the LYF Maintenance Plan is combining fresh, whole, living foods with complete proteins, and high-quality complex carbohydrates. This synergy has been worked out for you, detail-by-detail, in your Marching Orders. Before we discuss exactly what to eat, I want to tell you a little more about this time-honored Maintenance Plan.

LYF Maintenance Works!

LYF Maintenance is based on a simple, yet profound three-step formula that will guide you to permanent weight loss. Most folks who are overweight are incarcerated by their weight gain as they get caught in a cycle of losing and gaining weight. This formula will give you the code to break free. It gives you the necessary skills you need to effectively maintain your ideal weight and end yo-yo dieting.

LYF MAINTENANCE THREE-STEP FORMULA:
1. Reprogram Your Attitude: Select for Smartness
2. Acquire Nutritional Know-How: Learn What to Eat
3. Take Action: Do it! Eat Smart.

- Remember: Attitude + Know-How + Action = Permanent Weight Loss

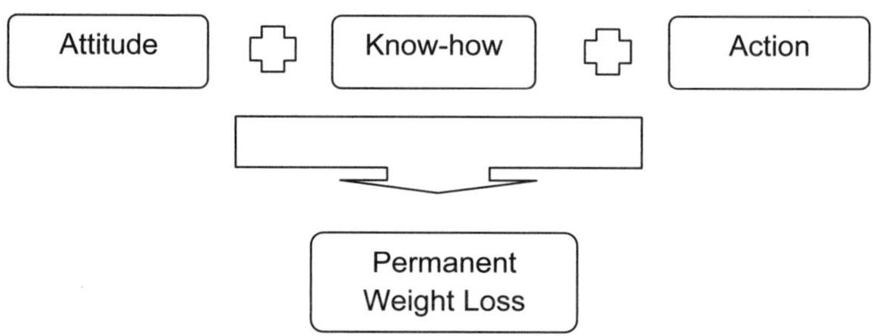

Step 1—Change Your Attitude: Select for Smartness

Your attitude is your frame of mind; it is the way you see things. Your nutritional attitude is the way you relate to food, the way you look to food, and the role food plays in your life. So what kind of nutritional attitude will lead you down the path to permanent weight loss? The attitude of choice is Nutritional Mindfulness. You will need Nutritional Mindfulness to achieve permanent weight control. Yes, the right nutritional attitude plays a huge role in your ability to maintain your new weight and your new look. Let the truth be known, Nutritional Mindfulness is necessary to support a lifetime of endless energy, good health, and ideal weight. Let me explain.

I want you to pause, take a moment, and take some time to reflect on your relationship with food. Are you a recreational eater or do you eat with Nutritional Mindfulness? That is, do you principally eat for pleasure or eat for wellness? This is an important distinction to make. Unfortunately, most of us eat for comfort and pleasure. We turn to food for entertainment and not for its health benefits. In other words, most of us eat for the wrong reasons. It is a matter of habit. We've been raised in a culture that turns to instant gratification in the here and now over long-term benefits. For our whole lives, we have looked to food for its reward, pleasure, and entertainment value. This is very much ingrained in our lifestyle. When we eat, we are typically responding to an impulse. When we think of something "good to eat," we only consider the immediate, sensual appeal of food, and not of the negative effects it may ultimately have on our health or metabolism. Eating for pleasure is an impulse-driven attitude. This does not work for permanent weight loss. It is the opposite of Nutritional Mindfulness.

Nutritional Mindfulness is defined by selecting items based on their nutritional and metabolic value rather than their initial taste or emotional appeal. Eating for wellness is smart and savvy eating. It is of utmost importance that we reprioritize our food choices.

Make the Shift

The right attitude requires a slight shift in outlook:

- Eat to live, don't live to eat.

When you eat to live, the focus is on wellness. When you live to eat, the focus is on pleasure. Eating for pleasure rather than wellness will ultimately let you down. I know how this sounds. Eating to live may seem boring to you. But let me assure you that eating for wellness can still be a lot of fun and very enjoyable! Eating for wellness can be tasty, appetizing, and appealing. By using a variety of herbs and seasonings, you can prepare Smart Food to fit your tastes. To tempt your palate, think of tomato-basil-mushroom pasta; rich minestrone soup; thick guacamole, chunky salsa, and creamy hummus dips; rainbow fruit salads; bean tostadas; nutty soy spreads; veggie pizzas; plus an assortment of Indian, Mexican, Italian, Greek, and Chinese dishes. Yes, eating for wellness can be very pleasurable as well!

Karen Knows Best

Karen and Barbara are exercise buddies. They are both in their early forties and are almost identical in height at 5'7". Five years ago, they both weighed approximately 170 pounds. Five years later, Karen is 135 pounds whereas Barbara still weighs 170. Despite the same workout routine throughout the week, Karen has been successful in maintaining her ideal weight for several years whereas Barbara has been trying to lose thirty-five pounds with little success. Barbara's weight fluctuates as she goes in and out of fad diets and can never sustain any of her weight loss. So why has Karen been successful in maintaining her weight whereas Barbara has failed? It's not her genetics. It's not her exercise habits. It's not her religion, and it's not her marriage. It's Karen's nutritional attitude!

After their morning jog, they usually pass by a pastry shop. Barbara can't wait to reward herself with a treat. Within seconds, she succumbs to the bakery's sweet aromas and buys the brightest goodies on display. Karen sees and smells the exact same items, but she is not lured by the fragrance of fresh brewed coffee and sugary doughnuts. She anticipates the fruit salad and bowl of muesli and soy milk that await her at home.

Karen, of course, has the Smart Food attitude. She eats for wellness. That's why she lost the weight and was successful in keeping it off. Karen won't sabotage her daily jog for muffins and croissants. When Karen and Barbara lunch together, Karen typically has a soup and salad whereas Barbara enjoys a sandwich with the works, french fries, and a diet coke in addition to her salad. When they dine out with their husbands, Karen sticks to a salad and an entrée whereas Barbara tends to overeat. Barbara is known to finish a basket of bread before her meal and is the first to order dessert. The point is, Karen eats to live whereas Barbara lives to eat.

Karen respects her body and wants to look and feel her best. It took her a little time. Like most of us, she was raised on the SAD—Standard American Diet. She gradually found herself gaining weight through her thirties; by her late thirties, she was thirty to forty pounds overweight and feeling more and more fatigued. She decided to take a stand, made fitness and health a priority in her life, and devoted her attention to nutrition and the healing arts. As she started making better food choices, she noticed an interesting transformation. Not only was she starting to lose weight, but she had more energy; she was more productive at work, and she saw herself develop more self-confidence. Karen began to really value how the food she ate made her look and feel. Her food preferences began to change to a point that she was no longer attracted to food that wasn't good for her. She now knows that sugary desserts and caffeinated coffee drain her energy, and she finds colorful, seasonal fruit salads and leafy green salads more appetizing and appealing. She would rather eat some fresh pineapple than a glazed doughnut any day.

Barbara, on the other hand, was never able to change her impulsive attitude toward food. She lives to eat and feels she is at the mercy of croissants, pizzas, pastas, fried foods, and rich creamy desserts.

Free Your Mind: Thoughts Lead to Action

Thought precedes action. Thought leads to action. Let me explain. It is ingrained in our culture to look to food to satisfy our palate. We've all been programmed to eat what is popular, and the most popular items are those that are most heavily advertised, most readily available, and most pleasing to the palate. Over time, these thoughts lead to a self-indulgent attitude of eating for pleasure. Unfortunately, as discussed, this is the wrong attitude for managing your weight and sustaining good health. This is shortsighted and doesn't address the big picture. It is important to enjoy your meal but not at the expense of your well-being. It doesn't make sense to sacrifice your health.

So how do you go about converting from a recreational eater to a health-minded eater? First, you have to understand that your attitude about eating and your actual eating habits are inextricably interwoven. Therefore, you need to change your thoughts before you can change your eating habits. Here is a simple thought process that I want you to adopt. This new way of thinking needs to take into consideration the impact the food is going to have on you long term. When you are deciding what to eat, I want you to think about how the food is going to make you feel later, *after* you have finished eating. For example, having fruit and nuts for breakfast is going to keep you feeling energized, healthy, and looking good throughout the day. Alternatively, indulging in bacon, sausage, and eggs may seem more appealing at first glance. When you stop and think about it, it is not as appealing when you know the breakfast of bacon, sausage, and eggs contributes to long-term fatigue, sluggishness, health problems, and excess weight.

I want you to keep this in mind. Nothing tastes as good as feeling good. Nothing tastes as good as looking good and feeling sexy and attractive. Nothing tastes as good as being energized and feeling well. This is the necessary thought process to eat for wellness, as opposed to eating for pleasure. This will lead you to Nutritional Mindfulness and permanent weight loss.

I've observed an interesting transformation take place with countless patients of mine. As they adopt a new attitude and begin to value how a food is going to make them look and feel over the long term, their food preferences begin to change. Over time, the bowl of fruit with nuts actually sounds more appealing to them than the doughnut and coffee.

Lyin', Cheatin', Lowdown, Dirty, Good-For-Nuthin' …

Let's say you're single, and you meet someone you find physically attractive, so you embark upon a relationship. Yes, you like the person's personality, but let's also say that this certain someone doesn't tell the truth and you often catch this person lying. What if that person was also stealing your valuables behind your back? How long would you stay in that relationship? What is the benefit of continuing it?

The same holds true for food selections. Junk foods and comfort foods may have some superficial sizzle, but they're bad for you. They're all flash, no substance; and they often stress you out. As humans, we are blessed with free will. We can change our attitudes about the emotional and entertainment value we attach to food. It is within our power to select wholesome nutrition that is still enjoyable. Ask yourself, what's holding you back?

Change Your Attitude for Food, Change Your Attitude for Life!

One final point about attitude: When you change the way you think about eating, you don't just change your appetite for food. There's a ripple effect that impacts your appetite for excellence and appetite for life. Great health transforms everything—from your performance in sports, to your stamina when the flu fells everyone else at the office, to your energy level at the end of the day when your kids need help with their homework. By feeding your body, you're also feeding your soul.

As you develop a taste for Smart Foods, I guarantee that you'll also look forward to and enjoy these foods. In fact, you'll take pride in them. After all, Smart Foods are the real thing—wholesome, fresh, colorful, and sensual. They have not been pressed, bleached, or chemically altered.

Step 2—Acquire Nutritional Know-How: Learn What to Eat

Acquiring Nutritional Know-how is the second step in the LYF Maintenance formula for permanent weight loss. So what is it you need to know? You need to know what to eat to maintain your ideal weight. There are two fundamental components to learning what to eat.

LYF MAINTENANCE NUTRITIONAL KNOW-HOW
1. Smart Food Selection
2. Combining Smart Foods to Create Metabolic Balance

Smart Food Selection

The first step of Nutritional Know-How is knowing how to select Smart Foods. I'm confident that you know how to do this given our discussion of Smart Foods in LYF-Style Factor #2. In way of review, Smart Foods are those that are fresh, whole, living foods that are high-fiber, high-alkaline, phytonutrient- and antioxidant-rich. Smart Foods are free of trans fats and are not a significant source of saturated fat. Choosing foods based on these qualities will enable you to select the best carbohydrates, the best proteins, and the best fats for your metabolism and overall health.

Smart Food selection is based on applying the benefit-to-risk ratio; that is, choosing foods with the most nutritional benefits and least metabolic risks. For example, the media would like you to believe that eggs are the perfect protein. But eggs are sky-high in cholesterol and extremely mucus-forming. They put the consumer at risk for everything from the common cold to respiratory problems to clogged arteries. In other words, the risks of egg consumption far outweigh the benefits, especially when you can substitute scrambled tofu sautéed lightly in olive oil with onions and mushrooms and gain the equivalent protein value without the saturated fat, cholesterol, or phlegm. Whenever in doubt, use the benefit-to-risk ratio to help you make your Smart Food choices.

By now you are well versed in the ins and outs of Smart Food selection. The next step in Nutritional Know-How is knowing how to combine these Smart Foods appropriately and in what general proportions they should be eaten.

Combining Smart Foods

Maintaining your weight is based on balancing your body chemistry once you have lost the weight. This comes down to combining the right Smart Foods.

- ***LYF Maintenance offers you a variety of choices that combine fresh, whole, living foods with complete proteins and high-quality complex carbohydrates.***

This is the essence of achieving nutritional balance, sustaining Metabolic Fire, and maintaining your ideal weight.

Honor the Four Real Food Groups

Smart Food combining is based upon honoring the Four Real Food Groups. Smart eating, therefore, balances the right combinations and proper proportions of vital nutrients and Smart Foods from the four most important food groups. Based on people's eating habits, you might think the four food groups are meat, dairy, breads, and dessert. This is not the case. For optimal nutrition, adhere to the four *real* food groups in these general proportions:

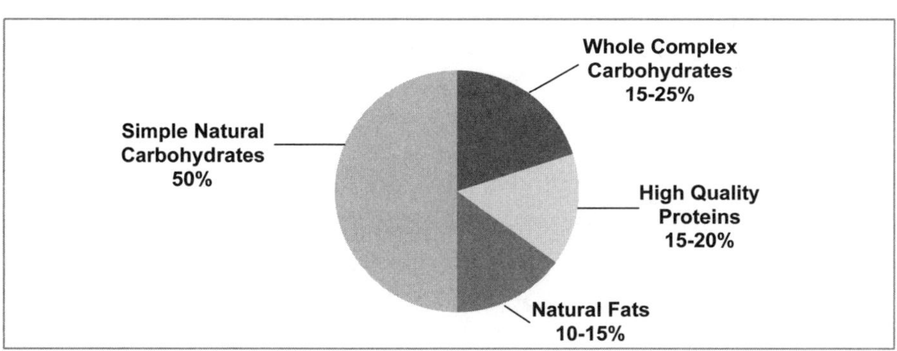

I. **Natural, Simple Carbohydrates** (50%) Fresh fruits, fresh vegetables, and their natural juices are good carbohydrates. They are the best simple carbohydrates. Fruits and vegetables are high-fiber, low-fat, nutrient-rich food. These are the paper, twigs, and kindling wood of your Metabolic Fire.

II. **Whole, Complex Carbohydrates** (15–25%) Whole grain breads, whole grain pastas, whole grain cereals, brown rice, corn on the cob, baked potatoes, and other whole grains are all good carbohydrates for maintenance. In fact, they are the best complex carbohydrates. They are the "bigger logs" in the metabolic food chain. Therefore, they are omitted in the Power Cleansing and Nutritional Detox regimes and are added once the fire is established and you want to keep it burning.

III. **High-Quality Proteins** (15–20%) Plant proteins, such as beans, legumes, tofu, tempeh, lentils, peas, and veggie burgers are all good proteins. They are the best proteins for your metabolism because they are high in fiber and low in fat, are not a significant source of saturated fat, and have a higher alkaline chemistry. Choosing predominantly plant proteins is a great option for your health and metabolism. Although the LYF Power Cleansing and Nutritional Detox diet is strictly vegetarian, the maintenance program offers you the option to go vegetarian or not. What's important, however, is to emphasize plant proteins as a staple to LYF Maintenance. It is preferred that at least 80 percent of your maintenance protein is of vegetable or plant origin. As you will see, combining complex carbohydrates with the right protein sources is what identifies this plan as your maintenance program.

IV. **Natural Fats (unsaturated fats)** (10–15%) Unsaturated fats found in avocados, nuts, nut butters, seeds, and vegetable oils are the best kind of fats for your liver, your metabolism, and your overall health. They are the right fats for your LYF Maintenance Plan.

Maintenance Has Enough Protein

The LYF Maintenance Plan has a substantial amount of complete protein. It is carefully constructed to provide anywhere from thirty-five to sixty grams of complete protein daily to match your needs. In general, most adults require forty to fifty grams of complete protein, at least five days per week, to sufficiently maintain their protein requirements. This does not apply to children;

teenagers under eighteen; competitive, high performance athletes; or pregnant or lactating females who made need more***.

*** If you have increased protein requirements, high-protein smoothies can be included between meals. Smoothies can include almond butter, brewer's yeast, soy yogurt, and Re-Vita to increase protein intake.

Complete Proteins

What does it mean to be a complete protein? Let's take a review of protein chemistry for a moment. Amino acids are the building blocks of protein. There are eight essential amino acids that must come from your food supply that cannot be synthesized by the human body. When all eight essential amino acids are present in your protein source, it qualifies as a complete protein. Complete protein sources are necessary for growth, development, and good health. There are two categories of complete sources of protein:

1. Single Food Source: as the name implies, single food source complete proteins provide all of the eight essential amino acids in one food source. Animal protein, such as the protein found in meat, dairy, and eggs are all single food sources of complete protein.
2. Combined Food Source: typically, plant proteins do not provide a complete protein within one food. Not to worry. By combining one or more plant foods, you can provide all of the essential amino acids and achieve complete protein nutrition. For example, beans and rice are a combined food source of complete protein.

By consuming a simple variety of plant proteins that we encounter every day, the full range of essential amino acids can be easily met with a plant-based diet. We can grow just as tall, just as strong, and just as fast with plant-based proteins. Therefore, it's not important whether your protein comes from a combined food source or a single food source. What matters is you have a complete protein.

You can be sure you are getting enough complete protein when you feel good, look good, and are energetic. Your body needs just the right amount of protein; that is what nutritional balance is all about. Too much protein, particularly acid-forming animal protein, predisposes you to health problems such as arthritis, kidney disease, and cancer. Not enough complete protein causes malnutrition, fatigue, and muscle wasting. LYF maintenance provides the right balance of high-quality, complete protein to suit your needs.

What are the Best Sources of Protein?

As Americans, we tend to have an obsession with protein. We've been taught that protein makes us big, strong, and healthy—the more quantity, the better. Interestingly, in deciding the best source of protein for your health and metabolism, it is the *quality* of the protein source that matters most. How do you go about judging the quality of a protein source? It is smart to use the benefit-to-risk ratio to decide. You see, it is important to select quality proteins with the most benefits for your health and the least risks to your body and taxes to your metabolism.

In fact, determining which nutritional program is right for you and your metabolism will often come down to the prevailing type of protein choices in your diet. That is, whether your protein comes primarily from plant sources or animal sources. Historically, we have been guided to think that animal proteins were a superior form of protein. Why is that? Because animal protein is a single source complete protein. Alternatively, plant proteins have been looked down upon because each individual plant food typically does not have a complete set of essential amino acids. It is necessary to combine one or more plant foods to get the same complete protein.

So is the complete protein argument sufficient to crown animal protein as the superior form of protein? Keep in mind that complete protein is complete protein. If plant proteins are equivalent to animal proteins when combined—and it is a simple task to do so—the more compelling argument lies in the disparity in health risks of plant vs. animal proteins.

Plant-Based Protein Is the Safest Protein

Evidence based research and scientific studies over the past few decades have linked animal foods and animal protein as a primary cause of heart disease, cancer, stroke, and many other widespread chronic and degenerative diseases afflicting the U.S. and other developed nations. (For further reading on this subject matter, *The China Study*, by T. Colin Campbell, and *Diet For A New*

America, by John Robbins, provide in depth research and studies on nutrition and its role in the promotion and prevention of chronic disease.) Conversely, plant proteins and plant-based foods have been shown to help prevent these same diseases. While these trends have been establishing themselves for the past twenty-five years, physician organizations within the medical community are just beginning to take action. For example, the latest nutritional education from the California Academy of Family Practice (July, 2008) supports these findings and is encouraging its primary-care physicians to emphasize a plant-based diet. These actions are well advised. When you consider the ease in which you can get complete plant protein alongside the hazardous health risks associated with animal proteins, the benefit-to-risk ratio clearly points in favor of plant proteins as the safest proteins. You can get all of the quality protein you need through plant proteins and avoid the tax on your health, your metabolism, and your well-being.

My patients often ask me why plant proteins help prevent disease whereas animal proteins, over time, contribute to chronic and degenerative illness. The answer is, it is likely due to a multitude of factors. Let me explain.

First, let's look at plant proteins. Plant proteins, such as those found in beans, legumes, tofu, whole grains, nuts, and seeds, are accompanied with a host of metabolically stimulating nutrients and health-promoting compounds. These include fiber, antioxidants, and phytonutrients. Plant proteins are also low in saturated fat, free of cholesterol, and promote a more alkaline body chemistry. The combination of the nutrients provided by plant-based foods and the nutritional pollutants and toxins not present in plant foods have been shown to promote long-term health, prevent disease, and sustain a healthy metabolism. In fact, in forty years of practicing Preventive Medicine, I have found that a plant-based diet is the most effective way to prevent chronic and degenerative disease such as heart disease, cancer, stroke, Alzheimer's, arthritis, and diabetes. I've also observed that plant-based foods and plant-based proteins are the best for losing weight and maintaining weight loss.

Animal-based proteins—such as those found in beef, pork, chicken, fish, eggs, milk, and cheese—have a much different long-term effect on the body. As we've discussed, diets high in animal proteins have been linked to significantly increased rates of cancer, heart disease, stroke, and a host of other chronic and degenerative diseases. Why is that? Again, it is likely due to a confluence of factors. Animal products are zero-fiber foods, are the only source of dietary cholesterol, are a significant source of saturated fat, and can be a source of pro-oxidants rather than antioxidants. This doesn't bode well for your health, your metabolism, or your weight-loss goals. Animal proteins also promote a more acidic body chemistry, which I believe plays a role in promoting disease and metabolic dysfunction.

Taking an anthropological approach is also helpful in better understanding why plant and animal proteins have a different impact on the body. When you compare the human anatomy and digestive system to that of other carnivores, omnivores, and herbivores, it helps shed some light on what the most natural food is for our bodies. Contrary to what most people would think, our digestive system most closely resembles that of other herbivores and is notably different from that of omnivores and carnivores. For example, the length of the human small intestine is ten to eleven times the length of our body, similar to those of other herbivores; carnivores and omnivores have much shorter small intestines at three to six times their body length. (Milton R. Mills, M.D., *The Comparative Anatomy of Eating*.) The length and structure of our intestines have many implications as to the transit time, absorption, and general processing of our food as it moves through our body. For the human body and other herbivores, this process favors that of high-fiber plant foods as opposed to zero-fiber animal foods. Other comparisons—such as stomach acidity, digestive enzymes in saliva, and jaw motion—all distinctively associate the human digestive system with that of other herbivores. The anthropological approach, similar to the latest nutritional studies and evidence-based research, also points to plant foods as the most natural food for the human body.

While the health benefits are enough to get some people to adopt a plant-based diet, it may not be the prevailing reason why most people adopt this lifestyle. Eastern philosophies teach that a plant-based diet is a stepping-stone to a higher consciousness. Others are motivated for environmental, spiritual, and moral reasons. In fact, I personally made the switch to a vegetarian diet over thirty-five years ago when I realized I didn't need to sacrifice animals when I could get superior nutrition from a plant-based diet.

Make the Shift

The point is, an emphasis needs to be made to include more of your protein from plant-based sources than animal-based sources. When applying the benefit to risk ratio, you get the benefits of plant-based proteins without the health consequences and troublesome risks that are continuing to stack up against animal-based proteins. Simply put, the more you transition to plant protein, the easier it will be to maintain your weight and sustain good health. With that said, the LYF Maintenance Plan is designed to give you flexibility around your protein options. In addition to a Vegan and Vegetarian Protein Plan, there is a modified protein plan that gives guidance for the inclusion of animal protein. I like to call this the Modified Plant-Based ("P.B.") Plan, because it still puts an emphasis on plant-based proteins.

LYF MAINTENANCE PROTEIN OPTIONS

	Vegan	Vegetarian	Modified P.B. Plan
Protein Sources	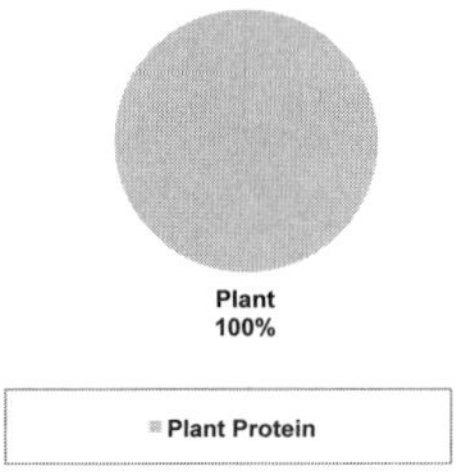 Plant 100% Plant Protein	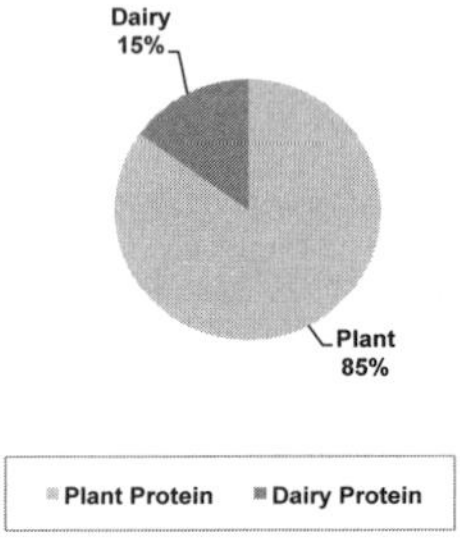 Dairy 15% Plant 85% Plant Protein, Dairy Protein	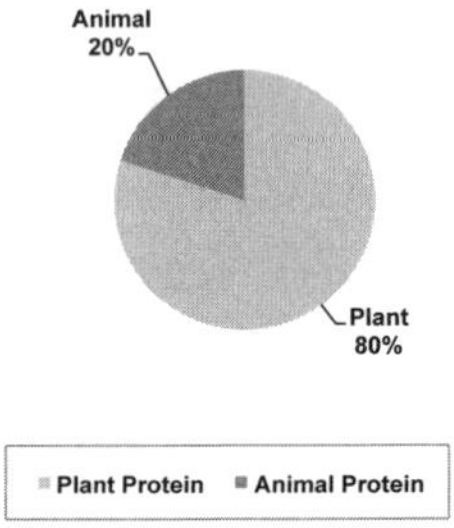 Animal 20% Plant 80% Plant Protein, Animal Protein
Plant Proteins	• 100% Plant Protein • Beans, Lentils, Peas, Tofu, Tempeh, Veggie Burgers, Soy Products, Whole Grain Breads, Whole Grain Rices, Nuts and Seeds, Soy Milk, Nut Milk, Spirulina, Brewer's Yeast	• 85–100% Plant Protein • Beans, Lentils, Peas, Tofu, Tempeh, Veggie Burgers, Soy Products, Whole Grain Breads, Whole Grain Rices, Nuts and Seeds, Soy Milk, Nut Milk, Spirulina, Brewer's Yeast	• 80–100% Plant Protein • Beans, Lentils, Peas, Tofu, Tempeh, Veggie Burgers, Soy Products, Whole Grain Breads, Whole Grain Rices, Nuts and Seeds, Soy Milk, Nut Milk, Spirulina, Brewer's Yeast
Animal Proteins	N/A	• 0–15% Protein from Dairy • Cottage cheese, yogurt, milk and cheese. • Rennet-free dairy is the dairy of choice.	• 0–20% Protein from Meat and Dairy • Broiled fish or salmon is meat of choice. • Rennet-free dairy is the dairy of choice.
General	N/A	• Include dairy in up to three meals a week, but not twice a day and not two days in a row.	• Include fish protein or dairy protein in up to four to five meals a week, but not twice a day. • Including fish protein or dairy protein in one meal every other day is a good target.

Combine Your Foods Wisely

Now you know ***the LYF Maintenance Plan is based on combining fresh, whole, living foods with complete proteins and high-quality complex carbohydrates.*** This is the key to providing everlasting energy, optimal health, and permanent weight loss.

All the homework needed to give you complete protein meals in combination with complex carbohydrates and fresh, living food is worked out for you in the following tables. With the proper combining, you can consistently create smart nutritional meals.

As we've discussed, vegetarian nutrition does require a simple variety of plant foods throughout the day to make sure you get a sufficient balance of all of the essential amino acids. I don't want to overcomplicate the issue because it is a relatively simple task to combine foods effectively to achieve complete proteins. It is good practice and most effective to get in the habit of combining foods to get all the essential amino acids at one meal. As a general rule of thumb, as long as you have any two of the following groups of foods in every meal you will be getting plenty of high-quality complete protein:

I. Legumes (beans, soy products, peas, lentils, etc.),

II. Whole grains (whole grain bread, whole grain rice, whole grain pasta, etc.),

III. Nuts and seeds (almonds, peanuts, nut butters, sunflower seeds, etc.).

Some easy examples can be beans and rice, a peanut butter sandwich, or hummus and pita.

Find Your Rhythm!

You can Cleanse with Smart Foods, you can Detox with Smart Foods, and you can Maintain with Smart Foods. Depending upon your appetite and your activity level, you have a variety of choices at each meal. Some days you may feel lighter and want a Cleansing "Lightweight" lunch and a Detox "Welterweight" dinner. On these days, you would leave out some of the denser, more long-lasting complex carbohydrates like the whole grain breads, whole grain pastas, or potatoes. Another day you may choose to have a Cleansing "Lightweight" breakfast, a Detox "Welterweight" lunch, and a Maintenance "Heavyweight" dinner. The beauty is that it is up to you and your metabolism. It will be up to you to find your rhythm based on your hunger, energy level, and activity level. As you master your eating habits (the subject matter of Part II), you will guide yourself to the proper Maintenance choices to maintain superior weight control and excellent health. To get you in the habit of maximizing the right mix of complete proteins, complex carbohydrates, and fresh foods, I have outlined the vital food combinations in your prescribed maintenance meals. Now it is time to take action!

Step 3—Take Action!

A Typical Day in the Life of Your Maintenance Plan:

Morning (7:00–8:00 AM)	• Orange Juice with Re-Vita • South American Tropical Fruit Salad – ½ cup papaya – ½ cup banana – ½ cup pineapple • Almonds (7–10) with whole grain cereal or oatmeal
Afternoon (12:30–2:00 PM)	• Garden-Green Chlorophyll Salad with herbal dressing, and – 2 teaspoons unsalted sunflower seeds – 5-6 garbanzo beans • Avocado sandwich with whole grain bread
Night (5:30–7:00 PM)	• Fresh carrot, carrot-celery, or carrot-celery-beet juice • Spice-of-Life Spinach Salad with herbal dressing • Vegetarian Lasagna

Nutritional Supplementation

- Re-Vita, as described above.
- Liquid Nutrition as needed.
  - Fresh orange or grapefruit juice with Re-Vita and / or Brewer's Yeast can be used if you are hungry between meals or as a meal substitute when you feel like having a light meal.
- Additional supplementation
  - VEMMA is recommended as a great all-purpose super-nutrient for your health and energy. (Refer to LYF-Style Factor #7 for additional details on VEMMA.)

Exercise

- Refer to your LYF Exercise Plan in LYF-Style Factor #2.
  - Aerobic exercise in morning before breakfast
  - Additional workout before dinner (for optimal health)

Blueprint for Maintenance: Your Complete Nutritional Options

Part I: Maintenance Breakfast—Choose from the following Lightweight, Welterweight, and Heavyweight options.

Breakfast	• 8 ounces fresh-squeezed grapefruit or orange juice with 1 tablespoon Re-Vita • A seasonally based fresh-fruit salad combination (1–1 ½ cups) *** • In addition to a fruit salad, choose one of the following options to turn your breakfast into a complete protein meal. You have the option of going Light, Medium, or Heavy.
Lightweight Breakfast	**Options** 1. 1–3 ounces mixed nuts, ***or*** 2. 6–8 inch celery stalk with 1–2 tablespoons almond butter
Welterweight Breakfast	**Options** 1. 1 ounce unsalted almonds with 2 ounces low-fat granola, ***or*** 2. 1–2 tablespoons nut butter (unsalted almond butter is preferred) with 2 ounces granola

Heavyweight Breakfast	**Options**
	1. 1–2 slices whole multigrain bread ***or*** seven-grain sprouted flourless bread with 1–2 tablespoons nut butter, ***or*** 2. 1 ounce almonds with ½ to 1 cup serving of oatmeal, millet, or whole grain cereal, served with soy, rice or almond milk, ***or*** 3. Whole grain pancakes ***or*** waffles with 1–2 ounces mixed nuts, ***or*** 4. Scrambled tofu, or 5. Scrambled tofu and hash browns (on holidays), or 6. Whole grain bagel with rennet-free cheese (no more than 1–2 days a week, preferably on the weekends) Important Notes: • After a heavyweight breakfast, if you still feel full at lunch, you may choose to use your liquid nutrition and have some juice with super-nutrients instead, and pick up again at dinner. • Always work out before having a heavyweight breakfast. • If you have a heavyweight breakfast without working out prior to the meal, you are probably overeating.

***See table 12.1 at the end of the chapter for seasonal fruit salad combinations

Part II: Maintenance Lunch—Choose from the following Lightweight, Welterweight, and Heavyweight options.

<table>
<tr><td>Lightweight Lunch</td><td>Select one of the following Lightweight Lunch options.
Options
1. Select any option from your LYF Power Cleansing lunch options. This generally includes a leafy green salad + your choice of celery sticks with almond butter or vegetable sticks with guacamole.
2. A fresh fruit salad (1–1 ½ cups) with any one of the following will make lunch a complete protein meal:
a. ½ cup of soy yogurt, or
b. 1–3 ounces of nuts and seeds
3. Dr. Meltzer's Lightweight Power Smoothie
a. For a third lunch option, toss a seasonal fruit salad (1 cup) into the blender with: 1 table-spoon Re-Vita; 1–2 tablespoon brewer's yeast; 1 teaspoon bee pollen; 1–2 cups of fresh-squeezed fruit juice; 1 tablespoon of almond butter or ten unsalted, roasted almonds; and ice.</td></tr>
<tr><td>Welterweight Lunch</td><td>• Leafy Green, Phytonutrient-Rich, Low-Glycemic, Chlorophyll Salad*** with herbal dressing, and
– 2 teaspoons unsalted sunflower seeds (or 4–7 walnuts)
– 5–6 garbanzo beans or red kidney beans
• Add any one of the following lunch options to make a complete protein meal:</td></tr>
</table>

<table>
<tr><td></td><td>

Options

1. Any taco combination or veggie dip option from your LYF Nutritional Detox lunch options.
2. Side Salad Options
    a. ½ cup of tabbouleh
    b. ½ cup of tofu with celery, onions, and tomato
    c. ½ cup of eggless potato salad
    d. Whole grain pasta salad
3. Soup Options
    a. Lima bean
    b. Bean-vegetable
    c. Split pea
    d. Lentil
    e. Mushroom
    f. Carrot-onion
    g. Potato-leek
4. Additional Welterweight Options
    a. Guacamole (made from half an avocado) on carrot or celery sticks
    b. Vegetarian taco: fresh, raw, or steamed vegetables inside a warm corn tortilla; avocado optional
    c. Avocado sandwich: half an avocado spread on 2 slices of whole multigrain bread
    d. Mid-eastern garbanzo spread (hummus—2–3 tablespoons) with whole-wheat pita pocket bread

</td></tr>
<tr><td>

Heavyweight Lunch

</td><td>

- Leafy Green, Phytonutrient-Rich, Low-Glycemic, Chlorophyll Salad*** with herbal dressing, and
    - 2 teaspoons unsalted sunflower seeds (or 4–7 walnuts)
    - 5–6 garbanzo beans or red kidney beans
- Add any one of the following lunch options to make a complete protein meal:

</td></tr>
</table>

Options

1. Half an avocado on whole multigrain bread; mixed vegetable soup (8 ounces) on the side
2. Whole wheat pita stuffed with avocado, tomato, sprouts, and onions; mixed vegetable soup (8 ounces) on the side
3. Lentil soup with 1–2 slices whole multigrain bread
4. Guacamole with vegetable bean soup
5. Corn tortilla or whole wheat chapati stuffed with guacamole (no cheese); mixed vegetable soup (8 ounces) on the side
6. Quesadilla: corn tortilla with rennet-free or soy-based cheese; mixed vegetable soup (8 ounces) on the side
7. Falafel: whole wheat pita stuffed with garbanzo-bean patty
8. Veggie burger: mushroom, soy, lentil, garbanzo, or tofu burger on whole wheat bun; or without bread, but with vegetable soup on the side
9. Split pea soup with 1–2 slices whole multigrain bread or whole wheat pita bread
10. Bean vegetable soup with 1–2 slices whole multigrain bread or whole wheat pita bread

*** For variations of the Leafy Green, Phytonutrient-Rich, Low-Glycemic, Chlorophyll Salad, see table 10.1 in Power Cleansing.

Part III: Maintenance Dinner– Choose from the following Lightweight, Welterweight, and Heavyweight options.

Lightweight Dinner	• Choose any dinner option from the LYF Power Cleansing Plan.
Welterweight Dinner	• Choose any dinner option from the LYF Nutritional Detox Plan.

Heavyweight Dinner	• Leafy Green, Phytonutrient-Rich, Low-Glycemic, Chlorophyll Salad* with herbal dressing, and
	  • 2 teaspoons unsalted sunflower seeds (or 4–7 walnuts)
	  • 5–6 garbanzo beans or red kidney beans
	• For complete protein dinners, add any one of the options from the following six categories:

Complete Soy Bean Dinner Combinations	
Option 1	• Scrambled tofu with vegetables
Option 2	• Scrambled tofu with ½ cup brown or wild rice
Option 3	• Tofu chop suey with vegetarian egg rolls
Option 4	• Tofu lasagna (Use your favorite lasagna recipe but substitute soy cheese for cheese and scrambled tofu instead of meat.)
Option 5	• Tofu enchiladas**
Option 6	• Vegetable casserole (soybeans and vegetables on brown rice)
Option 7	• Soy burger on whole grain bun
Option 8	• Tempeh burger on whole grain bun
Option 9	• Soy grits with ½ cup of cooked brown rice and ½ cup of soy milk
Option 10	• Whole grain pasta with tofu and fresh tomato sauce**

Complete Bean Dinner Combinations	
Option 1	• Organic tostada: corn tortilla, ½ cup cooked beans (kidney and pinto), sprouts, tomato
Option 2	• Falafel: ¼ cup garbanzo beans made into a patty combined with mushrooms, onions, green bell pepper, and sesame seeds, with or without pita bread
Option 3	• Hummus Lebanese dip: ½ cup cooked garbanzo bean spread, 1–2 slices whole wheat pita
Option 4	• Beans and rice: mung beans, adzuki, lima, kidney, and pinto beans with brown or wild rice, ½ cup each
Option 5	• Vegetarian enchiladas, burritos, or tamales
Complete Soup and Grain Dinner Combinations	
Option 1	• Lima bean vegetable soup with 1–2 slices whole grain bread
Option 2	• Lima bean vegetable soup with brown rice
Option 3	• Split pea soup with ½ cup brown or wild rice
Option 4	• Split pea soup with 1–2 slices whole grain or whole wheat pita bread
Option 5	• Minestrone bean vegetable soup with ½ cup brown rice
Option 6	• Minestrone bean vegetable soup with 1–2 slices whole grain bread
Option 7	• Mushroom soup with whole grain pasta noodles and fresh tomato sauce
Option 8	• Vegetable soup with whole grain pasta noodles and fresh tomato sauce, mixed with scrambled tofu

Complete Lentil Dinner Combinations	
Option 1	• Lentil mixed vegetable soup with raw or sautéed mushrooms
Option 2	• Lentil-mushroom-vegetable casserole
Option 3	• Lentil-sesame-nut roast**
Option 4	• Lentil soup with 1–2 slices whole grain or whole wheat pita bread
Option 5	• Lentil soup with ½ cup brown rice or millet
Option 6	• Lentil burger on whole wheat bun
Complete Pea Dinner Combinations	
Option 1	• Steamed peas, steamed carrots, 1 baked potato
Option 2	• Vegetable casserole
Complete Dairy Dinner Combinations	
	Use soy or rennet-free cheese:
Option 1	• Vegetarian lasagna
Option 2	• Vegetarian pizza
Option 3	• Vegetarian enchilada
Option 4	• Eggplant parmesan
Option 5	• Zucchini-rice casserole (with or without cheese)

* For variations of the Leafy Green, Phytonutrient-Rich, Low-Glycemic, Chlorophyll Salad, see table 10.1 in Power Cleansing.

** Refer to Maintenance recipes.

Maintenance Plan: Basic Recipes

The basic recipes for Power Cleansing and Nutritional Detox will give you a good start for your Maintenance Plan options. In addition, we've included a few more dinner recipes to get you going. As you know, the big difference in Maintenance is the addition of a variety of complex carbs, such as whole grains and brown rice. The following information will give you a better idea of how to cook a variety of whole grains and how to cook brown rice. We've also included an overview on cooking times for a variety of beans. Again, make sure to utilize our website as a resource for additional recipes—www.maketimeforwellness.com.

COOKING TIMES FOR GRAINS		
Grain (1 cup dry)	**Water**	**Cooking time**
Barley, pearl	2 ½ cups	1 hour
Buckwheat groats, raw	3 cups	20–25 minutes
Cornmeal and corn grits	4 cups	30 minutes
Millet (sauté in 1 table-spoon oil for nutty flavor)	3 cups	30 minutes
Oats, whole	3 cups	1 hour
Oats, flaked or rolled	3 cups	30 minutes
Rice, sweet or short grain	2 cups	50 minutes
Rice, long grain	2 cups	40–50 minutes
Rye berries	2 ½ cups	1 hour
Rye flakes	2 cups	20 minutes
Triticale berries	2 ½ cups	20 minutes
Wheat berries	2 ½ cups	1 hour
Wheat, bulgur	2 cups	15–20 minutes
Wheat flakes	2 cups	20 minutes

For example, here is how to make your brown rice:

Short, medium, or long grain can be mixed together. Wild rice can be added and cooked with other rice for added flavor. Add one bay leaf with your favorite herbs, such as dill and onion; or add a vegetable bouillon cube to the rice. As a rule of thumb, one part rice to two parts water. Boil water, place all ingredients in baking dish and stir. Cover and bake at 350 degrees for 50 minutes, stirring occasionally. Cooked rice is two and one-half (2 ½) times the quantity of uncooked rice.

COOKING TIME FOR BEANS			
Beans (1 cup dry)		**Water**	**Cooking Time**
Black	Soaked overnight	4 cups	2–3 hours
Black-eyed peas	Not soaked	3 cups	1 hour
Garbanzos	Soaked overnight	3 cups	2–3 hours
Great Northern	Soaked overnight	3 cups	1 hour
Kidney and red	Not soaked	3 cups	1 ½ hours
Kidney and red	Soaked 1 hour	3 cups	1 hour
Lentils	Not soaked	3 cups	1–1 ½ hours
Lentils	Soaked 1 hour	3 cups	45 minutes
Lima	Not soaked	3 cups	1 ½ hours
Lima	Soaked 1 hour	3 cups	45 minutes
Navy	Not soaked	3 cups	1 ½ hours
Navy	Soaked 1 hour	3 cups	1 hour
Pinto	Not soaked	3 cups	2–2 ½ hours
Pinto, split	Not soaked	2 cups	45 minutes
Soybeans	Soaked overnight	4 cups	3 hours
Split peas	Not soaked	3 cups	45 minutes

Complete Lentil Dinner Combinations

Lentil Nut Roast

Ingredients:

1 ½ cups cooked lentils
1 ½ cups cooked brown rice
½ cup peas, cooked
Agar agar mix (1 cup water, 1 vegetable bouillon cube, 1 tablespoon agar agar)
½ cup whole grain bread crumbs
½ cup chopped nuts (raw almonds, cashews, pecans)
¼ cup rolled oats
¼ cup chopped onion
¼ cup chopped sunflower seeds
3 tablespoons safflower oil
2 stalks celery, chopped
½ teaspoon dried sage
1 teaspoon parsley, chopped
¼ teaspoon rosemary
¼ teaspoon thyme
2 tablespoons sesame seeds

Cooking Instructions:

Preheat oven to 350 degrees. Oil a 9x5-inch loaf pan.
Dissolve agar agar and vegetable bouillon cube in 1 cup boiling water and set aside. Heat 3 tablespoons safflower oil in large skillet and sauté celery and onions until they are soft and clear. In a large bowl, combine agar agar mix, sautéed celery and onions, lentils, rice, and all remaining ingredients (except sesame seeds). Mix until evenly distributed. Spoon the mixture into the loaf pan and then sprinkle with sesame seeds.
Bake until loaf is firm and top is lightly browned, about 45 minutes.
Serve topped with mushroom gravy (see below).

Mushroom Gravy

Ingredients:

½ cup brewer's yeast
¾ cup brown rice flour
2 shallots chopped
2 cups mushrooms, chopped
¼ cup or less tamari
¼ cup safflower oil
4 cups water or to desired consistency

Cooking Instructions:
Brown rice flour can be made from scratch, or purchased at the store. If made from scratch, place ¾ cup brown rice on cookie sheet and heat in oven at 350 degrees. Stir occasionally and let bake for 20-25 minutes. Remove cookie sheet from oven, let brown rice cool, and then blend brown rice in a blender to make brown rice flour. Set brown rice flour aside. Heat up safflower oil in a large skillet and sauté shallots and mushrooms. Mix rice flour with yeast and 4 cups water, and then add to skillet. Finally, add tamari and stir. Simmer over low heat, stirring frequently as mushroom gravy thickens.

Whole Grain Pasta with Tofu and Fresh Tomato Sauce

Ingredients:

Scrambled tofu (Refer to Nutritional Detox Recipe)
Whole Grain Pasta
Fresh Tomato Sauce

Cooking Instructions:
In a large pot, bring 3–4 quarts of water to rolling boil. Add pasta, stir with a fork to separate, and boil approximately 10–12 minutes. Test pasta by removing some from water, cooling under cool water and tasting to see if it's tender. Whole grain pastas usually have a heavier consistency. When pasta is done, remove from heat, drain off hot water, rinse pasta with warm water, and serve. Upon serving, add tofu (per recipe provided in Nutritional Detox) and fresh tomato sauce (your favorite homemade recipe or store-bought sauce).

Complete Soy Bean Dinner Combinations

Tofu Enchiladas

Tofu Filling for 12 corn tortillas

Ingredients:

- 3 yellow onions, sliced and quartered
- 3 tablespoons olive oil
- 4 cloves garlic, crushed
- 3 cups tofu (crumbled)
- 10 mushrooms, chopped
- 6 green onions, sliced

Seasonings of choice: Spike (to taste)

Cooking Instructions:
Heat oil in a large skillet. Sauté onion and garlic until golden brown, medium heat. Add tofu. Cover and steam in own juices, stirring often. Uncover, let brown, add mushrooms and seasonings. Cover and cook briefly. Uncover and cook until golden brown. Turn off heat and add green onions. Mix well; set aside.

Sauce for dipping tortillas and banking enchiladas

Ingredients:

- 6 ounces tomato paste
- 3 cups hot water
- 1 clove garlic, crushed
- 2 teaspoons chili powder
- ¼ teaspoon Spike

Cooking Instructions:
Mix ingredients for enchilada sauce in a large bowl and stir well. Set sauce aside. Pre-heat oven to 350 degrees. Place stack of tortillas inside aluminum foil and bake for 5 minutes, or until tortillas are soft enough to roll. Dip tortillas, one-by-one in sauce, and place in lightly oiled baking dish. Place tofu filling in center of tortilla and add a little sauce, and then roll up. Cover with remaining sauce. Garnish with sliced green onions and olives and bake at 350 degrees uncovered for 30 minutes.

Now you have it. Enjoy.

Before I close the chapter on LYF Maintenance, there are a few more practical things I want you to know. Let's start with the features of the LYF Maintenance Plan.

Features of LYF Maintenance Plan

LYF Maintenance was designed with several features in mind to promote permanent weight loss and long-term health.

• Maintain an alkaline nutritional chemistry	• LYF Maintenance heavily favors alkaline-forming over acid-forming foods. The result is a more alkaline body chemistry that is kinder on the liver, kidneys, and heart.
• Maintain a raw-to-cooked ratio of 1:1, and when Cleansing up to 4:1.	• A 1:1 raw-to-cooked ratio is achieved by including a fresh, living, raw fruit salad or vegetable salad with every meal.
• Eat at least twenty-five to thirty grams of fiber daily.	• Smart Foods are loaded with fiber. You can get all of your fiber needs without having to think about it.
• High-quality complete proteins	• LYF Maintenance is designed to provide a favorable plant-to-animal protein ratio to support long-term weight loss as well as long-term health.
• The best fats	• Unsaturated fats are the fats of choice in LYF Maintenance.
• Tasty, visually appealing meals	• Use herbs to flavor your food. • Colorful fruit and leafy green salads make for visually appetizing meals.

Now let's check out the guidelines for LYF Maintenance.

Guidelines for LYF Maintenance: What's In, What's Out

These are the recommended foods for LYF Maintenance.

What's In		
Seasonal Fresh Fruits and Fruit Juices	***Yes!***	All fresh fruits in season. Include a fresh fruit salad with breakfast. Fruit salad options available for lightweight lunch. Seasonal fruit salad combinations are referenced in table 12.1.
Fresh Vegetables and Raw Vegetable Juices	***Yes!***	All fresh vegetables with an emphasis on romaine lettuce, sprouts, mushrooms, cabbage, celery, carrots, avocado, cauliflower, spinach, tomatoes, red onions, cucumber. Steamed broccoli, zucchini, string bean, and eggplant are of significance.
Legumes	***Yes!***	These are the highest quality proteins with the best benefit-to-risk ratio. Tofu, tempeh, soy burgers, beans, peas, and lentils are all good staples.
Nuts	***Yes!***	These are the good unsaturated fats that will keep your metabolism and health in good running order. Almonds are a staple. Walnuts and cashews in moderation. Pecans, brazil nuts, and macadamia nuts for special occasions.
Nut Butters	***Yes!***	Almond butter, peanut butter, cashew butter, sesame-tahini butter in moderation. Make sure they are unsalted and not hydrogenated.
Seeds	***Yes!***	Seeds are a good way to round out your complete proteins. Sunflower, sesame, and pumpkin seeds are good choices for a garnish to your salad.

Whole Grains	***Yes!***	Whole grain breads, whole grain noodles, whole grain rice, and whole grain cereals are recommended. Eat whole grains for up to two to three meals a day. Whole grain cereals optional at breakfast. Whole grain breads optional at lunch. Cooked whole grain suggested at dinner.
Sprouts	***Yes!***	Emphasize sunflower greens and bean sprouts with your raw salads
Beverages	***Yes!***	Water. Herbal teas of choice. Fresh fruit juice, fruit smoothies, and fresh carrot juice or other fresh, raw vegetable juices.
Seasonings	***Yes!***	Cleansing herbs, basic herbs, salsa
Dairy Products	***Optional***	Dairy products are optional in the Vegetarian and Modified P.B. Protein plan. Rennet-free or soy cheese is the cheese of choice. Low-fat cottage cheese and low-fat soy yogurt are suggested in moderation (up to once a day, no more than two to three times a week).
Flesh Foods	***Optional***	Flesh foods are optional in the Modified P.B. Protein Plan. Salmon and broiled or baked fish (except shellfish) are the meats of choice. Not more than once a day and up to three times a week.

Take a Stand Against Commonly Available Foods

When you eat the right foods in the right proportions, you thrive! Nutritional balance means you are not eating too much or too little of any vital nutrient. Avoid harmful, inferior quality foods. Nutritional excess and low-quality, toxic fuel are very common triggers that cause metabolic dysfunction, fatigue, mental wasting, anxiety, and depression—all of which are symptoms of nutritional burnout.

High-Quality Fuel	Low-Quality Fuel
Fresh Fruit	Butters, Ice Cream, and Dairy
Fresh Vegetables	Saturated Animal Fats
Whole Grains	Refined Carbohydrates
Legumes and Beans	Beef and Pork Protein
Freshly-Squeezed Juices	Eggs
Sprouts	Coffee and Soda
Nuts and Seeds	Added, Refined White Sugars, and High-Fructose Corn Syrup
	Sugary, Refined Commercial Breakfast Cereals
	Heavily Salted Foods

When You Travel or Go Out to Eat: Keep it Light!

One final note before you are ready to take on part II and master your eating habits. When you are traveling, keep it light and keep an open mind. With seeing eyes, you can stay as close to the program as possible. Seek out the best natural foods restaurants. Ask around and look under specialized dining directories to find the best places to eat. When you go out to eat, especially when you are with friends, enjoy yourself! Be certain to place the highest priority on loving, sharing communication with those breaking bread with you. Have fun! The food you are eating is not the main reason you are out with friends and loved ones. When people ask you why you are not indulging in their kind of food and drink, simply respond that you feel like eating *light* today. With a smile on your face and light in your eyes, tell them you really enjoy what you choose to eat. Just be mellow and calm about it. With some creativity, persistence, and enthusiasm, you can generally find some high-quality restaurants.

Absolutely draw the lines on what you will not eat! Then within the boundaries of what you select to eat, enjoy! Don't be difficult. Most Italian, Chinese, Indian, Mexican, Greek, and Thai restaurants have a wide variety of vegetarian and plant-based entrees. Even the most traditional restaurants serve fresh salads, garden vegetables, and baked potatoes. One word about cheating while on this program: as we were taught in grade school, the only person you really cheat when you are cheating is yourself. To get the main benefits of this nutritional plan, the closer you follow it, the greater the results. As you get in touch with your own nutritional and emotional needs, you become more of an expert in determining what your optimal nutritional plan is. Continuity and consistency make all the difference. Keep cool. Be prudent and discriminatory. Stay relaxed and centered. Then you will know what to do.

Table 12.1: Seasonal Fruit Salad Combinations

Spring	
Tropical Fruit Salad	Papaya, pineapple, banana
Spring Salad	Pineapple, banana, strawberry
Cherry Supreme Salad	Cherry, peach, banana
Grape Delight Salad	Green, purple, and red grapes
Mango Salad	Mango, pineapple, banana
Summer	
Summer Melon Salad	Cantaloupe, watermelon, papaya
Nectarine Peach Salad	Nectarine, peach, cherries, plums
Hawaiian Fruit Salad	Papaya, mango, pineapple
Tropical Fruit Salad	Papaya, pineapple, banana
Apricot Salad	Apricot, peach, plum, grape, cherry
Mango Peach Salad	Mango, peach, banana
Berry Salad	Berries, peach, apricot
Cherry Plum Salad	Cherries, plum, nectarine
Summer Grape Salad	Grapes, cherries, banana
Autumn	
Mixed Apple Salad	Pippin, Macintosh, and Golden apples
Autumn Salad	Banana, papaya, apple
Waldorf Apple Salad	Apple, pear, banana
Grape Salad	Green and red grapes or any apple or pear
Pear Salad	Pear, papaya, banana
Winter	
Tropical Fruit Salad	Pineapple, papaya, banana
Winter Citrus Salad	Orange, pineapple, pink grapefruit
Grapefruit Salad	Pink grapefruit, orange, banana
Orange Salad	Orange, pineapple, banana
Papaya Salad	Papaya, orange, banana

Part II

Master Your Eating Habits

13

Introduction to Master Your Eating Habits

I have made an interesting observation over the years in working with people to improve their health, happiness, and well-being. Teaching people the right technique to achieve their wellness or weight-loss goals is often not enough. Even with the best technique, you must have the right strategy in order to follow through on the plan. So what are the techniques and strategies you are going to need to achieve permanent weight loss?

In part I, you learned the necessary technique to naturally accelerate your metabolism. You discovered what are the Smartest Foods to eat to lose your excess weight. Yes, knowing *what to eat* is the necessary beginning. But nutritional know-how in and of itself is not enough. Learning *how to eat* is equally important. This chapter provides the strategies you need to learn how to eat and, ultimately, how to master your eating habits.

The idea is simple. To achieve permanent weight loss, you must follow through on what you know is best. It is the *doing* that counts. You can know what the Smartest Foods are. You can even be dialed into how to ignite, build, and maintain your Metabolic Fire. However, until you become the master of your eating habits, you will have difficulty following through and achieving long-term success. When you fall victim to unhealthy eating habits, such as overeating, cravings, and food indulgences, you are at considerable risk for never losing your excess pounds or eventually putting the weight back on that you worked so hard to lose.

I want you to get the big picture. Permanent weight loss is not just about Smart Foods. It is also about the timely, relaxed eating of these Smart Foods. You see, your eating habits speak volumes about your nutritional lifestyle. In fact, your eating habits have a huge influence on your permanent weight-loss (PWL) plan. When your eating habits are solid, they become the nuts and the bolts that keep your metabolism working well. On the other hand, bad eating habits lead to poor food selection and metabolic dysfunction. Over the long run, destructive eating habits take their toll and sabotage permanent weight loss.

The Way You Eat Is the Story of Your Eating Habits

Not only what you eat, but how much you eat, when you eat, how quickly you eat, your hunger level and mood while eating, and *why* you eat are all important constituents of your eating habits. Let's take it one step further. It is important to get tuned in. Knowing what specific mood or circumstances trigger off overeating or food indulgences is part of the personality of your eating habits. Having positive eating habits and being the master of your eating habits are distinguishing characteristics that separate those who achieve and maintain their ideal weight from the 97 percent of dieters who do not.

Every human being, whether they are dealing with weight issues or not, is susceptible to giving in to hazardous or dysfunctional eating habits. I like to call these dysfunctional eating habits *food swings*. For some, it may be overeating. For others, it might be late-night indulgences when they are feeling emotional. And even others may give in to cravings or look to comfort foods and mood foods when they are stressed or upset. Let me share with you an observation that I see in my clinic all the time. Unless you have a method for identifying and addressing your common food swings and a system for overcoming those negative eating habits, it will be an uphill battle to lose weight, let alone maintain your ideal weight. Ultimately, poor eating habits that go unaddressed can unravel even the best weight-loss plans, undermine your weight-loss goals, and extinguish the fire you worked so hard to build up.

Learn a System for Mastering Your Eating Habits

Keeping your excess weight off can seem like a daunting task. It is up to you to resist temptation. It is up to you to not overeat. It is up to you to avoid junk foods, mood foods, sweets, and your favorite refined carbs. There are too many distractions, impulses, and temptations that can derail your weight-loss program. Your willpower, without the appropriate system or support, usually isn't enough to keep you on track. That's why you need a reliable strategy for approaching each meal. The Golden Rules of Smart Eating will empower you with the strategic tools to develop the right eating habits and overcome common nutritional pitfalls.

You see it wherever you go. There are seemingly infinite social and cultural factors that set off dysfunctional eating habits. These patterns of overeating are very much ingrained in our lifestyle. In the game of weight loss, this stacks the deck against you. The key is to learn how to identify the root causes of your food swings and to learn a system for overcoming them. This system, which I will teach you in the Golden Rules of Smart Eating, will stack the deck back in your favor. These rules will teach you how to be a master of your eating habits instead of being a slave to your eating habits. I don't want you to approach your PWL process alone. The Golden Rules of Smart Eating will stand shoulder to shoulder by your side. With these tools and strategies, coupled with your nutritional know-how, you will be well equipped to achieve permanent weight-loss success.

In this section of Master Your Eating Habits, I'll explain the following:

- The connection between stress and your eating habits;
- The connection between your emotions and your eating habits;
- Our propensity to relieve emotional tension (EMT) through negative eating habits; and
- The difference between your hunger, or your physiological need for food, and your appetite, your emotional desire for food.

You will also learn:

- How to honor your true hunger instead of your appetite;
- A crucial pre-meal approach: a system for approaching each meal that will enable you to establish the positive eating habits you need to achieve and maintain your ideal weight;
- A reliable system for overcoming the most common food swings, such as overeating, cravings, compulsive bingeing, snacking and nibbling, late-night indulgences, etc.; and
- A dependable system for overcoming the negative effects that stress and emotional tension have on your eating habits.

Let's get started!

14

Size Up Your Eating Habits

EVERY person has their own style of eating, just as everyone has their own personality. Your eating habits are about you and your most personal, social, and emotional relationship with food. Your eating habits describe your daily approach to eating. Have you ever given much thought to the way you eat—to the way you look at food? Are you clear about how you identify with your favorite foods? Are there certain foods that comfort you when you are feeling down? Just how important is your diet to you, and what role does nutrition play in your life? Your eating habits often tell the story of how you think, feel, and identify with the foods you commonly eat. This relationship with food becomes even more important in the face of stress, restlessness, anxiety, and emotional tension. Could you be an emotional eater? Do you eat when you are stressed or irritable? How about when you are bored? It turns out that your day-to-day eating habits are acquired repetitive actions that eventually become second nature to you. In this part of the book, I want you to identify and understand what is at the core of your eating habits. Once you have made that recognition, we will then outline the Golden Rules of Smart Eating. These rules will help you overcome your food swings, establish positive eating habits, and maintain superior weight control.

You really have just two choices. You can be the master or the slave to your eating habits. It is your choice. Take a moment to answer the following questions and get familiar with the personality of your eating habits.

- Do you sometimes eat even though you aren't really hungry?
- Is your food selection influenced more by the taste and emotional appeal of the food or the food's nutritional value?
- Do you find that your diet or your favorite foods are largely based on the foods you were raised on?
- Do you look to certain foods to improve your mood?
- Are you a recreational eater; that is, do you look to food for entertainment?
- Are your eating habits influenced by your friends or social calendar?
- Are there any eating habits that you know you need to improve?

15

Stress and Your Eating Habits

DID you ever stop to realize that there is a pivotal relationship between your stress levels and your eating habits? Have you ever noticed the influence stress has on the way you eat? In this chapter, I explain why it is necessary to manage your stress levels to enjoy healthier eating habits.

Stress and the Modern-Day Paradox

I find it very interesting that, in recent years, there has been an explosion of interest in health, nutrition, and the importance of weight loss. Today, the media is obsessed with being thin and fit. And yet, a puzzling paradox exists. At a time when we know, more than ever, about the positive impact of regular exercise and good nutrition, we as a society are more overweight than ever. We know so much, yet we choose food as though we are mindless. We eagerly gather information but are loath to apply it. Is it not ironic that simultaneous to the rebirth of organic food and the home gym craze, sweets, fats, junk foods, and artificial energy drinks dominate the airways and tyrannize TV? Yes, Americans, young and old, are plagued by the increase in obesity and the rise in chronic and degenerative diseases. High cholesterol levels, diabetes, and the hardening of the arteries all go hand in hand with excessive weight gain. Did you know that cholesterol-lowering agents are the number-one drug prescribed around the globe today? The actuarial tables predict that, at the current rate of increasing obesity, some 90 percent of the American public is expected to be overweight by 2025. What is going on?

Let me tell you what's going on. It's been going on like this for the last twenty-five years. Our fast-paced, high-tech lifestyle has left us computer literate but emotionally illiterate and nutritionally out of focus. We spend our time online, in line, but misaligned. As a society, we are more stressed, fatigued, and restless than ever. So how does this relate to weight gain? Let me give you the insight to solve this paradox of modern day obesity. ***There is a vital connection between stress levels and poor eating habits.*** Furthermore, buried and repressed emotions lead to self-defeating eating habits. Let's explore these relationships a little further.

Stress Plays Havoc with Your Eating Habits

A balanced emotional life is conducive to the right eating habits. On the other hand, when stress dominates our lifestyle, it is far more difficult to sustain a healthy relationship with food. Think about this for a moment. When you are under stress, do your eating habits have a way of falling apart? For most of us, the answer is yes. When stress acts up, we tend to look for some mood foods that we hope will make us feel better and lift our spirits. Unfortunately, stress is widespread. It wreaks havoc on our emotions and, by extension, our behavior, as witnessed by our eating habits. It is all too easy to turn to food for emotional comfort. Even the firmest New Year's resolutions to lose weight go to the wayside under the pressures of stress. After a tough day at work, what is your particular crutch? Is it beer? Pizza? Chocolate chip cookies? Ice cream? What foods do you turn to when you want a pick up or you want to fight off some situational anxiety or depressing thoughts?

Mood foods usually provide a temporary relief and tend to improve your mood at first. However, their long-term side effects are just the opposite. You tend to crash after eating sweets. Too many refined carbs leave you drowsy at work and send you off early to bed. Alcohol is an emotional depressant and has a way of eroding willpower and self-discipline. The wrong fats and added sugars can ruin your metabolism. Your momentary pleasure from your mood foods—we all have them—is typically followed by a debilitating low. For example, eating sweets may make us feel good in the moment. However, the sugar blues, which inevitably follow, increase stress on your metabolism, your thinking, and your mood. In fact, your favorite mood foods do not counter stress. They actually compound it!

Stress Dictates Your Eating Habits

The point I am trying to get across is simple—stress triggers bad eating habits. Stress triggers food swings like cravings, bingeing, overeating, compulsive snacking, late-night indulgences, and so on. ***Emotional stress, financial stress, and work stress usually serve as the driving force behind cravings and addictions.*** In fact, stress sets into motion a self-abusive cycle: stress leads to poor food choices, and poor food choices lead to weight gain, fatigue, and even more stress! What I have witnessed is that the majority of dysfunctional eating habits are responses to emotional stress. People who are overworked, financially stressed, love-starved, lonely, or bored commonly turn to food for comfort.

So how do you overcome stress-induced, dysfunctional eating habits? I will give you a system, detail-by-detail, in the Golden Rules of Smart Eating. Smart eating habits are the missing link between your diet and your emotions. They penetrate and reach down deep inside to the core of your values. Smart eating habits give you roots. They ground you to improve your ability to cope with the stressful curveballs life has a way of throwing your way. Smart eating habits give you strategies to manage stress instead of being managed by stress. With the Golden Rules of Smart Eating at your side, you will be empowered with the tools to conquer stress and avoid dysfunctional eating habits. Before we get into the Golden Rules of Smart Eating, however, let's review the other major factors that influence your eating habits.

16

Your Eating Habits and Your Emotions

ALTHOUGH we don't always think of it as such, diet is one of the most controversial and emotional issues in modern life—as emotional, in fact, as say, sex, religion, and politics. Today, many of us are dialing in to improve our self-awareness. Here's what you need to know. How we feel—our moods and our mood swings—affects what we eat. Yes, there is a mood behind each food.

- **Your mood affects what you eat and how you eat it**

I want this to be clear. It is crucial for you to understand that your emotions have a huge influence on your PWL plan. Emotional stress adversely influences our eating habits, and our negative eating habits, in turn, weaken our Metabolic Fire.

In other words, emotional stress, directly and indirectly is bad for your metabolism. In LYF-Style factor #6, we explained the direct connection between stress and a slower metabolism. In addition to this, when you are restless, stressed, emotionally volatile, emotionally drained, or burned out, it is the path of least resistance to indulge in your favorite foods. The end result, on both accounts, is weight gain.

Your Emotions Play a Crucial Role in Losing Weight and Keeping It Off

Moods and food choices touch each other in a myriad of ways. People look to their meals for more than just nutritional input—sadly, that's sometimes the last consideration if it's thought of at all. No, instead, we eat for comfort or companionship or to satisfy a craving. We focus on all the social aspects of eating: the most convenient meals to buy, the current culinary trends, the hottest restaurants. It's human nature—and it's an unhealthy force that leads to obesity.

Think about your favorite foods. They have an emotional appeal—maybe even a sensual and physical attraction, don't they? Undoubtedly, your favorites have a special taste, look, and smell. You profess your undying devotion to chocolate, french fries, ice cream, or sirloin steak. You can't imagine living without them. You cannot resist their smell, taste, or charm. You lick your fingers and smack your lips. Munching away on preferred foods is one of life's greatest pleasures. Pasta stuffed with cheese and swimming in red or cream sauce, salty tortilla chips dipped in salsa, submarine sandwiches stacked with deli meats, cartons of Chinese takeout, birthday cake topped with ice cream scoops and garnished with sparkling candy bits and cookie crumbles—if loving them is wrong, why does it feel so right? Our lives revolve around food. We live to eat. Events big and small, good and bad, are commemorated with special meals—breakfast in bed on Mother's Day, dinner out to celebrate a promotion, a pint of ice cream when the romance ends. Remember McDonald's™ old slogan? "You deserve a break today." We emotionally reward ourselves with food instead of choosing ingredients for their high-octane nutritive value and biological benefits. The short-term satisfaction that comes from indulging in our favorite foods, however, leads us down the primrose path of unsightly weight gain.

It's time for a détente. To strike a balance between emotions and eating habits is a sound, soulful aim. When your emotional, nutritional, and metabolic powers work together, permanent weight loss follows. But what good are tools if you don't know how to use them? Before you can fix a problem, you have to understand it. Let's explore the underlying fabric of your eating habits.

The Mommy-Daddy Diet

The seeds for your adult eating habits were planted in your subconscious mind when you were just a kid. How so? That's when you first experienced the emotional value of food as it relates to your family's dietary habits, rituals, or celebratory patterns. The foods you grew up with form your first diet. Oftentimes this is your only diet—your core diet, the meals you return to week after week, the foods you look for time and time again. I sometimes refer to it as the Mommy-Daddy diet. They represent the foods you remember eating while bonding to your mother and your father. You're familiar with these foods—they're like childhood friends. The barbecues, the birthday cakes, the thanksgiving roast, the mashed potatoes, your mother's apple pie—you know what I'm talking about! They remind you of your youth and of time spent with siblings, parents, and relatives. Little did you know that, in your adolescence, you were already being programmed for a particular pathology of eating that would come to dominate your adult life. And yet, looking back, didn't your favorite foods relate to a reward system? Didn't your parents treat you with ice cream or pizza if you behaved well? Didn't you get to choose the restaurant on your birthday?

Taste of the Town

Ours is also the culture of instant gratification. Instead of considering how we'll feel two hours after downing that bacon cheeseburger, we can only think of now—of how good that first bite is going to taste. In America, we swear by the motto "Work Hard, Play Hard"—and, by extension, "Party Hardy." For the majority of folks, food is a recreational drug. For heaven's sake, we're the home of the free, land of the hotdog eating contest! Of course, eating is a social activity and can be a wonderful way to relax with others. But problems result when eating becomes the focus of a get-together, not just a way to enhance it. Equally sad, overeating often occurs when you're alone—to remind you of when you did have a large, loving group around you. Mommy-Daddy foods become a major source of security in a high-stress, lonely, chaotic world. Dairy products, cheeses, meats, ice cream, pizza, bagels, and chocolates are popular and common Mommy-Daddy foods.

Did you ever stop to wonder that we have been conditioned to use food as an emotional reward system? We've been accustomed to turn to food to handle personal and professional frustrations. We use food as a coping mechanism to comfort ourselves. We've been unwilling guinea pigs, conditioned into such destructive behavior. Now our challenge is to break the cycle.

Constant Companion

Over-attachment to your mood foods and Mommy-Daddy diet sets the stage for undisciplined eating habits. Your eating habits can become a crutch. When you're hurt, depressed, or disappointed, you may reach for your favorite snacks, sweets, and sandwiches. When friends, family, or a spouse lets you down, food's a constant companion. There you sit TV remote in one hand, potato chips in the other, avoiding all the problems in your life. After a while, you become so mesmerized by your chosen foods that you may as well be having a love affair with them. You can't wait to see them; you rush home after a hard day to greet them. The first thing you do when you come home from work is to open the refrigerator and look for one of your favorite rewards. You conduct a clandestine rendezvous out in the garage or locked behind the bathroom door. Whenever they're not readily available, you start feeling irritated, angry, or deprived.

As you get to know your own emotional profile and the effect it has on your eating habits, you'll discover the simple truth: dietary patterns and, in particular, your most self-defeating eating patterns, help you temporarily cope with the conflicts in your life. They are coping mechanisms rather than coping skills. Put another way, your food choices are heavily influenced by mood.

Do You Look to Food for Emotional Comfort?

For most of us, when we are stressed, we look to food for emotional comfort. Rather than squarely facing our personal hurdles and making the appropriate adjustments, we numb the pain by filling our stomachs.

Are you using your diet as a pacifier? For most folks, eating habits and emotional reactions are interrelated. If your emotions are out of balance, your eating habits may very well be too. Early warning signs that your emotional register is off-kilter include anxiety, depression, insomnia, lack of focus, restlessness, and irritability. But have no fear. In the process of applying the Golden

Rules of Smart Eating, you can overcome your emotional overeating habits. Furthermore, smart nutrition balances your brain chemistry, equalizing your emotions. Nutritious meals keep you in a good mood and generate a sense of well-being; the calm that results encourages you to continue to make sound, conscientious food choices.

In order to master your emotional overeating habits, you'll need to be able to make the distinction between your feelings and emotions. Do you know the difference?

Feelings vs. Emotions

Let me give you some background. Since appetite, like mood, is emotionally driven, then one of the most critical steps toward establishing permanent weight control is to cultivate healthy emotional eating habits. To do this, you must become familiar with your feelings and your emotions. Most of us don't think to make a distinction between the two, but understanding the difference between them is crucial. It helps us to advance to higher levels of emotional fitness and gain control of our eating habits.

Feelings are an inside job. They are natural responses to events or experiences. They're about the sensations, impressions, and vibrations of your heart and soul. Feelings are facts, and as facts, they are neither good nor bad—neither right nor wrong. You know what it feels like to feel good. That's a fact. You know what it feels like to give and receive warmth and affection. You know when you're in love (when you're not sure, you're probably not!). Feelings rate in levels: okay, great, sensational. You know when you feel bad just as you know when you feel great. You know that stress does not feel good. It is important to discover the scope of your feelings so you can act responsibly and develop smart eating habits.

Self-Regulate Your Eating Habits: Stay Tuned into Your Primary Feelings

Here is an important observation I've made in my forty years as a physician. You can self-regulate your eating habits when you stay tuned into your primary feelings:

- **Emotional self-awareness—that is, knowing how you feel and**

> **how to deal with these feelings—leads to responsive, responsible behavior. This results in wholesome eating habits. Instead, lack of emotional self-attunement invites reactive, impulsive, over-reactive, indulgent, or self-defeating eating habits.**

So how do emotions differ from your feelings? Emotions are the expression of your primary feelings, or the reaction to your primary feelings. The movement of your feelings through your mind and body creates your emotions. Take a moment to reflect on this. I want to make sure you understand how this works. For example, you may feel let down or betrayed; those are your primary feelings. Yet, your emotional reaction is dominated by intense anger. That is why your emotions are called secondary feelings, because your emotional states are rooted in your feelings first. Like the plucked strings of a guitar, your emotions vibrate with their designated note. When you feel bad, you cry, sulk, and shout. When you feel good, you smile, sing, or laugh. Across the board, there's a reactive element to emotions. For example, disappointment is a primary feeling, yet you may bypass that feeling and shift into the emotional reactionary states of being agitated, angry, or upset.

From an emotional perspective, eating is a transient solution to emotional uneasiness or chaos. It is almost impossible to self-regulate your eating habits when you censor, lose touch with, or detach from your primary feelings—when you are dominated by your emotions. ***Remember, it is when you are emotional that you are more likely to act out on your immediate impulses, and compulsively eat or overeat.*** It stands to reason that being dialed into your feelings will lead you to behave quite differently, with respect to your eating habits.

Keep in mind that the stronger the primary feelings, the stronger the emotions. Strong feelings of trust and affection encourage deep loving gestures. Energetic, vital, enthusiastic feelings move you to the depths of passion and playfulness. Joyousness puts a smile on your face and a spring in your step. Conversely, primary feelings of fear and frustration can lead to anger, temper tantrums, and more and more negative outbursts.

Tune into Your Feelings

Before you can alter your eating habits, you have to be attuned to your feelings, whether they may be good or bad. Most of us use food as a way to detach from our feelings. Destructive eating habits occur as a consequence of bypassing our feelings. This kind of detachment causes negative food swings that impair your weight-loss plan. At the end of the day, being dialed in to your feelings is the very first step to prevent emotional overeating that ultimately results in weight gain. You will soon find out that is why, in the Golden Rules of Smart Eating, it is taboo to even consider eating when you are emotionally wound up. Rest assured, as you get into the Golden Rules, we'll give you a strategic process to work through your primary feelings.

Before we move on, I want to get back to avoiding how we feel. You know, it's not easy to shut off our feelings—but somehow we manage to do it. We've learned by watching our parents, and we do our best to carry on the family tradition. There's a price to pay for all this repression: it is called emotional stress. In some form or another, emotions have to find an outlet. When they can't be released in an open, positive way, then they'll find a more hazardous manner to work through our system. Don't be surprised to see these buried emotions show up as snacking, raiding the refrigerator, or bingeing on your favorite chocolates or ice cream. This is why it is so important to get a handle on how you feel. ***Your negative eating habits are emotionally driven, not feeling driven.*** This is important. Let me say it again. Your negative eating habits are emotionally driven, not feeling driven. When you stay in tune with your feelings, it gives you the control you need to manage your taste buds. Let me explain.

Emotional Self-Discovery Is Key to Mastering Your Eating Habits

Sometimes it doesn't feel good, but being disappointed, frustrated, or let down does not give you the license to get emotional. Remember that fear, emotional pain, frustration, disappointment, and anxieties are primary feelings. For example, when you suppress your hurt or pain, you begin to lose touch with yourself. All too often, this is due to being overly busy, caught up in your own narcissistic thinking, or obsessed with common addictions of our society (e.g., food, work, alcoholism, TV, etc.). When you deny, suppress, or lose touch with your primary feelings of fear, pain, frustration, hurt, and disappointment, secondary feelings of anger, resentment, and worry start to accumulate. When unresolved anxiety or fear mushrooms into agitation, that is when you are most vulnerable to a self-defeating food swing. It is necessary to address your anxiety or fears. You can learn to work through them in a drugless, foodless manner before they turn into agitation. Working it out is feeling-based. Overeating or acting it out is emotionally based. When you don't work it out and, instead, act it out, destructive eating habits can take over.

What is the conclusion I'm trying to draw? You are much less vulnerable or likely to act out and indulge in food from a feeling. You typically act out from your escalating emotions. Let me go over it one more time. Let's say you get your feelings hurt, and you avoid dealing with the emotional pain. You may very well start getting angry or resentful and act out from these defensive emotional states. This is an important point to grasp. Repressed emotions invite over-reactive eating, throw you out of balance, build up stress, drain your immune system, and impair your metabolism.

Emotional Literacy and Emotional Sobriety

I find it most interesting that, in spite of the advances in technology, intellect, and telecommunication, the majority of people—particularly those over the age of thirty—are emotionally disconnected and drowning in an ocean of drama, chaos, and confusion. Public schools focus on reading, writing, and arithmetic. Institutions of higher education emphasize mental development at the expense of emotional maturity. And while there's much to be said for academic acuity—the smarter we get, the broader the gap between our intellect and our emotions. It's a sign of the times that the higher our IQ, or Intelligence Quotient, the lower our EQ, or Emotional Quotient. This presents considerable risk for self-destructive eating habits and, eventually, obesity. What is the solution?

The Golden Rules of Smart Eating will guide you to stay in touch with your primary feelings. That way, any negative feelings that may arise will not be buried or hidden for days to weeks to years. The Golden Rules teach you to find a way to constructively express how you feel about being hurt, frightened, or rejected; how to respond, not react, to these feelings; and how to keep your emotional life balanced. Therefore, the Golden Rules will show you how to express how you feel, ask for what you need, work things out with respect, and stay in command of your eating habits. A balanced emotional life is the stepping-stone to mastering your eating habits. This is called emotional sobriety.

The process of emotional sobriety calls for knowing how to express yourself and how to respond calmly to all kinds of circumstances. This not only applies when things are going well but also when things are not going well. For example, when you have a quarrel with your lover or disagree about how you see things, it doesn't mean that you have to satisfy your cravings for pretzels or cheese and crackers and then scarf them down.

Similarly, a misunderstanding with a good friend needs to be openly discussed. When you feel taken advantage of at work—or if you do not like your job—get in touch with what it will take to do a better job and tell your employer what you believe will make your work more meaningful. Unresolved emotional wounds create fears and negative belief systems. Unresolved emotional conflicts set the stage for abusive eating habits that, in time, can destroy the quality of your life.

You Need an Emotional Compass

If you were lost in the wilderness, you'd need a compass to find your way back to civilization. This metaphor holds true for our inner landscape. If you're not comfortable and capable of embracing your feelings, you lack an emotional compass. You need an emotional compass to navigate your way out of the morass of your repressed feelings that have a way of triggering off your favorite food indulgences and compulsions. Our modern-day merry-go-round lifestyle can turn into a ceaseless spinning wheel of stress. In all the confusion, it's easy to lose perspective of our eating habits. By keeping track of your mood, how you feel when you eat, and how often you eat, you can get a grasp of your ingrained, unconscious emotional eating patterns.

Size Up Your Emotional Connection to Your Diet

Who wants to analyze their feelings while eating? Who knows what ugly creatures might crawl out from under that rock? If ignorance is bliss, then knowledge is power. The truth hurts, but it will help you to understand, for example, what it is about scarfing down a pizza that is more appealing than preparing a fresh meal. Self-assessment and making time to keep track of your eating habits are your initial call to action. If you want to lose weight, look good, and feel great, you need to understand your connection to your favorite foods, as well as the emotional and physical costs of your eating habits.

Your Hunger and Your Mood Tell the Story

Here's a new spin for you at mealtime. Approach each meal as though you are approaching the stop sign at the end of your roadway. Stop; look; listen—and then feel. Ask yourself, am I hungry? How hungry am I? What am I feeling? I want you to get good at this.

This is one of the very first steps in your pre-meal strategy that will be highlighted in the Golden Rules of Smart Eating. You are about to find out that your pre-meal strategy is everything to weight control. Permanent weight loss is not only about the meal itself; it is also about you and where your emotional state is at before and during the meal. That's right—permanent weight loss isn't just about the meal; it is about you as well!

Use the following chart to rate your mood and degree of hunger each time you eat or snack for the next several days. The results will give you a handy overview of your present emotionally driven dietary patterns. Remember, you can't fix a problem until you know it exists. Self-assessment leads to self-correction. If you don't recognize it, a bad eating habit can creep up on you at any time and sabotage your best intentions.

Eating Habits Survey

Here is an important link for you to understand your own individualized eating habits. Tracking your own dietary/emotional inventory will enable you to take charge of your habits instead of allowing them to control you. In the appropriate square, mark the time of day you eat, including snacks. In the upper half of the square, rate your feelings. Use the feelings listed below to track your mood. In the lower half, rate your appetite according to your perceived degree of hunger.

Feelings

(H) Happy
(S) Stressed
(A) Anxious
(C) Content
(E) Emotionally Upset
(R) Relaxed
(D) Depressed
(B) Bored
(L) Lonely

Hunger Level

0 None
1 Mild Hunger
2 Moderate
3 Extreme

For example, S/3 would signify that you are feeling extremely stressed and hungry, H/O if you're happy and not hungry at all, and B/2 if you are bored and moderately hungry.

Day 5	Day 4	Day 3	Day 2	Day 1	
					5–6 AM
					6–7 AM
					7–8 AM
					8–9 AM
					9–10 AM
					10–11 AM
					11–12 PM
					12–1 PM
					1–2 PM
					2–3 PM
					3–4 PM
					4–5 PM
					5–6 PM
					6–7 PM
					7–8 PM
					8–9 PM
					9–10 PM
					10–11 PM
					11–12 AM
					12–1 AM
					1–2 AM
					2–3 AM
					3–4 AM
					4–5 AM

In the following spaces, take some notes on what you have learned from this exercise.

******** What connection can you see between your emotions and your eating habits?
******** What are you usually feeling when you're hungry?
******** How does your stress level influence your eating habits?
******** Do you only eat when you are hungry?
******** Do you find yourself wanting to eat when you are emotional?
******** Do you find yourself relaxed or rushing and multi-tasking during mealtimes?

As human beings, we have to eat. There's no quitting cold turkey—the way we might with, for example, cigarettes or alcohol. An emotional involvement with your diet is inescapable, so why not strive to make the relationship a positive, nurturing one? Love your diet and gain respect for your eating habits the way you would a best friend. It will reward you with boundless energy, positive mental health, and superior weight management skills.

17

Emotional Tension "EMT" and Your Eating Habits

BY now it is apparent that to lose weight and keep it off permanently, your emotional eating habits can either make or break you. The pieces of the puzzle are starting to fall into place. In chapter 15, you discovered the relationship between stress and your eating habits. In chapter 16, you became familiar with the influence your emotional life has on the way you eat. In this chapter, we'll take a look at how prolonged stress and unaddressed emotions can lead to emotional tension, or what I like to call EMT.

The truth is, most folks have a difficult time dealing with emotional stress. Long-term stress antagonizes your eating habits and interferes with your weight-loss plan. Too many Americans subscribe to the puritanical notion that stress makes you a stronger, sharper person. Yes, short-term difficulties that get successfully resolved build character. Yes, short-term stress that teaches you to overcome hurdles and wrestle with adversity empowers you to face up to your life issues. However, chronic stress is a horse of a different color. Prolonged stress not only undermines the inner workings of your metabolism, but leads to poor food choices and negative eating habits. Stress is not the wind beneath your wings—it is the thundering storm that, in time, will tear off your wings.

When you're stressed, EMT accumulates. The more prolonged the stress, the greater the EMT. It's human nature to want to decompress the high level of EMT and thereby reduce tension, but we often rely on unhealthy food choices. And therein lies the origin of addictive eating habits and negative food swings. Bottled-up feelings and buried fears feed repressed emotions such as anger. Over time, this brings your EMT to a boiling point and presents a significant problem. The high emotional tension level triggers rotten moods. To cope, we search for comfort—a quick fix to relieve the stress. This need for relief is at the root of all addictions; food as well as alcohol, work, shopping, sex, gambling. We're often too preoccupied or self-absorbed to pick up on the emotional undercurrents that may be eating away at us. Recognizing these patterns is one of the first steps in allowing us to address escalating EMT.

Our favorite foods are custom-designed to relieve EMT and effect an immediate mood change. They're available right now at a drive-through window or grocery store or a shelf near you. More than likely, they're already sitting in your cupboard or refrigerator, waiting for your next craving. They don't require any advance preparation—no time for second thoughts. Just pop the lid, rip the wrapper, call for takeout; and you're good to go. Your hand-to-mouth reflex can clock in at less than ten seconds.

EMT and Fingerprint Food Swings

Each person handles escalating EMT in a unique way, shaped by his or her individual emotional profile, their Mommy-Daddy diet, and their emotional attachments to food. Each person has his or her own fingerprint food swings. The trick is to counter EMT by effectively resolving stressful issues instead of falling back on the familiar battery of dysfunctional eating habits.

Jennifer's Five Buttons

Let's look at someone who exemplifies this situation. Jennifer had been trying to lose weight forever. In the past few years, she had taken diet pills, water pills, and hormone shots. She had tried two high-protein crash diets and one low-carb diet, and she had been to no fewer than three weight-loss clinics. Nothing worked. The 5'9", thirty-nine year-old schoolteacher came to my office complaining of stress, fatigue, and weight gain.

"Dr. Meltzer," she said, "my glands aren't working anymore. I can't shake this fat loose." She weighed 205 pounds.

In spite of her self-diagnosis, there was nothing unusual about Jennifer's weight gain. She did not have a thyroid or a glandular condition. After taking a thorough history and physical examination, I determined she had destructive eating habits that were ruining her metabolism. She was overeating. And, she had an inadequate exercise program to boot. Jennifer pleaded that she was too busy to exercise. The way she described her life, she multitasked all day and was constantly climbing a wall of worry.

Aside from fighting the battle of the bulge, Jennifer found herself in the seventh year of a stressful marriage. Her eight-year-old daughter was driving her nuts. The only treadmill she found herself on was one of financial difficulties, marital discord, and work-related stress. She was contemplating throwing in the towel, quitting her job, and moving with her daughter back to her parents' home in Northern California.

Jennifer's eating habits revealed the root of her health problems. She admitted she had a set routine, so it wasn't hard to evaluate. At the end of her work day, she would pick up her daughter from school and head home. Once there, she would thumb through the mail, put her things away, and change out of her work clothes. At this point, it would be about four o'clock in the afternoon. She'd then look around to make sure no one in the family was watching and proceed to raid the refrigerator. She would take food to her bedroom, and a tremendous sense of relief would wash over her as she indulged behind closed doors. For the climax of her daily feast, Jennifer would down her favorite desserts from deep within the recesses of her closet. Indeed, Jennifer was a certified closet binger, burning herself out in a three-way tug-of-war between her husband, her daughter, and her job.

Despite the obviously destructive nature of her eating routine, Jennifer was reluctant to think of it as an emotional crutch. Moreover, she wasn't sure she was ready or willing to give up her daily ritual. At the same time, she said she was desperate for an answer to her predicament. I explained that her abusive eating patterns were ruining her metabolism, and they had put her on a collision course with chronic illness—premature aging, heart disease, diabetes, and obesity. I advised Jennifer to inventory her eating habits for five days. She recorded the frequency with which she ate, the amount of food she consumed, her appetite at the time she ate, and her moods. I also emphasized that she pause to take account of her real feelings whenever she was compelled to overeat. Just as 2 + 2 = 4, overeating equals high EMT. Always. Yes, emotional tension is the trigger that inevitably activates overeating. Whenever you find that your emotional needs are not being met, you are at risk for an emotional food swing. On the other hand, you'll find that you won't overeat when you are at one with yourself.

At the end of her self-survey, Jennifer and I concluded she had five broad buttons that set off her abusive food swings. She would eat when she was one of the following:

1. Tired
2. Bored
3. Frustrated
4. Lonely
5. Depressed

Over the course of the next three months, Jennifer committed herself to conquering her negative food swings and mastering her eating habits. She dug deep and confronted her personal problems in all their complexity. It became clear to her that food was her best friend. She took a stand against emotional overeating. She carefully adhered to the Golden Rules of Smart Eating and, in particular, the pre-meal eating strategies. She closely followed the LYF Cleansing, Detox, and Maintenance Plans. Within six months, she'd lost thirty-five pounds. Over the next six months she lost another twenty-five pounds. That was three years ago. To my delight, Jennifer continues to maintain her weight at145 pounds.

Who's the Boss?

Jennifer experienced an "a-ha moment" when she realized that, by following the Golden Rules, she could relieve her EMT. She discovered that healthy emotional eating habits had a positive influence on her weight-loss program and well-being. She realized that positive eating habits brightened her attitude, sharpened her willpower, fired up her motivation, and energized her mind and body. With these tools in hand, she was able to maintain her ideal weight.

Jennifer's experience is something we can all learn from. Unhealthy eating habits can spread like weeds, insidiously undermining your weight-loss plan. Stubborn, undisciplined eating habits create arthritis of the mind as well as stiffness of the body and the grinding of the gears in your metabolic machinery.

What's the moral of the story? Ongoing, self-abusive eating habits mushroom into destructive patterns whereby stimuli—such as anxiety, fatigue, boredom, or depression—may automatically provoke a binge. Do not allow yourself to become anaesthetized to your own emotions. Fight back. Follow the Golden Rules. You can count on the strategies presented in the Golden Rules to provide the necessary support to your PWL plan. Remember that, like Jennifer, you're in charge of your own eating habits. You're the boss.

The Red Light Theory of Dysfunctional Food Swings

Even though disappointments, frustrations, and disturbances are a very real part of life, we are not usually prepared for these unhappy surprises. After all, few of us have been blessed with emotional mentors. Consequently, emotional ignorance becomes the norm. When you suppress or shut out bad feelings, you're vaguely aware that something's not right; but beyond that, you may find yourself clueless. You probably can't even define the problem, much less address it. You may be too distracted by the more immediate, tangible difficulties in your daily life, whether it be work, money, marriage or family issues. Your anxiety festers; your EMT escalates; and you rely more and more on your mood foods and Mommy-Daddy diet for comfort—even though it seems to be helping less and less. What happens if you run a red light at a busy intersection? Clearly, you put yourself at the very real risk of serious damage from oncoming cars. Stopping your car at a red light is a learned behavior. We're even tested on it before we're granted a driver's license. A red light is easy to spot, and its message is clear: do not proceed until the light turns green. If you decided to quit stopping at red lights, you'd be deemed reckless and a menace to yourself and society, and your license would be revoked.

The human body does not come with traffic signals. Our nose does not light up at the first sign of stress. But EMT does alert us to rising stress. We just have to learn how to recognize our mind-body signals—the red lights of EMT—which, admittedly, are more subtle than crossing guards and traffic cops. If we ignore or overlook our internal stop signs, then, like a careless car driver, we're headed for a crash.

When you feel tense, stressed, rushed, or pressured, your EMT warning signal is flashing. As if you were driving a car, you need to slow down to a stop and think about your next course of action. Go through the red light, and you end up gorging late at night or snacking as soon as you get home from work. Emotional stress and EMT can masquerade behind a variety of bad moods. Look for these warning signs: impatience, irritability, restlessness, hostility, defensiveness, frustration, forgetfulness, and anxiety. Others may accuse you of rudeness, insensitivity, or a short temper. In conversations, you may come across as distracted, disruptive, or overly aggressive. The sudden onset of irrational or hypercritical behavior is a sure tip-off that you're suffering from EMT.

We're all familiar with the general malaise caused by emotional stress: exhaustion, depression, insomnia, inability to concentrate, loss of self-confidence, low self-esteem. But prolonged unresolved stress turns into EMT that undermines your eating habits. In the Golden Rules, I'll discuss in detail how to respond to emotional red lights and resolve emotional conflicts.

Let's be honest. Stress is here to stay, so the challenge is to keep EMT at a minimum. To resist the temptation of overeating, you must begin by taking full responsibility for your feelings. Calmly accept them. Don't stuff them into temporary silence. Experience your cravings, but don't indulge in them. They will pass. The honest admission that you are hooked on your unhealthy behavior, that you have chosen this behavior, and that you have the power to change this behavior is an essential step toward overcoming dysfunctional food swings.

Avoid the Vaccination of Nutritional Mediocrity

Imagine the anguish of waking up one day to realize you're old before your time. Your world is in pieces; life's passing you by. Why willingly subject yourself to such agony? You deserve better. You deserve a more energetic, fulfilling existence. So ask yourself what you're holding on to. Then let it go. Up to a point, excessive weight gain is reversible. Start now, and avoid the vaccination of mediocrity that immunizes the unexamined self. Will it be tough? Yes, occasionally. Sometimes you have to climb a couple of mountains and cross raging rivers to get to where you want to go.

Take a few minutes and complete the following survey, so you may inventory the relationship you have with your eating habits. Keep in mind, they are what they are. Be honest with yourself. Everyone can improve their eating habits. These questions will help you identify what components of your pre-meal, mealtime, and post-meal approach need the most attention. Upon completion, total your score and see how you fare!

Eating Habits Survey: Your Pre-Meal, Mealtime, and Post-Meal Approach

	Always	Usually	Sometimes	Rarely	Never
1. I center myself and make a point to take a timeout and slow down before each meal.	5	4	3	2	1
2. I get some physical exercise before breakfast.	5	4	3	2	1
3. I get some physical exercise before dinner.	5	4	3	2	1
4. I only eat when I am truly hungry.	5	4	3	2	1
5. I make a point not to eat when I am emotional, stressed, or rushed.	5	4	3	2	1
6. I usually stop eating when I'm no longer hungry, even if there is still food left on my plate.	5	4	3	2	1
7. I make certain that I am truly relaxed in mind and body while eating.	5	4	3	2	1
8. I set aside worries and problems at meals.	5	4	3	2	1
9. I create a peaceful, healing ambience at mealtime.	5	4	3	2	1
10. I allow myself a half hour to sit down and get completely involved with my meals.	5	4	3	2	1

11. I have a regular time each day that I eat breakfast.	5	4	3	2	1
12. I have a regular time each day that I eat lunch.	5	4	3	2	1
13. I have a regular time each day that I eat dinner.	5	4	3	2	1
14. In social settings, I emphasize intimate conversation and good company at mealtime instead of overindulgence.	5	4	3	2	1
15. I chew each morsel of each food individually, one mouthful at a time, and avoid gulping and inhaling my food.	5	4	3	2	1
16. I avoid watching TV while eating breakfast, lunch, or dinner.	5	4	3	2	1
17. I appreciate and enjoy my meals.	5	4	3	2	1
18. I make a point to sit down at every meal.	5	4	3	2	1
19. I avoid eating on the go, while standing up, or in my car.	5	4	3	2	1
20. I stay active, mentally and physically, after eating a meal.	5	4	3	2	1

Total Points	Grade	
90–100	A	• Your eating habits are a major support to your LYF Program! Keep up the good work.
80–89	B	• You have a good foundation for your eating habits but still have room to improve. Check out our Golden Rules of Smart Eating, and you'll see where you can improve.

70–79	C	• You have some good eating habits, but too many bad ones that can undermine your PWL plan. Suggests that your eating habits can be improved across the board. Pay close attention to the Golden Rules of Smart Eating, and you will be well on your way to mastering your eating habits.
69 and below	D	• Suggests that your eating habits need an overhaul. Not to worry … we will give you step-by-step strategies in the Golden Rules of Smart Eating that will work your eating habits into shape in no time.

Now that you have finished evaluating your pre-meal, mealtime, and post-meal eating habits, take a moment and complete the following Food Swings Survey. This will help you identify any specific problem areas or food swings that may be sabotaging your weight-loss plan.

Food Swings Survey

	Always	Usually	Sometimes	Rarely	Never
1. I overeat at least one time a day, whether it is breakfast, lunch, or dinner.	1	2	3	4	5
2. I look forward to and eat a big breakfast every morning.	1	2	3	4	5
3. I clean my plate every time and sometimes go back for "2nds" at breakfast.	1	2	3	4	5
4. I clean my plate every time and sometimes go back for "2nds" at lunch.	1	2	3	4	5
5. I clean my plate every time and sometimes go back for "2nds" at dinner.	1	2	3	4	5
6. By the end of the day I've usually eaten more than I had intended.	1	2	3	4	5
7. When I am emotionally upset, I usually eat.	1	2	3	4	5
8. When I am irritable or stressed, I usually eat.	1	2	3	4	5
9. When I am lonely or bored, I usually eat.	1	2	3	4	5
10. When I am depressed, I usually eat.	1	2	3	4	5
11. When I am in a bad mood, I usually eat.	1	2	3	4	5
12. When I am tired, I usually eat.	1	2	3	4	5

13. I typically indulge in my food cravings.	1	2	3	4	5
14. I find myself craving breads and carbs at least once a day and sometimes more often.	1	2	3	4	5
15. I find myself craving chocolate or sweets, such as ice cream, doughnuts, candy, or cookies at least once a day and sometimes more often.	1	2	3	4	5
16. I find myself craving salty foods, such as potato chips, pretzels, and party snacks at least once a day and sometimes more often.	1	2	3	4	5
17. I find myself craving dairy products at least once a day and sometimes more often.	1	2	3	4	5
18. I find myself craving protein at least once a day and sometimes more often.	1	2	3	4	5
19. I snack between meals every day, and sometimes several times a day.	1	2	3	4	5
20. I snack on sweets or cookies between meals.	1	2	3	4	5
21. I usually snack after dinner or before I go to bed.	1	2	3	4	5
22. I snack on salty foods between meals, such as chips, pretzels, salted nuts, or popcorn.	1	2	3	4	5
23. The first thing I do in the morning when I wake up is think about food.	1	2	3	4	5

24. I often think about eating lunch while going through my morning activities.	1	2	3	4	5
25. I often think about eating dinner while going through my afternoon activities.	1	2	3	4	5
26. I find myself indulging in ice cream, chocolate, cookies, or sweets at least one night a week and sometimes several nights a week.	1	2	3	4	5
27. I often indulge in chips and salsa, party foods, or mood foods at night.	1	2	3	4	5
28. I often raid the refrigerator late at night.	1	2	3	4	5
29. When I'm alone at night, I usually make myself dessert or something comforting to eat before I go to bed.	1	2	3	4	5
30. Within one hour of finishing dinner, I'm usually looking for something else to eat.	1	2	3	4	5

Total Points	Grade	
135 –150	A	• You have your food swings under control!
120 –134	B	• Your food swings are largely in check, but you have some fine tuning to do to upgrade your eating habits. We'll give you the strategies you need in "How to Overcome Appetitis," your trouble-shooting guide to the most common dysfunctional eating habits.

90–119	C	• Sometimes you can manage your food swings, but your food swings can often manage you. Troubleshoot your particular vulnerabilities in "How to Overcome Appetitis" and take action against your most hazardous eating habits.
90 and below	D	• Suggests that your eating habits need an overhaul. You are vulnerable to most, if not all, of the most common food swings that stand in the way of permanent weight loss. Start incorporating the strategies laid out in the Golden Rules of Smart Eating and pay close attention to "How to Overcome Appetitis," so you can troubleshoot each particular dysfunctional eating habit.

Making the connection between your EMT, your approach to eating, and your food swings enables you to map out a master plan—a counterattack that will help you to establish healthy food swings. In my Del Mar, California clinic, we have a saying: "Pay Now or Pay Later." Make a conscious decision to alter your eating habits now, and you will comfortably glide into a lifetime of superior weight control and good health. Otherwise, the consequences of obesity and disease may be knocking at your door.

Now that you've had a chance to assess your eating habits and understand how much stress and EMT influence your eating habits, do you know the answer to the following questions?

- What is your usual food reward when you are stressed or tense?
- What do you want to do about it?
- What do you plan to do about it?
- Are you the master or the slave to your emotional tensions and your eating habits?

Say Yes to Hunger, No to Appetite

Before we can move on to the Golden Rules and the strategies you'll need to master your eating habits, I'm going to ask you to do one final thing. I want you to be able to say yes to your hunger and no to your appetite. Do you know the difference between the two? Let's make sure you do.

18

Appetitis: Appetite vs. Hunger

OBESITY is at an all-time high. Appetites are more ravenous than ever. Why? Because stress and EMT have a way of influencing our appetite. When we are ambushed by EMT and fatigue, self-abusive eating habits are all too common. Faulty eating habits cloud the senses, dull the emotions, and tax the body. A closer look reveals that a common thread unites EMT and hazardous eating habits—an affliction I call *appetitis.*

Appetite vs. Hunger

Just as tonsillitis is an inflammation of the tonsils and hepatitis is an inflammation of the liver, appetitis refers to an inflammation of your appetite. What happens when your appetite becomes inflamed? You eat! The problem is, you very well may not be hungry.

Let's make a clear distinction between your hunger and your appetite. Your appetite is your desire for food. It is your emotional hunger. It is susceptible to innumerable factors that have nothing to do with your physiological hunger. Your mood, job stress, emotional stress, and EMT can all wreak havoc with your appetite and lead to appetitis.

Hunger is your need for food. When your fuel reserves have been depleted, the resulting physiological state is hunger. Hunger acts as a motivational survival mechanism that encourages you to eat in order to avoid malnutrition. To express its concern, your stomach growls. Prolonged hunger and a lack of food lead to under-consumption malnutrition. My point being, hunger originates from physical, rather than emotional need.

In summary, appetite is your emotional *desire* for food whereas hunger is your physiological *need* for food. Hunger is a state of body whereas appetite is a state of mind. Got it? Good! Let's move forward.

Have you ever taken a moment to slow down and try to make the distinction between your appetite and your hunger? When you are struggling with your weight, emotionally stressed, burned out, and off balance, you cannot trust what you think is hunger. You may think you're hungry for a fourth slice of pizza—but you're not. You've already had too much to eat. In fact, you may not have been hungry for the first slice, never mind the next three. The craving you feel for that candy bar is very real. Unfortunately, it's coming from your mind and your mood—not your stomach. You may think you are "dying" of hunger when more likely you're dying of fatigue, loneliness, depression, or boredom. In reality, you may be dying of appetite, or emotional hunger.

Emotional Hunger

The true purpose of eating is simple: we need vital nutrients to fuel our biological systems. That's it. But over time, food has taken on all sorts of secondary objectives. We usually eat certain foods based on our ethnic heritage or to celebrate a specific situation. For example, as children, we associate cake with birthdays from the very first time we go to a party, or sweets for Halloween trick-or-treating.

By far the most destructive, self-defeating reason we eat is to fill an emotional void. Yes, everyone does it. We use food to lift our mood. ***Emotional hunger is one of the biggest obstacles on the path to permanent weight loss.*** Most of us know Smart Food is better for our bodies than fast food and junk food. So why do we still succumb to the lure of greasy, fried, fatty foods, steak, cake, creamy fillings, and takeout? The answer has to do with the emotional value we ascribe to the food we eat. When we're anxious, depressed, or under pressure, our level of contentment is threatened. Instead of facing the situation, we often feel an overpowering urge for the quick fix that Mommy-Daddy foods can be counted on to provide support. We know in our heads that this kind of false comfort has negative consequences, but our emotional needs overrule logic. Yes, emotional hunger can take over our lifestyle.

When Doug is feeling frustrated at the end of the day, he believes he deserves crackers and cheese before bed. As far as he's concerned, the amount of food he's already consumed for dinner is irrelevant because he's focused on consoling, rewarding, and entertaining himself—especially late at night. Metabolic balance does not factor into Doug's equation. Nor does his obesity: At six feet and 262 pounds, he's at least 75 pounds overweight. Doug is a coronary waiting to happen, but the food fix comes first.

Marcy also indulges at night. She is 5'5" and weighs 175 pounds. Her drug of choice is ice cream. She desperately wants to lose weight, but like Scarlet O'Hara, she always vows to think about it "tomorrow." Today, she's under too much stress at work. Deep down, Marcy knows that her stress feeds her emotional hunger. She is impulsive as well as compulsive, and her negative late-night food swings continue to feed her stress. She desperately wants and needs to lose weight, but she can't muster up the self-control to stop the vicious cycle and overcome her cravings for chocolate ice cream.

Too Much of a Bad Thing

Many Americans suffer from overconsumption malnutrition—eating too much of the wrong things. This dysfunctional tendency is appetite-driven, influenced by sight, smell, sound, and thought. Taste buds can rule. Let's be honest. Food can be very "appetizing." Everything from social circumstances, to sexual innuendos, to the sound of burgers grilling on the barbecue can prompt the appetite.

In the simplest of terms, appetitis is a mood disorder in which emotional needs dictate food choices, and the body can hardly recognize genuine hunger any more. Fatigue and food rituals can be underlying and contributory causes; but in most cases of appetitis, EMT is the culprit. EMT results in a bad mood. To ease the unpleasant feelings, those in the grip of appetitis reach for food to counter their emotional hunger.

Emotional Deprivation
Emotional Stress
Increased EMT
Emotional Hunger
Appetitis
Food Swings

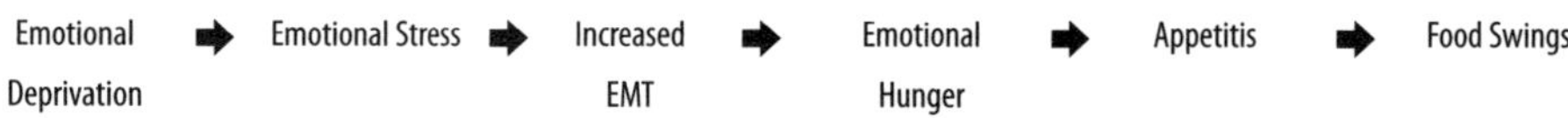

Learn How to Distinguish between Appetite and Hunger

Learning how to distinguish between your appetite and your hunger, and honoring your true hunger, are fundamental principles to mastering your eating habits. Stress, emotions, and EMT all have a way of overstimulating your appetite. It will be your job, by applying the strategies set forth in the Golden Rules of Smart Eating, to combat these forces. We will outline a pre-meal strategy that will give you the tools to do this. The pre-meal strategy will help you establish a clear mind and relaxed body, which are crucial components to distinguishing between appetite and hunger.

Now that you have made all of the necessary connections between stress, emotions, EMT, your appetite, and your eating habits, it is time to apply this knowledge. Let's move on to the Golden Rules.

19

The Golden Rules of Smart Eating

IT is time to connect the dots. You've gone through the thought process of linking healthy eating habits to permanent weight loss. Thought precedes action. Healthy eating habits are the call to action; positive eating habits get results. Think about the slimmer waist and smaller dress and pants size. Think about the increased quality of life. Think about all the attention you will get. Then put those thoughts to work!

The Golden Rules of Smart Eating serve as your operating manual for how to eat, just as the DMV has a driver's manual outlining the basic rules of the road. Follow the Golden Rules, and you'll soon develop the necessary eating habits that will keep you fit, trim, and looking good! When you deliberately repeat the same positive actions, eventually they'll become dominant lifestyle habits—the norm, not the exception, and as natural to you as breathing. Taking control of your thoughts and mood foods leads to permanent weight loss. Taking charge of your eating habits pays huge dividends!

Emotionally comforting foods like carbs, crackers, cheese, salted nuts, chips, candy, and ice cream exploit the hand-to-mouth reflex. They trigger a primitive reaction, a basic instinct to comfort and soothe the wounded child within. For many, food is an emotional crutch, especially your favorite foods. To resist your most preferred mood foods, it's vitally important to adopt a system—one that you can adapt to the adversity or vicissitudes of everyday life.

Follow the Golden Rules and Get Results

I have a reliable system that will give you the strength to own the most constructive eating habits and apply them under all circumstances. The Golden Rules will clear up any confusion about what constitutes positive eating habits. These rules give you the necessary strategies to consistently eat smart and lose weight. They also provide you with practical tools to overcome dysfunctional food swings that can undermine your PWL plan. The Golden Rules of Smart Eating is comprised of three important parts. There is the Pre-meal Str*eat*egy, Mealtime Str*eat*egy, and Post-meal Str*eat*egy.

THE GOLDEN RULES OF SMART EATING	
1. Pre-meal Str*eat*egy	• Strategies that make up your pre-meal approach
2. Mealtime Str*eat*egy	• Strategies to keep in mind while you are eating
3. Post-meal Str*eat*egy	• Strategies to apply once you are done eating

Adhering to this three-step process is especially important when you're most vulnerable—when you're tired, lonely, blue, stressed, bored, or anxious. Put your faith in my foolproof system and learn to master your binges, cravings, and emotional hunger.

It's All in the Approach: Your Pre-meal Strategy is Crucial

I'm going to share with you a little known secret in the weight-loss industry. Your pre-meal strategy is everything. You will soon learn that six of the Top Seven Golden Rules have to do with your pre-meal eating strategy. After working with thousands of patients, I have learned that the pre-meal approach is as important and sometimes more important than the meal itself. How can that be? Let me explain.

It is in your pre-meal approach where you gain the focus to solidify your eating habits. You see, your pre-meal strategy prepares you to be calm and centered in mind and body before eating. This will enable you to make the distinction between your appetite, or your emotional desire for food, and your true level of hunger. Your pre-meal strategy aligns your mind with your weight-loss goals and gets you ready to take action. The attitude you bring to the table is very, very important.

For example, one of the main rules I want to bring to your attention from the get go is the nutritional timeout before eating. The nutritional timeout, for three to fifteen minutes before meals, prepares you to eat well and safeguard your eating habits. It is your opportunity to check in with yourself and make the necessary adjustments before eating. It is in this nutritional timeout where you take note of your mood and your level of hunger. It is in this pre-meal quiet time that you can dial into your stress levels and apply the necessary strategies to overcome EMT. Without a nutritional timeout, it would be unrealistic to expect you to be in touch with your mood and level of hunger. It would be the equivalent of trying to navigate a ship without knowing which way the wind is blowing. A nutritional timeout gives you the support to make the distinction between hunger and appetite. As you know, getting in touch with your mood and true hunger at mealtime is critical to permanent weight loss. In summary, it will be necessary to pause, find your inner silence, and get your bearings before you eat.

With an enthusiastically positive attitude, Smart Foods, and the Golden Rules at your disposal, you can win the battle of the bulge. The Golden Rules are geared toward achieving permanent weight loss, of course, but they come with an added bonus. They'll teach you to resolve emotional distractions and dilemmas, instead of pacifying them with your favorite mood foods, comfort foods, or party foods.

Let me summarize what you will need to know to master your eating habits. To eat well, there are three vital steps.

1. You need to know ***what to eat*** and ***what to avoid.***
2. You need to understand ***when to eat*** and ***when not to eat.***
3. When you are eating, you need to be able to ***determine when enough is enough.***

You'll accomplish all three of these steps by following the Top Seven Golden Rules.

The Top Seven Golden Rules

Among all of the Golden Rules, there are seven rules that stand out. These seven rules are written in stone. Memorize them. Copy them down yourself, and carry them around in your wallet. Tape them to the kitchen refrigerator, or post them on your computer at work. Be consistent and unyielding with them. The only way to achieve metabolic balance and permanent weight loss is through mastering these top seven life-giving dietary guidelines and strategies.

TOP SEVEN GOLDEN RULES
I. Make the Commitment to Select Smart Foods.
II. Know What Not to Eat.
III. Earn Your Meals.
IV. Always Take a Nutritional Timeout before Eating.
V. Never Eat When You Are Emotional, Stressed, or Rushed.
VI. Only Eat When You are Hungry.
VII. Know When Enough Is Enough.

Let's go a little deeper.

I. Make the Commitment to Select Smart Foods

You have been given your nutritional Marching Orders in "How to Naturally Accelerate Your Metabolism." The closer you stick to the prescribed nutritional plan, the better your weight-loss results will be. When you are cleansing, be smart; only select the LYF Cleansing foods. When you are in Nutritional Detox, be smart; only select the LYF Detox foods. When you are in Maintenance and you are at your desired weight, only select the recommended LYF Maintenance foods.

II. Know What not to Eat

Knowing what not to eat and which foods to stay away from is as important as knowing what to eat. This comes down to avoiding foods with the lowest benefit-to-risk ratio. Review the Top Ten Stress Foods on page 447 and eliminate—or at a minimum, minimize—your consumption of these foods. What do you believe you eat too much of?

III. Earn Your Meals

Earning your meals is a fundamental building block in establishing healthy eating habits. Earning your meals with regular exercise has two main benefits. Earning your meals:

1. Regulates Your Metabolism
2. Regulates Your Appetite

Earning Your Meals Regulates Your Metabolism

To begin with, exercise is a necessary tool for accelerating your metabolic rate and establishing an active, healthy metabolism. We've reviewed this in detail in LYF-Style Factor #1. Working out before eating prepares your metabolic machinery to burn fat and generate energy. That's not all. Exercise is also a pre-digestive aid. Working out coordinates your circulatory and digestive processes. Exercising before meals tunes up your digestive enzymes and gets your digestive system ready to consume and effectively metabolize carbohydrates, proteins, and fats. Furthermore, it improves your body's ability to effectively absorb, utilize, and assimilate the nutrients you consume.

Earning Your Meals Regulates Your Appetite

The second major benefit of exercise is that it helps you regulate your appetite. By now, you well know the impact that stress, emotions, your mood, and EMT have on your eating habits. Exercise is an important part of your pre-meal approach that will help you calm your mind and body and relieve any built-up stress and EMT.

When you refresh your mind and body before eating, you work up a natural hunger and can avoid nervous, appetite-driven overeating. Furthermore, regular exercise has a way of shrinking your appetite. A regular fitness routine also releases endorphins—feel-good natural neuropeptides—into the bloodstream. Their presence contributes significantly to a prolonged positive mental outlook. Yes, exercise elevates your mood and thereby suppresses your appetite. Exercise is also a natural antidepressant. As we've discussed, when you feel content, calm, and centered, it's easier to eat well. Over the long haul, earning your meals will guide you to better food selection and better eating habits.

The Timing of Your Workout Counts

To earn your meals, work your body and exercise before most, if not all, meals. As a result of your effort during your workout, you then earn your meals. It's imperative to get your metabolism off to the right start by working out before breakfast. In the morning, get the blood pumping with at least twenty minutes of cardio or aerobic exercise. Under optimal circumstances, exercise precedes dinner, too. To really get your metabolism going, I have found that breaking two sweats a day is important. For example, in the evening, condition muscles and joints through at least twenty minutes of yoga, gym work, Tai Chi, or a brisk walk.

In summary, the major benefits of exercise include:

- Exercise regulates your metabolism.
  - Accelerates your metabolism.
  - Tunes up your digestive system.
  - Maximizes your assimilation of nutrients.
- Exercise regulates your appetite.
  - Relieves built-up stress and EMT.
  - Shrinks your appetite.
  - Releases endorphins and elevates your mood.

*** Be certain to earn your meals. At the very least, take a brisk walk before breakfast and preferably before dinner.

Earning your meals teaches us to value our body and understand its relationship to food. The body is designed to work hard, play hard, and stay in shape. In fact, neglecting your body could be considered a form of disrespect, even self-abuse. Earning your meals is about deserving your meals. It teaches us not to take meals for granted. Eating without a pre-meal exercise plan is a self-defeating strategy.

IV. Always Take a Nutritional Timeout before Eating

Your nutritional timeout is a vital component to your pre-meal strategy. Your nutritional timeout will help you get in touch with your mood, lift your mood, and relieve EMT. Furthermore, your nutritional timeout will help you dial in to your true level of hunger and regulate your appetite. What do I mean by taking a nutritional timeout? It is necessary to take a few minutes to check in with yourself before each meal. I want you to take a few moments to relax and get centered before eating. This can range from a three-minute breathing drill with affirmations to fifteen minutes of meditation or prayer. Your nutritional timeout is an important part of your pre-meal approach that will regulate your appetite. Let me give you an example of a practical three-minute drill.

NUTRITIONAL TIMEOUT—THREE-MINUTE DRILL

1. Find a quiet place.
2. Close your eyes and then steady your eyes with a slight upward gaze at the center point between your eyebrows. This central point between your eyebrows is often referred to as your "third eye."
3. Take seven cleansing breaths.
   a. Inhale deeply and then pause.
   b. Exhale deeply and then pause.
   c. Be certain to do the following:
      i. Pause between breaths.
      ii. Keep your gaze gently centered on your third eye.
4. Use simple affirmations to bring yourself into the moment.
   a. Return to normal breathing and repeat each one of the following affirmations three times.
      i. I love life. (3x)
      ii. I love the miracle of life. (3x)
      iii. I love the miracle of my life. (3x)
   b. Try to experience the impact of these affirmations from deep in your heart.
5. Evaluate your hunger and mood.
   a. Tune into your level of hunger and your mood.
   b. Ask yourself, "What is best for me to eat?"

*** Note: when you have time, it is best to extend your nutritional timeout to fifteen minutes of meditation. We detail our preferred meditation drill in part III of the book, "The Inner Strengths of Permanent Weight Loss." Please refer to pages 378-381 for a complete description of this technique.

Relaxation Counts

Keep in mind, relaxation is a necessary complement to your pre-meal exercise routine: it's just as important to calm your mind as it is to condition your body before a meal. To downshift from the exercise-induced endorphin high, take some time to get quiet. As discussed, at a minimum, do three minutes of cleansing breaths and affirmations. When you have the time, take fifteen minutes and go into silent meditation or prayer. You'll need a few moments to really unwind. America was founded on the Puritan work ethic; to this day, most of us are afflicted with relaxation-deficit disorder and choose to ignore it. Pre-meal relaxation keeps you calm enough to control your appetite and enables you to get in touch with your true level of hunger. You'll notice that, when you take time to relax before each meal, you'll be less inclined to overeat and will know when enough is enough. Furthermore, like exercise, relaxation before eating increases the assimilation of nutrients and aids the digestive system. Remember, breathing is key to relaxation.

When mind and body are in a state of balance, digestive enzymes, nerves, and hormones can cofunction efficiently. When nervous, many people speak of "butterflies in the stomach" or complain of a stomach ache and indigestion. When relaxed, the opposite is true. Relaxation via breathing exercises, meditation, or prayer creates an inner climate of peace. It also promotes liver, pancreatic, and intestinal wellness.

Your nutritional timeout prescribes active relaxation as a way to reduce anxiety. "Active relaxation" is not an oxymoron. There's a big difference between collecting your thoughts in fifteen minutes of silent meditation and slouching on the couch "relaxing," while watching television before eating. You know that stress triggers harmful food indulgences, addictions, and compulsions. Setting aside some quiet time before each meal helps reduce your level of stress, thereby increasing your capacity to eat right and effectively digest your food.

Rules #3 (Earn Your Meals) and #4 (Nutritional Timeout) Work Together

Ideally, I recommend that patients incorporate the full mind-body combination before both breakfast and dinner in the following manner:

	Exercise	Nutritional Timeout
Sunrise Cleanse	• Morning routine of aerobic exercise • Minimum of twenty minutes • Make sure to break a sweat.	• Start with the three-minute drill outlined on page 265. • Add one minute of meditation each week until you reach fifteen minutes.
Sunset Recharge	• Evening routine of aerobic exercise • Minimum of twenty minutes • Make sure to break a sweat.	• Start with the three-minute drill outlined on page 265. • Add one minute of meditation each week until you reach fifteen minutes.

The Sunrise Cleanse refreshes the mind, strengthens the body, opens the heart, and awakens the soul—all within the first hour of the day. The Sunset Recharge does all of the same things, before dinner. The Sunrise Cleanse and Sunset Recharge, coupled with a nutritional timeout before lunch, will keep your mind and body calm and centered throughout the day. This will help you regulate your appetite and master your eating habits.

Think of how powerful these two rules are. For example, how often would you fall victim to a dysfunctional food swing if you were relaxed and had worked out beforehand? Not very often. You see, physical and psychological stress weaken your resolve. Nervous energy turns to negative food choices as an outlet for emotional tension. Golden Rules #3 and #4 work to overcome EMT and bad eating habits by giving you peace in mind and body before meals.

V. Never Eat When Emotional, Stressed, or Rushed: Know When Not to Eat

Golden Rule #5 is crucial. It defines your boundaries. Don't eat when you're nervous. Avoid eating when you're upset or anxious. Eating when you are upset invariably sets a dysfunctional food swing in motion. As we have discussed earlier, emotional eating lends itself to overeating, impulsive snacking, and compulsive bingeing. When you are stressed before meals, please cool down, let down, and take a few minutes to unwind. Please do not eat when you are emotional. In fact, in these times, it is more essential than ever to de-stress and take a nutritional timeout. In your timeout, you can rely on your affirmations and breathing drills to get you back in control. This is why you go through the pre-meal process. The idea is to fully relax and let go so you are not stressed, rushed, or worried at mealtime. You see, you use your pre-meal timeout to let go of stress, quit worrying, and decompress EMT. This will help you stay in control and in charge of your eating habits. Calm yourself before you eat, so you can be in harmony with healthy eating habits.

VI. Only Eat When You Are Hungry

It is of the utmost importance to only consume food when you are hungry. Your body has its own natural wisdom. It pays huge dividends to listen carefully to your body. You know when you are not hungry. There is no value in eating when you are not hungry. For many, eating is knee-jerk reflex. When mealtime shows up, so does their palate.

The purpose of the pre-meal strategy is to give you the insight to ***identify*** and ***honor*** your true hunger. Golden Rules #3 and #4 (Earn Your Meals and Take a Nutritional Timeout) help you alleviate your appetite and ***identify your true level of hunger.*** Golden Rules #6 and #7 ("Only Eat When You Are Hungry" and "Know When Enough Is Enough") are about ***honoring your level of hunger***. Therefore, Golden Rules #6 and #7 are the follow-up and follow-through to your pre-meal strategy and nutritional timeout.

In your effort to lose weight and keep it off, only chow down when you can validate your hunger. This serves two fundamental purposes. First, it establishes an important principle: honoring your hunger. This is a self-discipline that, once acquired, will be a pillar of support in achieving and maintaining your ideal weight. Second, when you are not hungry, your body isn't ready to be consuming food. Therefore, you are doing your metabolism and your body an injustice by eating at these times.

Be Sure to Follow Through

Follow Golden Rule #6 and only eat when you are hungry. It will serve you well. This rule will give you the self-control you need to master your eating habits. Every time you approach a meal, it is not a given that you have to eat. It is a given to ask yourself at mealtimes whether you are hungry or not. You do this during your nutritional timeout. You might feel very light and not be in the mood or have much desire for food. That's okay. I see this in my clinic all of the time. It is not uncommon for folks actively involved in our LYF Plan to find themselves not hungry after going through their pre-meal approach. Learn to trust what your body tells you. When you are hungry, you eat. If you are not hungry, you don't.

Meal Skipping Is Not Recommended: Use Liquid Nutrition

In other words, do not force yourself to eat when you are not hungry. It is not required to eat three meals a day to lose weight permanently. ***It is required, however, to be well nourished at regular intervals with the appropriate essential nutrients.***

How do you accomplish this when you find yourself not hungry at mealtime? The answer resides in *liquid nutrition*. I recommend Re-Vita LiquaHealth, mixed with fresh-squeezed grapefruit juice, as a complete, living, whole-food, meal replacement. Re-Vita provides you with essential nutrients. It supplies you with necessary vitamins and minerals, essential amino acids, essential fatty acids, and a high concentration of phytonutrients and antioxidants. You can also add brewer's yeast to the juice and Re-Vita for additional high-quality protein, vitamins, and minerals. As we noted in LYF-Style Factor #7, the spirulina in Re-Vita is a natural appetite suppressant. When you add brewer's yeast to juice and Re-Vita, it has a way of taking your appetite away even further. Other liquid nutrition options include the potassium-rich vegetable broth. (see Power Cleansing recipes). Finally, you can complete your liquid nutritional meal with a soothing, warm herbal tea.

What if your natural appetite returns an hour or two later? Repeat another serving of liquid nutrition until the next designated mealtime. This way, you'll be able to keep it light, stay energized, and stick to your daily agenda.

VII. Know When Enough Is Enough

Knowing when enough is enough is pivotal to eating well. Golden Rule #7 ("Know When Enough Is Enough") picks up where Golden Rule #6 ("Only Eat When You are Hungry") leaves off. When you don't feel hungry after your pre-meal strategy, Rule #6 outlines what to do. If after your pre-meal strategy you do feel hungry, follow Rule #7 and you will be in control of your eating habits. Sometimes you may have some hunger, but not much. Other times, you may be legitimately hungry. "Knowing When Enough Is Enough" will help you understand how to honor different degrees of hunger. This final step is a major key to permanent weight loss. It allows you to regulate your food choices according to your true level of hunger.

It is Crucial to Become a Mindful Eater

Systematic, mindful, skillful, relaxed eating habits are the antidote to the villain of overeating. Eating can be more than fun and rewarding, as long as you know when it is time to quit. Often, we eat whatever is in front of us without thinking much about it. It might never even occur to you that you don't have to finish the pizza, the pasta, the sandwich—or get to the bottom of the bag of chips. Instead of stuffing your system with the Mommy-Daddy foods you think it wants, why not slow down, listen to your body, and fuel it with what it needs?

"Knowing When Enough Is Enough" describes the art of skillful, balanced eating. Knowing when you've had enough to eat often defines the line between a balanced diet and indulgence. Skillful, balanced eating allows your body to get the most out of the food you eat. By feeding it just right, you're giving the digestive system the key ingredients it needs to focus on—not a quagmire of overload or anti-nutritional gunk to slog through. If you're assigned a project at work, you do a better, more thorough job when you can really focus your attention on it. But if you're overwhelmed with a million other responsibilities, it's likely that the best you'll do with the new assignment is just manage. The body is no different.

There are two fundamental components to "Knowing When Enough Is Enough."

1. Honor Your True Level of Hunger from the Beginning of the Meal.
2. Put Down Your Fork When You Are No Longer Hungry.

Let's review the first component.

Honor Your True Level of Hunger from the Beginning of the Meal

Once you have gone through your pre-meal strategy and have gotten in touch with your true level of hunger, I want you to honor that level of hunger from the beginning of the meal. There are varying degrees of hunger. After your nutritional timeout, you may feel mildly, moderately, or very hungry. Prepare yourself to eat in accordance to your level of hunger. For example, when you feel light and not very hungry, I want you to fix yourself a light meal, such as a Cleansing lunch or Cleansing dinner. When you feel moderately hungry, you may want to have a salad and soup, a Detox lunch, instead of a heavyweight Maintenance lunch. The point is, I want you to respond to and honor your degree of hunger from the beginning of the meal. It's easier to avoid eating extra portions of food if they are not there in the first place.

Put Down Your Fork

The second major component to Rule #7 takes place during your meal. "Knowing When Enough Is Enough" emphasizes putting down your fork and getting up from the table when you are no longer hungry. It has been said that many people dig their graves with their forks and knives. It is a difficult social ritual. Nearly everyone overeats. Practicing skillful, balanced eating is a self-discipline. It will help you find a middle ground, one where you're eating just the right amount.

Periodically throughout the meal, I want you to get in the habit of asking yourself, "Have I had enough to eat?" Listen for the answer. When you think you might be overeating, you probably are. Ask yourself, "Am I still hungry?" If you are not, or are not sure, stop right that second! Put down your fork. Don't take another bite.

Take an Herbal Tea Timeout

At the moment you put down your fork, some find it helpful to get up and go for a walk. I also encourage my patients to go ahead and make a warm cup of tasteful herbal tea. Sometimes I like to call this the herbal tea timeout. It warms up your belly. After a brief walk or a cup of warm herbal tea, you may very well realize that you aren't hungry for more food; and you will have foregone the extra portion that you otherwise would have likely eaten.

The body is equipped with an internal alarm that goes off when the brain realizes you've had too much to eat or drink. The problem is, many of us have learned to tune out this alarm. In order to tune back in, it's important to relax and listen. This is why I recommend a nutritional timeout before each meal. It dials you into you, at that moment in time. When you pay attention, you will hear the signal go off that tells you that you have had enough to eat. You cannot hear it when you are multitasking, watching TV, or surfing the Internet at the same time you are devouring your meals. Under these circumstances, you will not be able to accurately regulate how much you eat. When your radio dial is off in your car, you don't hear the messages in the airways. When you are absorbed with too much going on outside of yourself, you will not be tuned in to your inner voice.

Many of us are actually frightened by the prospect of hearing what our body has to say—we often stuff ourselves to silence it, afraid to face the truth-telling. But even if you've been abusing your body, it is always on your side! It's your greatest ally and, along with mindful eating, gives you the capacity to make changes in your attitude and adjustments in your behavior.

Think of skillful, balanced eating as moderating what you eat. It's an incredibly powerful tool. It is a liberating feeling when you can comfortably, confidently say no to that extra serving. It makes good nutritional sense to stop eating once you have had enough. Knowing when enough is enough is key to permanent weight loss.

Sally and Her "See-Food" Diet

Sally, a nurse, had been working the graveyard shift at her hospital for the past seven years. She would punch in at 11:00 PM and punch out at 7:00 AM five days a week. Sadly, she had become so obese that she actually preferred to work these desolate hours. She reasoned that, as long as she worked while the rest of the world was sleeping, fewer people could see just how heavy she had become.

Sally had the proverbial "pretty face," but, at 5'8" and 200 pounds, she was about 60 pounds overweight. She'd become so isolated and self-loathing that it took the constant prompting of her best girlfriend to get her to my clinic.

With a blank look on her face, the first thing Sally said when she met me was, "I have no willpower, Dr. Meltzer. I enjoy eating all the time, under any circumstance."

> "When do you eat?" I inquired.
> "Oh, maybe two to three times...."

I was about to ask her just what she ate those two to three times a day when she continued, "... two to three times in the morning, two to three times each afternoon, and two to three times at night."

> "So you'd estimate you eat up to seven to nine times a day?" I asked, trying to downplay my concern.

> "Actually, I'm so stressed out that I eat whenever I get the opportunity, and I don't stop until I feel so bloated I can't take it anymore."

In Sally's world, "opportunity" equaled any time food was in sight. She followed the *see*-food diet. Whenever she saw food, she ate it. On her way to work each night, she would stop by one of the many fast-food chains. At the hospital, she made frequent visits to the cafeteria and hit the vending machines in between. On her way home in the morning, she looked forward to pancakes and eggs at one of the local diners before she went to bed. Eating was the most important, most interesting thing in her life.

I took a thorough medical history. In the process of describing her health, Sally revealed how lonely and socially frustrated she was at the age of 41. Although I sympathized, I also gently explained to her that her emotional attachment to food was not only hurting her health but also compounding her personal problems. I told her about the benefits of skillful, balanced eating and that "Knowing When Enough Is Enough" was key to her PWL plan. Sally protested that she was too overweight to be able to accurately assess when she had had enough. But I assuaged her fears.

> "It's simple," I told her. "When you're uncertain if you're eating too much, ask yourself, 'Am I eating too much?' Then listen to your body for the answer. If you are still unsure, take an herbal tea timeout to resist overeating."

Although the prospect of *talking* with her body terrified her, Sally took my program to heart. She soon learned when enough was enough. Within three months, she found herself satisfied by a salad and a cup of soup when previously she had gone through three to five plates per meal. Sally learned to say no. Sally gave up her see-food diet and followed the LYF Nutritional Plan. Sally lost sixty-five pounds. She is still looking good with a new outlook on life.

The Golden Rules Feed Nutritional Common Sense

Every day hundreds of physicians send thousands of patients to their local pharmacies to purchase drugs. Furthermore, every day millions of Americans add over-the-counter aids to their shopping carts full of prescriptions. But there's one item that cannot be bought or sold: nutritional common sense. However, you can acquire nutritional common sense by adhering to the strategies outlined in the Golden Rules.

Nutritional common sense clicks on when you're about to eat something you don't need or even want to eat—commonly items that can be categorized as one of the Top Ten Stress Foods. It also kicks in when you realize that there is no benefit to subjecting yourself to self-defeating emotionally driven eating. Knowing when to abstain from food is an important principle of wholesome nutrition. Nutritional common sense is defined by the boundaries of knowing how to eat well. To acquire nutritional common sense, you need to understand three vital steps:

- You need to know *what to eat* and *what to avoid.*
- You need to understand *when to eat* and *when not to eat.*
- When you are eating, you need to be able to *determine when enough is enough.*

Nutritional common sense is the dietary equivalent of your conscience—it's the little voice inside your head telling you that maybe what you're about to eat isn't such a grand idea. It encourages you to avoid unhealthy, emotionally biased food swings, just as your good judgment encourages you to avoid unhealthy relationships.

The Golden Rules for Smart Eating are simple and clear. Count on them. They are reliable. When the traffic light is red, you don't drive through the intersection. When the sign says stop, you don't go. When a school bus brakes, you don't pass it. These are basic rules of the road that you must learn to avoid accidents. The same holds true for successful eating. Follow the Golden Rules, and you'll avoid the metabolic traumas that accompany emotional overeating.

The Streategy—Your Complete Pre-Meal, Mealtime, and Post-Meal Eating Strategies

The Top Seven Golden Rules shape the destiny of your weight-loss plan. There are some additional Golden Rules that will guide you to superior weight control. It is worthwhile to become the master of your eating habits. All you need to do is follow our strategies and your eating habits will fall into place.

As we've explained, the Golden Rules are divided into three sections:

1. Pre-Meal Str*eat*egy	• Strategies that make up your pre-meal approach
2. Mealtime Str*eat*egy	• Strategies to keep in mind while you are eating
3. Post-Meal Str*eat*egy	• Strategies to apply once you are done eating

We have emphasized the importance of the pre-meal strategy. This is where most of the legwork is done to make sure you have your stress, emotions, mood, and appetite in check. All three phases, however, are considerably important in fighting off weightiness. Let's take a look at all three segments and see how they fit together.

The Pre-Meal Strategy

1. Make a Commitment to Select Smart Foods.***
2. Know What Not to Eat.***
3. Earn Your Meals.***
4. Always Take a Nutritional Timeout before Eating.***
5. Never Eat When Emotional, Stressed, or Rushed.***
6. Only Eat When You Are Hungry.***
7. Drink Fresh-Squeezed Juice Fifteen Minutes before Breakfast and Dinner.
   a. Fresh-squeezed fruit juice with super-nutrients before breakfast.
   b. Fresh-squeezed carrot or other fresh vegetable juice medley before dinner, at least three times per a week. (This applies only to Nutritional Detox and Maintenance stages.)

***Signifies a Top Seven Golden Rule

The Mealtime Strategy

1. Know When Enough Is Enough.***
2. Relax While You're Eating: Find Your Rhythm.
3. Create a Peaceful, Healing Ambience at Mealtime.
4. Allow Yourself a Half Hour to Sit Down and Get Completely Involved with Your Meal.
5. Schedule Your Meals at Regular Times throughout the Day.
6. Substitute Intimate Conversation and Good Company for Overindulgence.
7. Chew Slowly, One Bite at a Time.
8. Appreciate and Enjoy Your Food: Keep a Positive Mental Attitude.
9. Posture Counts: Sit Up Straight.
10. Be Soulful While Eating.
11. Know the Fundamental Don'ts of Smart Eating Habits.

***Signifies a Top Seven Golden Rule

The Post-Meal Strategy
1. Keep Mentally and Physically Active.

Let's get more acquainted with the rest of the Golden Rules.

The Pre-meal Streategy

As we've discussed, the pre-meal approach plays the biggest role in forming positive eating habits. This is a time for you to get in touch with your attitude, mood, and hunger. It helps you resolve any stress and EMT prior to eating, which will help you overcome emotional overeating and dysfunctional food swings. Following the pre-meal strategy will help you establish peace in mind and body, enabling you to honor your true level of hunger. Most of these rules have already been discussed in the Top Seven Golden Rules. We will fill in the rest so you have a complete picture of the strategies you have at your disposal before mealtime.

Please refer to the Top Seven Golden Rules for pre-meal strategies 1–6.

1. Make a Commitment to Select Smart Foods.	4. Always Take a Nutritional Timeout before Eating.
2. Know What Not to Eat.	5. Never Eat When Emotional, Stressed, or Rushed.
3. Earn Your Meals.	6. Only Eat When You Are Hungry.

7a. Drink Fresh-Squeezed Juice Fifteen Minutes before Breakfast

Start the day right by drinking freshly squeezed fruit juice after exercising and before your nutritional timeout or pre-meal meditation. Make sure to add super-nutrients in the form of Re-Vita to your fresh-squeezed juice. Drinking juice with your super-nutrients before breakfast will energize you and help moderate your appetite. It will also give your digestive enzymes a gentle wake-up call and prepare your digestive system for the upcoming meal.

The Re-Vita goes best in fresh-squeezed grapefruit juice or orange juice.

For those that find citrus juices to be too acidic, pear or papaya juice with the Re-Vita is the second best option; watermelon juice can work as well.

7b. Drink Fresh-Squeezed Vegetable Juice Fifteen Minutes before Dinner

This rule calls for drinking fresh-squeezed carrot or mixed vegetable juice fifteen minutes before dinner, at least three times per week. You are well advised to precede your vegetable-based meals with fresh vegetable juice. Carrot juice is especially effective but is moderately higher-glycemic than most other vegetables. That is why I suggest carrot-celery, carrot-celery-parsley, or carrot-celery-beet as the juices of choice in the Detox stage of the LYF Plan. In addition to these vegetable juice combos, wholesome carrot juice by itself is a great option during Maintenance.

As with fresh-squeezed fruit juice in the morning, freshly prepared vegetable juice in the evening—after you exercise and before your pre-meal meditation or nutritional timeout—stimulates your digestive enzymes and helps moderate your appetite. The alkaline chemistry of carrot and mixed veggie juice helps balance the chemistry at work in the stomach and liver, thereby improving digestion, assimilation, and waste disposal.

The Mealtime Streategy

The pre-meal strategy is designed to give you the tools to distinguish your appetite from your hunger. The mealtime strategy is your chance to follow through and honor your true level of hunger. In addition, the better your mealtime eating habits, the better your digestion. Use these strategies to improve your mealtime eating habits.

1. Know When Enough Is Enough

Please refer to the Top Seven Golden Rules.

2. Relax While You're Eating: Find Your Rhythm.

Relaxation is a cornerstone to smart eating habits. Relaxation starts before the meal. It's important to maintain that calm composure throughout the meal itself. Without a full relaxation response at mealtimes, you can still fall prey to overeating and dysfunctional food swings. Furthermore, when nerves are calm, your stomach, digestive enzymes, intestines, liver, and pancreas are best prepared to digest. On the other hand, when you are in an anxious mood, your digestive efficiency is decreased because your body is diverting its attention elsewhere.

3. Create a Peaceful, Healing Ambience at Mealtime

Creating a peaceful, healing ambience at mealtime will help you carry forward the calmness and relaxation that you have created in your pre-meal strategy all the way through the meal. Why not make your meals one of your most respected daily rituals? Your mealtimes are an opportunity to self-nourish, self-nurture, and self-express.

Eat your meals in the most serene, aesthetically soothing setting you can create at the moment. Ideally, have flowers or plants nearby. In the morning, if possible, sit in a sunlit room; if weather permits, eat outside, on the porch, or in the yard. Fresh air and a scenic view have a calming effect on mind and body. At night, lower the lights and spark a few candles for a warm ambience. Avoid eating in the car, in front of the television, or when you're talking on the phone. Think of your dining area as a sanctuary—as a place where you can seek refuge from all the chaos of the outside world. Don't bring that chaos into the sanctuary by, for example, watching TV or surfing the Web while you eat.

4. Allow Yourself a Half Hour to Sit Down and Get Completely Involved with Your Meal

Slowing down enables you to get the most out of your meals. It allows you stay in touch with your true level of hunger. Slow down with slow food. Slow foods are the opposite of fast food. They take a little time to prepare, a little time to consume, and, once swallowed, are fully digested for all their nutritional potential. Brown rice with tofu and green vegetables is an example of a slow meal. Chicken in a bucket with a side of fries is not.

Designating thirty minutes to meals gives your body a solid opportunity to assimilate nutrients. It also gives your mind and soul a chance to unwind. At first, you may protest that you can't afford the time. The truth is, you can't afford not to slow down. The key is to make your meals a priority, as important to you as, for example, your favorite television programs.

5. **Schedule Your Meals at Regular Times throughout the Day**

   Timing your meals is one of the secrets of sound eating habits. Why? Because to stay well, it is necessary to be well nourished at regular intervals with the appropriate essential nutrients. How do you get your timing right for breakfast, lunch, and dinner?

Breakfast

When it comes to breakfast, the earlier the better—ideally right after your Sunrise Cleanse. Plan to eat breakfast by no later than 8:30 AM in the warmer months and by 7:30 AM during the shorter days of winter.

Lunch

Eat lunch between noon and 1:30 PM. Later lunches can throw off your timing for the rest of the day.

Dinner

Dinner is best metabolized right after sunset (and the Sunset Recharge). Eating too late in the evening can turn into a disruptive eating habit. It can slow down your metabolism and interfere with sleep by overtaxing your digestive organs. The net effect of eating too late is that it can drain you of valuable energy the next day. Be certain to have things to look forward to after dinner. Keep your evenings filled with events and activities that are personally and socially rewarding so that you feel less of a need to depend on dinner for emotional fulfillment.

For a three-meal day, work within this time frame:

- Breakfast: 6:30–8:30 AM
- Lunch: 12:00–1:30 PM
- Dinner: 5:30–7:30 PM

The importance of biorhythms is often overlooked, but your digestive organs function best as creatures of good habits. Eating at set intervals establishes order and continuity in the liver, bile, stomach, and intestines. It also regulates waste elimination. Spacing meals about six hours apart allows your body to engage in the entire cycle of nutrient absorption and waste elimination and then recover in time for the next feeding. Consider the opposite, but more common scenario: many of us eat breakfast late and lunch too soon afterward, so that the body's processing of the first meal is interrupted by the arrival of the second. By the afternoon, we're stuffed and sluggish, and postpone dinner until late in the evening. And that's not even considering what it is we're actually eating.

A regular meal schedule also helps you to stay balanced and in control of your lifestyle. Knowing when you plan to eat each day helps you to avoid many pitfalls, such as resorting to candy, caffeine, or energy drinks for an energy rush in the late afternoon because you've somehow neglected to have lunch.

When you find yourself out of sync and off schedule—particularly when you've eaten a late breakfast—use liquid nutrition for lunch to get back in rhythm for dinner.

6. Substitute Intimate Conversation and Good Company for Overindulgence

They say laughter is the best medicine. Companionship at mealtime is good for the soul, and it actually curbs your appetite by shifting the focus from eating to socializing. There are times when it is quite healing to enjoy breakfast or lunch alone in a relaxed natural environment. But at dinner, permit yourself some esprit de corps by spending time with loved ones, friends, and family. Eating together with intimates promotes emotional balance which, in turn, keeps emotional hunger at bay. The celebration of people takes precedence over the celebration of the palate.

7. Chew Slowly, One Bite at a Time

Extend the relaxation principle by maintaining a slow, steady pace when you eat. Remember that meals are opportunities to put your busy schedule on pause. They may be your only chance during an otherwise hectic day to take a break from responsibilities and chores. Pace yourself for a thirty-minute meal the same way you'd pace yourself for a three-mile run. Start slowly, one bite at a time. Don't inhale (or, as we say in California, "hoover") your food. Fully taste each forkful you put in your mouth. Relish it. If it helps, eat one food at a time: for example, don't mix carrots and broccoli in the same bite.

At dinner, start with crispy, raw salads. Chew thoroughly so that you grind out the water in the leafy greens. Crunch seeds and nuts. Masticate. The activity of the jaw reveals a lot about a person. Some people chomp nonstop, jowls jiggling, from the beginning to the end of a meal. The bottom line is to eat slowly and enjoy your meals.

8. Appreciate and Enjoy Your Food: Keep a Positive Mental Attitude

Ours is such a prosperous society that we often take food for granted. We think of it as a form of entertainment. Try to recognize the real, earthy magnificence of whole food and the important role it plays in your life. Are you grateful and thankful that you can see, smell, and taste food? Treat food with respect. Instead of pausing to appreciate nature's great gifts, most of us rush through our meals. Saying grace aloud, silently affirming, or simply holding hands are all ways to express gratitude for the aesthetic, emotional, and nutritive value of food. You can also show your consideration for food by selecting organically grown produce and preparing wholesome dishes.

During our first consultation, many of my patients state—sometimes with embarrassment and resignation—"I love to eat." Of course you love to eat! Everyone does. Eating is one of the great joys in life. We should not deny ourselves this pleasure, or be ashamed of it. We just need to shift the balance back to where it belongs so that food fulfills its maximum potential to nourish without being an emotional crutch.

9. Posture Counts: Sit Up Straight

Your posture makes a difference at mealtimes. Your best option is to sit in a chair that offers firm back support. When you are seated, circulation to the digestive organs and glands improves because, due to gravity, blood pools in the digestive system. Avoid hunching your spine. In fact, I encourage fledgling yogis to sit cross-legged, lotus or semi-lotus style, at a low table. However, here's one exception: sitting in your car—even if you're sitting up straight—and stuffing down takeout while driving does not count as a Smart Food move. (Not to mention it may be hazardous to your fellow motorists!)

Standing up while eating and eating on the go are bad habits of our modern-day, hectic lifestyle. It does not work to our benefit. When we stand, blood pools in the veins of the legs instead of the digestive region; this doesn't do us any digestive good. Furthermore, standing while eating encourages a myriad of negative food swings. For example, raiding the refrigerator. How many times have you opened the refrigerator door not to take out whole food items needed to prepare a planned meal but just to check out your snacking options? You don't really know what you're looking for when you open the door; you're just hoping to find something to munch.

What happened to your nutritional timeout? If it's not a designated mealtime, don't hang out in the kitchen.

10. Be Soulful While Eating

Acknowledge the blessing of being alive and having the privilege to eat healthy, wholesome food. Converting whole, living food into fuel for work and play is no less than a divine process. Many religions use food as a central focus to sacred rituals. Our body is a temple, our own personal cathedral, and we have the honor of maintaining it. Every day offers us a chance to come fully alive through our choice of food.

Acknowledge the divine in yourself and your diet. In a manner that corresponds to your own personal belief system, bless your kitchen and dining room and recognize them as healing centers. Most of us think of soul food as a Southern variety, deep-fried and smothered with gravy; but when you stop to consider it, fresh, whole, living food is the real soul food because it promotes life.

11. The Fundamental Don'ts

Take note of the fundamental don'ts of smart eating habits.

- Don't be a victim of nervous eating habits!
- Do not overeat.
- Do not eat when emotionally upset, anxious, or depressed.
- Do not snack, double up on servings, indulge in "just a taste," or raid the refrigerator.
- Do not binge on cheese, crackers, nuts, fruits, or dried fruits.
- Do not overdose on any food item from any food group.
- Do not snack while you are cooking.
- Do not eat dinner after 8:00 PM.
- Do not eat when standing, driving, or working.
- Do not take your diet for granted.
- Do not mix fruits and vegetables in the same meal.
- Do not indulge in cycles of feasting and fasting.

The Post-Meal Streategy: Keep Mentally and Physically Active.

The point of the post-meal strategy is simple: move on. Do not make a career out of your meals. After you eat—especially in the evening—take a brisk, fifteen-minute walk. Otherwise, it's very easy to get drowsy after dinner. This also holds true for late afternoons at the office. If you eat at your desk and then go right back to business without ever having gotten up, changed locations, or moved about, I guarantee your head will begin to droop. Those whose jobs keep them on their feet during the day, whether it's because they're store clerks or schoolteachers or hospital doctors, often succumb to the post-supper couch-potato syndrome. I understand the exhaustion, but sinking into the sofa after dinner stalls the metabolism. After you've enjoyed a smart meal, move on to a physically and mentally stimulating activity. Keep your feet moving.

20

How to Overcome Appetitis and the Eight Most Common Food Swings

BY now you've come to understand the power that stress has over your eating habits. You've itemized your Mommy-Daddy diet, identified your emotional attachment to food, and recognized how EMT triggers hazardous eating. You have also learned that by incorporating the strategies of the Golden Rules, you can overcome any bad eating habits. But keep in mind that even those well trained in the Golden Rules have to deal with life's ups and downs, disappointments, distractions, and challenges. Dysfunctional eating habits have reached epidemic proportions. Everyone is exposed to them; no one is completely immune. There is no vaccination against bad eating habits.

This chapter is about troubleshooting; it is the part of the book that helps you identify your most vulnerable food swings. It is also the part of the book that will help you outfox and correct common problems that can get in the way of your weight-loss program. Understanding the nature of your negative, self-defeating eating habits will help you disarm them forever.

As our society prides itself in its growing self-awareness, we've all become familiar with the term "dysfunctional." It's the psychologist's way of saying that something "sort of functions"—but in an adverse, damaging, unhealthy manner. A dysfunctional family, for example, is still a family. But its problems prevent it from being a healthy, happy, communicative unit. Dysfunctional or bad eating habits wreak havoc not only on your emotional well-being but also on your physical health. Dysfunctional eating habits, also called dysfunctional food swings, are not good for you. They disrupt your lifestyle, sabotage your weight-loss plan, and create and keep recreating emotional instability. In fact, in time, dysfunctional food swings can go on to cause you bodily harm.

Weeds in the Garden

Out-of-control overeating, compulsive bingeing, mindless snacking, or late-night indulging promote poor health, metabolic burnout, accelerated aging, serious illness, and morbidity. Like weeds, these dysfunctional food swings spread stealthily, choking off the roots of healthy plants and ultimately consuming an entire garden. Dysfunctional food swings feed off stress, and stress feeds off moodiness and dysfunctional eating habits. It's a murderous merry-go-round. Take a look at how emotional distress turns into a repetitive cycle of destructive eating habits and destructive food swings.

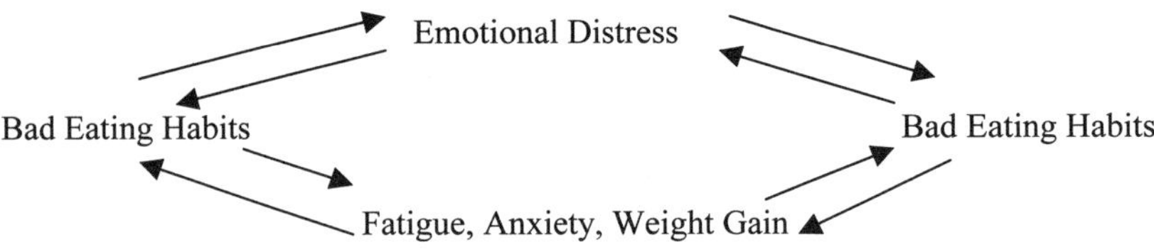

For the vast majority of Americans, destructive eating habits seem almost unavoidable. In the morning, you're late for work and have no time to make breakfast, so you stop at a local deli to get a bagel with cream cheese and a tall mocha frapuccino. At lunch, you're too busy to leave the office, so you order in a pizza, buy a caffeinated energy drink to pick you up at the vending machine, and down them at your desk while returning phone calls and e-mails. By nighttime, you're too exhausted to cook anything that requires more effort than pushing the buttons on the microwave. The next day, you get up and do it all over again. What can be done to stop the cycle of self-abuse and nutritional toxicity?

Like any other troublesome condition, hazardous eating habits can be approached in two ways. We can prevent them, or we can treat them. Prevention is always preferable. That's the purpose of the Golden Rules; to prevent bad eating habits.

An Ounce of Prevention ...

An ounce of prevention ... is worth a pound of cure. There's a lot of wisdom in that homespun adage. The active, intentional prevention of illness keeps disease from occurring. You get it before it gets you. The best way to prevent disease is to be well. It's basic logic; if you have wellness, there's no room for illness. The two can't coexist simultaneously in the same body.

So what is the best way to prevent dysfunctional food swings? The best way to prevent dysfunctional foods swings is to establish and acquire healthy eating habits. Again, that's what the Golden Rules are all about. But keep in mind, human behavior is consistently inconsistent. People's eating habits can fluctuate. Bad habits have a way of creeping into your lifestyle. Bad habits often become so ingrained on so many levels—physical, mental, emotional—they're almost impossible to break. That's where this part of the book comes into play. In this chapter, I address how to troubleshoot, ambush, and treat specific, common dysfunctional eating habits.

Eight is Enough: The Eight Most Harmful Eating Habits

The eight most common forms of *appetitis* are listed below. Keep in mind, in most cases of appetitis, emotional tension, also known as EMT, is the culprit. Appetitis has a way of taking over your life. The mind becomes fixated on crackers and cheese, a box of doughnuts, a rack of barbecue ribs, or other favorite foods; until you answer the craving, it dominates your thinking. The manifestations of chronic appetitis can vary, but the eight most common dysfunctional food swings are the following:

EIGHT MOST COMMON FOOD SWINGS
1. Overeating
2. Food Addictions
3. Cravings
4. Snacking and Nibbling
5. Food-on-the-Brain Syndrome
6. Late-Night Indulgences
7. Compulsive Bingeing
8. Poor Food Choices

Appetitis demands aggressive treatment. Because of its cyclical, recurrent nature, it can be difficult to reverse. Natural therapies such as nutritional and emotional detox can be of great benefit. We will show you how to overcome each one of these food nemeses.

There Is a Cure for Appetitis

The cure for appetitis is to enrich and glorify your appetite for life. The greater your ambition, the greater your love for life and will to love is—the less prone you are to appetitis. The more you look forward to every day, the more you are involved with life, and the greater your appetite for life, the lower your appetite for food. When you are fully connected to your soul, you are too busy living, thinking, and absorbing what is going on around and inside you to be obsessed with your appetite. Smart Foods and my Golden Rules of Smart Eating are also invaluable tools in the quest for appetite control. By following the Golden Rules, your mind and body become well nourished at regular intervals. This creates a balanced chemistry that helps you keep a handle on your appetite.

Patients of mine that have gone through the LYF Program and are now healthy, productive, and fit experience hunger—and appetite—all the time. They exert a lot of energy and require top-quality fuel to maintain their peak level of performance. They earn their meals with hard work and vigorous exercise. When faced with a flare-up of appetitis—for example, a craving for salted chips or popcorn—they put out the fire. They can do this because they're in charge of their emotional life. Over time, they've learned to recognize that food cravings are the signs and symptoms of EMT. They summon up their self-determination and emotional self-discipline to douse the flames and stick to the Golden Rules. Instead of using food to elevate their mood, they seek other, healthier forms of emotional gratification.

Never lose sight of the eternal truth that your health is a cornerstone to your happiness. Your well-being dictates your capacity for love and joy. The better your well-being, the more infinite your love and joy. Your well-being also fuels your desire to serves others. Without the well-being of a healthy, vital metabolism, you will be curtailing the time you spend in creating love and spreading joy. The more and more time you spend struggling with your weight-loss issues, the more your mind becomes preoccupied with losing weight and the less time you have to spend on other important issues.

It's challenging to live a balanced lifestyle when it seems as if everyone around you is under the spell of stress and inflationary consumerism. At first, curing appetitis and establishing positive eating habits may appear to go against society's grain and be too radical a departure from the frantic, frenzied norm. But the benefits of smart nutrition soon compensate for the initial effort required to make smart eating and the Golden Rules your personal standard. It's a wise investment.

The Cure: IBM—Intellectual Behavior Modification

Which is better—a lifetime of preventing problems or a lifetime of treating problems? The choice is obvious. But if you're already past the prevention phase, don't despair. As you positively alter your eating habits, and thereby treat your problems, you'll be able to work back to the prevention position.

I have treated thousands of cases of appetitis. There is a way to repair the damage and put a stop to hazardous eating habits that stand in your way. I'm going to break down the "Eight is Enough" dysfunctional food swings, so that you can take a targeted plan of attack. But remember that—whatever the food swing, whatever the style of appetitis—they are all characterized by obsessive-compulsive tendencies. They must be treated behaviorally with intelligent behavior modification, or IBM. Let's get started with the #1 form of appetitis.

Dysfunctional Food Swing #1: Overeating

Overeating is the single most common destructive eating habit. In fact, it's one of the greatest health hazards facing modern society. Overeating has dominated many a lifestyle. My simple definition of overeating is this: you are eating too much food, more than you need. Overeating comes into play at mealtime as well as between the meals. Consuming food you don't need, especially when you know you do not want to be eating, is an all too common form of overeating. Overeating results from a loss of food boundaries.

Overeating is a sign of the times and plays a role in many social rituals. Being well-fed is considered a sign of success, prosperity—the good life. Most parents encourage their kids to eat and be sure to clean their plate. "Children are starving in Africa," is a baby-boomer catchphrase. Oftentimes parents use food as a way of silencing and calming their children. Grandparents court affection with snacks. Furthermore, as we've already discussed in detail, for many of us food equals love. We down our Mommy-Daddy diets in a desperate attempt to soothe ourselves.

Less Is More

The malignant end point of overeating is obesity, which, as you know, increases the risk for coronary disease, cancer, diabetes, arthritis, hardening of the arteries, and stroke. In rare cases, obesity is caused by glandular conditions and genetic predispositions, but the majority of the time it's due to plain old overconsumption.

There is more to food indulgence than meets the eye. Did you know that emotional overeating is a mood disorder? Have you ever stopped to wonder that overeating is a substitute for love and affection? Overeating can show up when you are not getting enough attention. The root cause of overeating is emotional deprivation. As anxiety, depression, loneliness, feelings of emptiness, and low self-esteem mount, the overeater turns to food for a mood change. Appetite takes over. Impulsiveness sets in. Overeating becomes a compulsive, involuntary action. Appetitis is in control. Sometimes, you just want to eat to your heart's delight. It's your birthday or a special occasion, or you just feel like sitting down and going for it. Of course, I don't encourage this type of marathon recreational eating, but it can be looked at as a voluntary "discretionary indiscretion." It is chronic overeating that I want to declare war against. Chronic overeating is marked by its regularity—the self-destructive binge-fests that occur on any given day or the daily late-night food extravaganza. What's the point? After all, feeling stuffed and drowsy after you overeat only inhibits your mental and physical performance.

Terry in the Handicapped Zone

Terry was the head cashier for a large supermarket in Southern California. She liked to think of herself as a pleasant and charming person, but over the past six months, she had become increasingly moody and irritable. During this time, her hands and knees had swollen up, and her joints ached so much that she had to stop working. "Doctor," she confided. "I feel handicapped. I can't vacuum my house, make the beds ... and now I'm unable to keep up with my job."

At home, Terry had become quite inactive. She did little more than eat, sleep, read, talk on the phone, and watch TV. Since the onset of her arthritis, her husband had taken over kitchen duty. She ate whatever George served her, and he could be counted on to cook up all his favorites: fried steaks, mashed potatoes, ice cream, and cookies to accompany the night's television viewing. At work, Terry sat at her register most of the day. When she wasn't ringing up sales or supervising employees, she sat at her spot and ate. She had ravenous appetitis, downing everything in sight. At forty-two, 5'7", and 215 pounds, she was about 80 pounds overweight.

I concluded that Terry's arthritic condition was a result of her obesity. When she came to see me, she was motivated to change. She didn't want to be crippled for the second half of her life. By following the techniques I'll outline in this chapter, she quickly began to make progress. In three months, her joint pain began to diminish. In six months, she had lost fifty pounds, was pain free and back at work. By the end of a year, Terry had lost all of her extra weight. She continues to do well today.

Terry is a perfect example of how overeating can prematurely age the body and cause chronic illness. She discovered that the cure for overeating was the RIEXA technique. You can do the same. Here is how you can put an end to your overeating habits.

The RIEXA Technique

Overeating is a bad habit. Typically it is the result of an inability to deal effectively with personal frustrations. It's a cry for help. IBM (intelligent behavior modification) can answer the call. The RIEXA behavior modification technique will help you take back control. By learning the RIEXA technique, you will be able to overcome overeating as well as other bad eating habits. I'll be referring to this important formula again throughout the rest of the book, so let me spell out exactly what it is. Make a note of this page, as you may want to refer back to it again. Before we get to the RIEXA technique, however, let's review one important prerequisite.

Take Full Responsibility for Everything You Eat

The very first step in eliminating overeating or any negative eating habit is taking full ownership for everything you eat. Here is the good news. When it comes to your eating habits, you're the boss. You are in the driver's seat; you, and only you, select and consume your body's fuel. No one else is to blame. It's easy to come up with excuses: "It was my cousin's wedding," "I had a hard day," or "I've followed my diet for two weeks; I've earned a break."

Let's face it. Food is everywhere—at parties, wedding receptions, corporate functions, little league games. It's inescapable. Just because, for example, you go to the movies, it doesn't mean you have to eat a tub of popcorn. At the point of purchase, you are in charge. It is also vitally important to end the blame game and stop pointing fingers at your spouse, friends, and family whenever you indulge. The only person who can make certain that you eat well is you.

Take full responsibility for your eating habits. This important governing principle fuels the RIEXA technique. Taking full responsibility for your eating habits is one of the unwritten laws of permanent weight loss.

The RIEXA Technique

Each letter stands for an important component in the technique.

R: Recognition

Recognize when you are about to overeat. Right before you overeat, you typically have three to five seconds between your urge to eat—or the urge to continue eating—and the time you actually put food in your mouth. I call this the red zone. It is imperative to recognize the telltale warning signs that you are in the red zone and are likely to overeat. Common red-zone warning signals include times when you feel:

- Bored
- Upset
- Irritable
- Moody
- Frustrated
- Stressed

Most folks exhibit one, if not several, of these signs before overeating. However, each person has his or her own mood and pre-indulgent patterns. In other words, it is key to inventory your overeating habits.

You have come to terms with being accountable for your eating habits. Now, recognize THAT you overeat, recognize WHEN you overeat, recognize WHAT you overeat, and recognize HOW MUCH you overeat. Furthermore, recognize your state of mind before you overeat. Write it down. Teach yourself to recognize your own particular food traps.

I: Identify

Just as you've recognized your food traps, you must also identify your emotional state when you are about to, or are in the process of, overeating. To cure the overeating food swing, you have to be connected to yourself. This means you have to track how you feel right before and during your overeating experience. For example, I feel bored, lousy, left out, or lonely. Always take the time to identify your true feelings right before you make the move to execute your hand-to-mouth reflex. Overeating can be a knee-jerk reflex to moodiness. That is why the foods you typically overeat are called mood foods. Unless you take a momentary nutritional timeout to identify your emotional state, you may very well miss the opportunity to reverse the food swing. When appetitis has the upper hand, you typically will not stop to identify the mood you are in. You are too busy getting ready to enjoy your food. Eventually, you'll come to realize that, when you are overeating, it's probably because food is available and that you crave comfort or an emotional reward. Sometimes it can be that someone is expecting you to eat, and you feel obligated.

Get to Know Your Overeating Patterns

Identify if you eat to entertain yourself. Is food the main event or the most important part of your day? Do you eat for fun? Do you use food as a recreational drug? It would be optimal at the time of your binge that you stop to ask yourself:

- Am I really hungry?
- Do I really need to eat or continue eating?

Ask yourself these two questions every single time you eat until you know the difference between genuine hunger and deceptive appetitis. Self-discovery goes a long way in fighting off overeating habits. Before you begin another eating binge, identify the nature of your appetitis with this quick quiz:

APPETITIS QUIZ
• What is overeating doing for me? • Why do I need to eat at this exact moment? • What is the benefit of eating too much food? • What is the benefit of eating unhealthy food?

Use these insights to help you identify how you are feeling when you overeat. It is up to you to identify the predominant mood that triggers your overeating.

EX: Express and Experience

The minute you catch yourself overeating, put your fork down. Yes, you have recognized you are about to overeat. Yes, you have identified how you feel. Now express your feelings. Say it out loud if that will make it more real. If it involves another person, let him or her know. For example, if you reach for the chocolate-covered pretzels whenever you're frustrated with your kids, the next time your aggravation escalates take a deep breath and calmly say—to yourself or your children—how you are feeling. Tell it like it is, but say it calmly and without raising your voice. If that type of unedited self-expression feels too unnatural to risk, then start by writing it down in a journal.

The other dimension to the letters "EX" is experience. You've just said how you feel: now live it. Experience the sad, discouraging, enraging, or boring sensations that make you reach for the onion rings or fries. Make the distinction between your primary feelings and your emotions. When you engage your primary feelings, your emotional tension decreases, as does the likelihood that you'll be driven to indulge. Stay with your primary feelings, even when they're painful. Work through them to a place of inner peace. Take a nutritional timeout, breathe, meditate, and go deep. Find your center of tranquility and notice how the tensions recede. As you allow yourself to experience your emotions, ask the following questions:

- What will it take to make me feel better?
- What will it take for this feeling to go away?
- What kind of feelings can I recruit to make any unpleasant feelings go away?
- What can I do to let go of this tension?
- What will it take for me to let go of my preoccupation with food?

You'll likely find that overeating is an escape mechanism, developed to help you avoid harsh emotional realities.

A: Action

Get on the bus, Gus. Make a new plan, Stan. You may not need fifty ways to let go of your bad eating habits, but you've got to take meaningful action. The "A" stands for alternative action. You will need to substitute a new form of behavior to replace overeating and constructively deal with your emotional distractions. In fact, I want you to have a plan of action when you are vulnerable to overeating and find yourself in the red zone. I have found that it is helpful for my patients to rehearse this plan of action frequently in their mind. I want you to think through the action steps you will take when you are about to overeat. For example, when you know that boredom triggers overeating, practice in your mind what you will do the next time you are bored as a substitute for reaching to food. Maybe you will respond by taking a walk or calling a friend to jog on the beach. Other common action steps include the following:

COMMON ACTION STEPS

• Move Your Feet
  – Change your physical space—if you're at home, change rooms or walk outside; if you are at work, walk down the hallway.
  – Go for a walk around the block.
  – Exercise.
• Exercise Your Mind.
  – Take a nutritional timeout—do some cleansing breaths and affirmations.
  – Meditate.
• Find Some Social Support.
  – Turn to a loved one for emotional support.
  – Call a friend.
• Hydrotherapy
  – Take a shower, alternating hot and cold water for a few minutes.
  – Jump in a pool, Jacuzzi, or natural body of water.
• Do Something Creative.
  – Play a musical instrument.
  – Write some poetry.
• Move Your Hands and Fingers.
  – Repress the hand-to-mouth reflex by doing something besides eating with your fingers.
  – Write a thank-you note.
  – Punch a punching bag.

In addition to the action steps listed above, you can use liquid nutrition to help you satisfy your hunger and alleviate your appetite. Liquid nutrition serves as a substitute for biting, chewing, and swallowing.

LIQUID NUTRITION OPTIONS
• Make a glass of warm herbal tea.
• Have a glass of juice with Re-Vita and/or brewer's yeast.
• Have a cup of potassium broth soup. (See Power Cleansing recipes)
• Drink some ice water with a twist of lemon or lime.

Putting It All Together

While everyone may have a slightly different action plan, here is a common sequence of action steps I recommend to my patients.

First off, I suggest that you change your physical space when you feel like you may fall victim to overeating. This can be as simple as walking outside, changing rooms in your house or office, walking around the block, or walking down the hallway. Oftentimes, going for a quick walk and changing your physical environment are all you need to do to alleviate your appetite.

If you still feel hungry, I encourage taking some super-nutrients, such as a glass of fresh-squeezed juice with Re-Vita and/or brewer's yeast. Supernutrients are a great way to curb your hunger, increase your energy, and provide your body with essential nutrients it may be looking for.

Finally, if your appetite or desire for food persists, having a glass of warm herbal tea goes a long way in alleviating your appetite.

This is a powerful sequence designed to satisfy both your hunger, your physiological need for food, and your appetite, your emotional desire for food.

Positive Reinforcement—The RIEXA Technique Works!

The RIEXA technique gets results. It is the essence of effective cognitive behavior therapy. The cognitive phase is your becoming aware of your eating habits. Once you internalize this new reality, you can then take action and change your behavior. In time, with consistent repetition, it will help you distinguish appetitis from true hunger, cure emotional overeating, and establish constructive food habits. It's all about positive reinforcement—as I said earlier, a behavioral approach. You think new and then you act new! You decide to take control of your eating habits, and your actions back you up!

Here's a summary of the RIEXA technique—you may want to photocopy this and stick it on your refrigerator door or carry it with you and use it as a reminder when you're fighting the urges of appetitis.

The RIEXA Technique Gets Results!

R: RECOGNIZE that you're about to indulge. Recognize the need to change and take charge of your impulsive nature.

I: IDENTIFY any negative mental attitude or mood that feeds overeating. Identify what you are truly feeling. Please do not edit or censor your primary feelings. Your feelings count.

EX: Honestly **EXPRESS** how you feel about your situation and allow yourself to **EXPERIENCE** the full range of feelings you've been suppressing. Ask yourself what it will take to make you feel better.

A: Take **ACTION** and make the necessary adjustments in your attitude and behavior to affect positive change.

Dysfunctional Food Swing #2: Food Addiction

Overeaters can often be identified by their obesity, but anyone can get caught up in getting attached to their favorite foods. Everyone wants to feel good. One of the great ironies of food addiction is that junk-food junkies usually eat food to feel better, but that very food ultimately makes them feel worse. A compulsive quest for a mood change, brought on by taking pleasure in permissive eating, defines the hazardous eating pattern of the food-addiction food swings.

Food addicts have a lot in common with alcoholics, shopaholics, sexaholics, workaholics, TVaholics, and compulsive gamblers. They eat in spite of themselves and the adverse consequences of their actions. This is the hallmark of classic obsessive-compulsive behavior. Food obsession is an early symptom of food addiction. If you're always thinking of your next meal, completely preoccupied by thoughts of eating, you're officially obsessed. Eventually, this mind-set manifests itself in an inability to resist tasting the culinary objects of your desire—sweets, salty snacks, starches, breads, cheese, or whatever it may be.

Food Addiction Leads to Bingeing

Jane loved glazed doughnuts. They were the highlight of her day. Yet the whole time she was indulging, she knew it was food insanity—chocolate-covered madness. But she couldn't stop herself, even when she'd start to feel a headache coming on from all the sugar consumption. Instead, she'd continue eating, then take a variety of aspirins, and ride out the pain until it subsided a few hours later. By evening, when the stress of preparing dinner for her family began to take over, she'd start fantasizing about doughnuts again.

As a food addiction progresses, sneaking food becomes more commonplace. Jane kept an emergency box of doughnuts hidden in her linen closet, where no one else in the house would ever think to look. Psychologically, this behavior is doubly damaging. Not only is the food addict still indulging in the preferred junk items, but now he or she is also deceiving family and friends. Addicts become very uncomfortable when their preferred foods are not available. They begin manipulating people and situations to ensure access to their favorite items. Common patterns include the following:

- Eating "out of sight": in the bathroom, closet, car, or backyard
- Eating food secretly and stashing it in hard-to-find places
- Not eating at parties or dining out with others; only eating at home later
- Buying food supposedly for your spouse or kids when you really intend to eat it yourself

Excuses, exclusions, and exemptions mark food addiction. Addicts see food as the perennial pick-me-up and are prone to blaming their obsession on stressful life circumstances. Food is their main source of security although, in actuality, their dysfunctional food swings lead to fatigue, irritability, and depression. The clandestine behavior of food addicts—all that sneaking around—adversely impacts their personal relationships, too.

Roxy's Road

Roxy considered herself the life of the party. A friendly, caring, forty-five-year-old, she got a kick out of being the center of attention. And she was accustomed to having a man in her life. But when she met me for her first consultation, she was in the middle of some emotionally traumatic experiences. She had decided to end a seven-year relationship with her lover, Grant. She had previously been married, but the eighteen-year union ended in divorce. Her only child, Doug, was a senior in high school and living at home. Grant was still married to his second wife and had three children from his first marriage. Over the course of their relationship, Grant floated back and forth between Roxy and his wife. To me, the situation sounded like an emotional train wreck, but Roxy considered her relationship with Grant the closest thing to true love she had ever experienced. She and Grant could talk all night long, and he brought out in her a creative side she never knew she had.

Whenever Roxy was with Grant, she felt whole. Whenever he returned to his wife, she was devastated. After seven years of this wrenching pattern, and some intense soul-searching, she finally decided that they had no future. So she gave Grant an ultimatum, and he chose his wife.

Roxy was 5'10" and 240 pounds. She had gained twenty pounds just in the last two months over the course of ending her affair. She explained her habits to me with exasperation.

"Doctor Meltzer, I am addicted to food. I've tried every diet out there, and I can't take it anymore. I'm tired of playing the social butterfly. In my job as a bookkeeper, I have a lot of deadlines to meet. I'm not big on sweets, but I eat peanut butter and crackers all day long at work. I love rice and potatoes. Sometimes I can't stop eating them."

To counter Roxy's zealous overeating, I started her off with the LYF Cleansing diet and also recommended a daily exercise routine. Within the first week, I had expected Roxy to lose at least three and up to seven pounds. But when she returned for her second appointment, she'd gained seven pounds.

"Roxy," I mused, "on this diet, there is no way in the world you could have gained weight. What happened?"

"Well, Doctor Meltzer," she confessed, "food has always played a soothing role in my life, and this has been a particularly tough week for me. I've been hungry practically all day long. In fact, I've never felt so low. I have no strength. I tried to follow your diet during the day; but in the evening, when I'm lonely and depressed, I eat. On Tuesday, I 'spaghettied it' all night long. Then I felt too down to go to work the next day. I called in sick and stayed in bed until noon, with the shades drawn so that I wouldn't know how late it was."

"Eventually, the phone rang. It was Martha from the escrow company. I'd been planning to move into a new condominium with the money I was going to make from selling my house, but problems came up."

"The phone rang again. This time it was Grant. You know how it is when a relationship is over and you talk in its final stages. We ended up it an ugly argument. I slammed down the phone and started weeping like a baby. All I wanted was something to eat."

"So I conjured up the idea of spaghetti with onions and cheese sauce. Once I started eating it, I couldn't stop. My son came home from school late in the afternoon, and we decided to make it a pasta party. I ate everything in sight for a few days. I didn't get back on your cleansing diet until Friday."

Roxy's food addictions were ruining her life. I convinced her to study the RIEXA technique. It took her some time to stick to the program. Gradually, she began to identify the moods that triggered her binges, she addressed her emotional deficiencies, and she took alternative action.

I'm so proud of Roxy, and of the way she taught herself to deal with her frustrations without resorting to food, that I'm going to use her experience as an example of how to employ the RIEXA technique. What follows is practically a transcript of how Roxy and I worked through the steps. A caring friend or family member can play my role in the scene. But even if you play both parts, in the privacy of your own kitchen, it is a conversation you must learn to have with yourself. Rehearsing the RIEXA technique will improve your abilities to combat overeating.

The RIEXA Technique: "Roxy's Scene"

Dr. Meltzer: Roxy, I want you to take full responsibility for your eating habits. You know that food binges and indulgences are destroying your self-image, depleting your energy, increasing your weight, and putting you at risk for a heart attack. They're ruining your life. Are you prepared to take back control?

Roxy: I'm scared, but ready to be responsible.

Dr. Meltzer: It does require courage, but you have the power within you to change your eating habits.

Roxy: I truly want to tap into that power. I feel like I'm out of touch with it.

Dr. Meltzer: Be patient with yourself. It will take a little time, but if you dedicate yourself to abolishing your negative, harmful eating habits, your body will start telling you the difference between appetitis and hunger.

Roxy: Come what may, setbacks and all, I'm committed to the process.

R: Recognition

Dr. Meltzer: In your opinion, what are your food addictions?

Roxy: I recognize that I have a particular weakness for overeating dairy, starches, and carbs. I find all sorts of creamy, cheesy pastas—ravioli, spaghetti carbonara, manicotti, lasagna—comforting. I also love peanut butter and ice cream.

Dr. Meltzer: Good. Now you know what your refrigerator enemies are.

I: Identify

Dr. Meltzer: Is there a particular time when you feel most vulnerable to bingeing?

Roxy: I'm most vulnerable when I long for touch, comfort, and companionship. But it's especially bad when I come home from work and have to face another night alone.

Dr. Meltzer: How are you feeling when you are bingeing?

Roxy: Usually, I feel depressed and uptight, tired and lonely.

EX: Express and Experience

Dr. Meltzer: Tell me, what do you think it is that may make you feel this way?

Roxy: My seven-year relationship is over—he was married, and the whole thing was one long disaster. I mean, he brought out a lot of my good qualities; but at the same time, the fact that he wouldn't leave his wife was ... eating away at me. Literally, I guess! And the sale of my house is in limbo, which is completely screwing up my bank accounts. And, the tuition for my son's first semester of college is due.

Dr. Meltzer: I'm listening.

Roxy: I guess I just feel overwhelmed by all these responsibilities. I feel like I'm drowning. I can't keep on top of the bills, and I'm a total failure at relationships. Sometimes I wonder if I've ever done anything right in my life.

Dr. Meltzer: It must be very painful, but let yourself heal through feeling love for yourself. You can come to your own emotional rescue. Ask yourself what you can do or what it will take to make yourself feel better. I suggest applying the RIEXA technique as the first step to your recovery. Furthermore, your relationship with spirit and feeding your soul, feeding your heart, and feeding your mind will cure you. Unlike physical wounds, which heal with time, emotional wounds do not heal by themselves. It takes work. Allow yourself to experience your pain by crying, shouting, singing, or exercising. Let it out. Work it through. Ride the tumultuous wave. Write it down. Talk to a trusted friend. Do whatever it takes. Just don't eat.

Roxy: I'm working on it.

A: Action

Dr. Meltzer: What's your alternative to indulging in food?

Roxy: I have to catch myself when I'm on the brink of a binge. To blow off steam, I've been jogging. I'll even stop and do ten sit-ups just to regain my focus.

Dr. Meltzer: That's a great start. It also helps to take a nutritional timeout and meditate when you feel you're about to lose it emotionally. Find your center, open up your soul, and get in touch with positive vibrations.

Roxy: Sometimes I can do that. It depends where I am, if I can find a peaceful spot.

Dr. Meltzer: Even if you're stuck at your desk at work, summon up a happy memory. And if you're not able to truly meditate, end the moment with some creative visualization. Can you do that?

Roxy: Yes. I love to look for pretty shells in the sand; so if I can't actually get out and go to the beach, then I imagine it. It always makes me feel better.

Dr. Meltzer: Finally, you can also turn to liquid nutrition in the form of super-nutrients and herbal tea to curb your desire for food and alleviate your appetite.

Practice Makes Perfect

Rehearse this exercise with yourself until you have mastered the RIEXA technique. Put yourself in the role of both doctor and patient. Of course, when you play the part of Roxy, add your own dialogue and information that's true to your particular situation. Use the cues as a way to analyze your most recent food fiasco. Relive the experience and your emotions at the time and give yourself a distinct plan of action. The next time you're confronted with similar circumstances, you'll be better prepared to deal with them constructively.

Be vigilant. Depending on the degree of your food dependency, you may have to go through this self-inquisition five times an hour—some days more, some days less. Stick with it. Pay attention to whatever's missing in your life and acknowledge that your bingeing is just a form of compensation.

Roxy became a student of the RIEXA technique. She was able to put her life in a new, positive perspective. Roxy successfully lost all of the weight she set out to lose. You can do it too!

Dysfunctional Food Swing #3: Cravings

Specific cravings can dominate your mind. The first step on the road to recovery is to realize that whatever it is you crave, it's almost guaranteed not to be good for you. It doesn't take a rocket scientist to figure out that buffalo wings are loaded with salt and fat. And ironically, oftentimes the foods that you crave are the ones that you are allergic to.

Just as there's a difference between hunger and appetite, and a difference between a healthy attitude and a hazardous obsession toward diet, so, too, is there a difference between food preferences and food cravings. You can prefer certain items over others, but there's a range of flexibility to your choices—and you maintain control. When you crave food, however, the intensity of your appetitis overwhelms everything else, and you cannot rest until you feed the beast within. You have to have that candy bar right now. Until you do, you can't think, talk, work, sleep, whatever.

Food cravings are frequently caused by emotional and physical imbalances. For example, a craving for candy usually belies low blood-sugar levels or candidiasis. I've also observed that adrenal burnout, liver stress, and diabetes also spark cravings. Check out the following trigger foods to see if any of these examples sound familiar.

- **Bread:** common for those carboholics in need of hugs, physical comfort, and emotional support; a food staple that offers emotional security.
- **Chocolate:** panacea of the love- and sex-starved; PEA (phenylethylamine), present in chocolate, seems to promote a sense of relaxation and well-being; the effect it produces is similar to the feeling of being in love.
- **Crunchy Foods:** an outlet for anger and frustrations.
- **Salt:** counters feelings of depression by stimulating the system.
- **Sweets:** a substitute for affection and a stress-reliever.
- **Meat:** more common in men; indicates a lust for power; a classic Daddy food, associated with male authority.
- **Milk or Cheese:** more common in women, especially those hungry for a deeper emotional connection with Mommy; milk, cheese, and ice cream are common crutches during such female hormonal states as PMS, pregnancy, and menopause.

One of the tricky characteristics of cravings is they often trigger additional food dysfunction. In other words, cravings not only answer to emotional hunger, but they often precipitate—or trigger—compulsive overeating and all the other dysfunctional food swings. It is common that once you indulge, you want more. That's why it's so important to use the RIEXA technique to recognize your trigger foods and identify the feelings that accompany them. Next time you crave sugar, bread, cheese, or whatever your particular crutch is, be certain to go through your RIEXA technique. Recognize, Identify, Express and Experience, and finally, take Action. It takes willpower and emotional self-determination, but the RIEXA technique is the cure for food cravings.

Dysfunctional Food Swing #4: Snacking and Nibbling

Snacking is about nervous, hurried, compulsive eating. Weak, stressed, and tense nerves like to snack. People who are bored also like to snack. Snacking can become a crutch and is often seen as an emotional reward system. In fact, snacking and nibbling are so commonplace that we hardly even recognize them as nervous habits. How could anyone be expected to enjoy the Super Bowl without a buffet full of finger foods? But incessant snacking is a blatant way of releasing nervous energy. Almost everything we snack on is ready-made—just open the bag or flip the lid, reach in, grab a handful, and pop the microwaved food into your mouth. Snacking is the dysfunctional food swing that most exploits the hand-to-mouth reflex and, by extension, what Freud would call our oral fixation. We revert to an infantile stage, and find comfort by replicating an act that reminds us of breast-feeding. The problem is, we're all supposed to be grown-ups.

Whether it's hors d'oeuvres at a wedding reception or hot dogs at the ballpark, snacking is unavoidable in the average American lifestyle. To begin the process of change, start with moderation: decide before an event that you will not eat more than x-number of nachos and then stick to your limit. Try to substitute salty and fatty snacks with healthier counterparts—fruits and vegetables. As for the dysfunctional extreme of snacking—the compulsive, semiconscious nibbling that takes place all day long, at home or in the office, in the car or in front of the TV—well, that's a dead-end food habit. Unless you suffer from diabetes or hypoglycemia and have been prescribed a schedule of snacks to regulate your sugar levels, snacking serves only adverse purposes in your diet.

Compulsive snackers are just as out of touch with their emotions as over-eaters and bingers. The difference is that, instead of gorging themselves, they just nibble, nibble, nibble all day long in order to quiet the anxiety within. But grazing is not good for you. You are not a cow. You are a human being, and constant eating imbalances your metabolism. Snacking confuses your natural hunger mechanisms. Your body never has time to engage the full digestive cycle, because it's always receiving new deliveries into the stomach.

After the initial high of the snack attack subsides, you feel tired. Snacking promotes weight gain: the most common snack foods are high in fat—cookies, potato chips, candy bars, etc.—and snackers overeat these items.

If you are a compulsive snacker, refer back to Roxy's Scene on pages 303-306. Put yourself in the role of Roxy, but apply the dialogue to your snacking and nibbling between meals. The RIEXA technique can combat snacking's misguided emotional reward system by helping you figure out what drives you to indulge. Finally, the RIEXA technique will help you find a healthy alternative to this obsessive behavior.

Dysfunctional Food Swing #5: Food-on-the-Brain Syndrome

All of the dysfunctional food swings I've discussed so far—overeating, addiction, cravings, and snacking—are characterized by food-on-the-brain syndrome. Those afflicted are fixated by thoughts of shopping for, preparing, and consuming food. They are over-attached to their diets. They use food as an emotional crutch. Life revolves around eating. They go to bed at night thinking about what they'll eat in the morning. During breakfast, they're planning lunch; at lunch, they're planning dinner. In the middle of other activities—even exercise—their thoughts wander to food.

Do you spend more time thinking about food than about how to improve your relationship with your spouse, how to be more creative at work, or how to accomplish long-term goals? Does your appetitis take precedence over your family life, your relationships, your intellectual growth, or your emotional stability? The ideal mind-set is one in which, when you eat, you fully enjoy the meal; and when the meal is over, you do not think about food again until the next scheduled mealtime.

Morning, Noon, and Nina

My patient Nina had an interesting, though not uncommon, strain of food-on-the-brain syndrome. A forty-year-old, overweight homemaker, she took pride in her highly nutritious food selection, but complained, "Doctor, I am hungry all day. I'm thinking about food from the moment I wake up each morning."

I instructed Nina to write down everything she ate for one full week and to include the time and location of her meals. I also asked her to make note of how hungry she felt each time, what her mood was, and what she was doing. Even though her mealtime food selection was quite healthy, she snacked on cold cuts, cheese sandwiches, or chips and dips throughout the day.

Nina had food on the brain. Nina obsessed about eating all of the time. I introduced her to the RIEXA technique. She found action steps that fed her mind, fed her heart, and fed her soul. She overcame food on the brain and lost her excess weight.

Dysfunctional Food Swing #6: Late-Night Indulgences

It's the end of another day. You've worked hard; weathered the usual ups and downs. You're tired of the red tape, the rules and regulations, the convoluted bureaucracy of contemporary living. At last, you're home, safe for the night behind locked doors. You can finally let down your guard and indulge.

Some people are completely in control during the day, but then eat from the moment they get home from work until they go to bed. The usual suspects—ice cream, cookies, chocolate, pizza, beer—are popular with late-night indulgers, who often suffer from boredom or sexual frustration. The late-night indulger rewards him- or herself at the end of the day. Like all other dysfunctional food swings, late-night indulgence is a mood-altering behavior. Applying the RIEXA technique will reveal that the late-night eater most likely lacks emotional support and comfort. He or she may carry the burden of responsibility for the rest of the family and be the person everyone else relies on. Meanwhile, he or she relies on food.

If you're a late-night food addict, give yourself a break. When you find yourself on the brink of bingeing, take a deep breath and ask yourself, "What's really missing in my life?" Recognize that food is acting as a dysfunctional substitute for other flawed or nonexistent relationships.

In terms of the action step of the RIEXA technique, creative self-expression is often the key to curing late-night food indulgences. Frequently, people don't want to be bothered putting the effort into an after-work activity. They complain that they're tired, and would rather watch television than, for example, take a yoga class, play the guitar, or study African dance. But creative expression can be very stimulating. It has many benefits—you learn something new, you meet new people, you get away from food, and you show self-respect by treating yourself to something positive. If you're married or in a relationship, a shared interest can bring you and your partner closer together. Think about it. You deserve something better to look forward to than food. The RIEXA technique can be relied on to remedy late-night indulging.

Dysfunctional Food Swing #7: Compulsive Bingeing

Extensive food indulgence is the landmark of food addictions. Compulsive bingeing is an extension of food addiction. This eating disorder is especially common among young women, who may get caught up and trapped in the cycles of bingeing and purging that characterize bulimia. Compulsive bingeing and purging can cause serious damage to the kidneys and digestive system, and depletes the body of real nutrients and valued electrolytes. Bulimics get hooked on the notion that they can eat as much of whatever they want without gaining weight. They reason that, after they've enjoyed the taste of the food, they throw it up. As with other dysfunctional food swings, compulsive bingeing is dictated by obsessive-compulsive behavior. At first, it allows the addict to feel in charge, but soon he or she becomes a victim of the syndrome, torn between a preoccupation with food and a desperate desire to stay thin. People in the grips of the condition describe their lives as chaotic. They rationalize that food intake is the only thing they can control when, in fact, their eating habits are as out of control as everything else.

Vomiting or using diuretics or cathartics only worsens the food addiction. It tricks the body into thinking that it's starving—which, in a way, it is, for true nourishment. The more a binger vomits, the more food the body tries to accommodate the next time around, in a futile attempt to retain nutrients before they are regurgitated.

If you are bulimic or a compulsive binger, I recommend that you first seek some counseling in order to understand your own specific control issues and the ways in which you apply them to food. Professional support systems are needed to untangle the psychological roots of the disorder; then, the RIEXA technique can be used to change this behavior.

Dysfunctional Food Swing #8: Poor Food Choices

I include this dysfunctional food swing to remind you of the importance of Smart Foods and the Golden Rules of Smart Eating.

Junk foods, mood foods, and stress foods make you feel heavy—physically and mentally. They dampen your mood and wrap you up in negative routines, such as the sugar cycle. Once you indulge in a poor food choice, it sets a pattern in motion that becomes much harder to break than if you'd never started. Think of the hamster on the wheel, running to stand still.

Fresh, whole, living, Smart Food enriches body and soul. Move forward with the help of the RIEXA technique. Transform your poor food choices into smart ones. It will serve you well.

Part III

The Inner Strengths of Permanent Weight Loss

21

Introduction to Inner Strengths of Permanent Weight Loss

I have coached, counseled, and guided thousands down the path of permanent weight loss. I have been witness to dramatic success stories and devastating failures. So what have I figured out? People need a simple and reliable system to count on. The LYF Program is this system. As you know, the LYF Program is composed of three necessary pillars that support permanent weight loss.

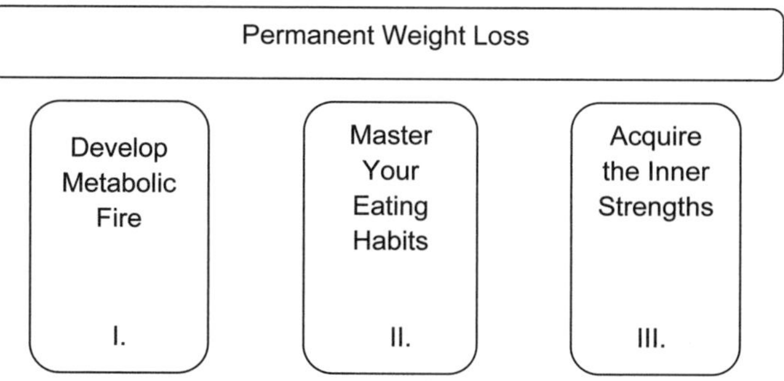

All three parts work together. Establishing Metabolic Fire and Mastering Your Eating Habits, parts I and II, are the nuts and bolts of the program. In combination, these first two pillars to permanent weight loss are incredibly powerful and effective. Even still, there is a third support system to the bridge of permanent weight loss (PWL) that is a must. It will fortify and give lasting power to your PWL plan. Let me explain.

Over the years, I have observed that there are a variety of personality, emotional, and social factors that influence one's ability to achieve permanent weight loss. Yet, there is one interesting feature common to all individuals who are successful in their conquest over the battle of the bulge. What might that be? There is an inner strength that is the source of their long-term success. They have the inner strength to stick to the program and turn their approach to PWL into a lifestyle.

You see, there is an important inner journey to achieving PWL. This journey is guided by your inner strengths. In this section of the book I will teach you how to develop and apply these inner strengths. These inner strengths will help you cultivate the intrapersonal support systems that you can rely on to achieve and maintain your weight-loss goals. With these support systems in place, you'll have the consistency you need to achieve PWL. My patients that have been able to develop Metabolic Fire, master their eating habits, and acquire the essential inner strengths, have lost their excess weight and have never looked back.

Awaken the Power Within!

Keep in mind, there is an important relationship that governs PWL strategies. It is the most important relationship in your life. It is the relationship you have with yourself! You see, success does not come from the outside. The seeds of successful weight management are within you. There is an inner strength to most all achievements, and make no mistake about it— the ability to maintain your weight at healthy levels is an achievement. It is the same kind of inner strength that empowers professional athletes, corporate executives, as well as those successful at school or at work. Yes, folks who successfully lose weight and keep it off have an inner strength that permeates their being and guides their lifestyle choices.

Inner Strengths: The Antidote to Temptation

Life presents many challenges. There can be clusters of distractions, obstacles, and hurdles that can derail your weight-loss progress. That is why it is so important to have inner strength. The path to PWL can be elusive. How will your PWL plan hold up in the face of temptation, restlessness, and fatigue? You will need inner strengths. How will your eating habits fare when anxiety, moodiness, and frustration show up? You will need inner strengths. There are three key inner strengths.

The Three Inner Strengths of Permanent Weight Loss
• Mind Power
• Soul Power
• Mood Power

Your inner strengths will help you overcome the temptations and distractions of everyday life that can ruin your weight-loss plan. How so? They will give you the staying power to follow the Golden Rules. Equally important, however, is that the inner strengths are a form of preventive medicine. They will target the root cause of restlessness, temptation, and distraction, and nip them in the bud before they have a chance to flare up.

Hold Your Own: Your Inner Strengths Give You Holding Power

Your inner strengths give you the holding power to stay trim in a changing and unpredictable world. The stronger your inner strengths, the easier it will be to lose and maintain your weight. I often come across people who have lost weight, yet food and weight gain continue to be on their mind and dominate their thoughts. Sadly, their *waist* management will always feel like a lifelong struggle without developing their inner strengths. For the great majority of them, they are destined to gain back their weight. What's my point? It's simple. PWL is a hard path to forge without paying attention to your inner strengths. A lack of inner strength invites metabolic dysfunction and leads to weight-loss failure. Alternatively, when you acquire the inner strengths of permanent weight loss, weight management will be an effortless process that will no longer consume your thinking. How do you go about building your inner strengths? You learn how to *feed your mind, feed your heart,* and *feed your soul!*

Feed Your Mind, Feed Your Heart, Feed Your Soul

When you break it down to its roots, your inners strengths fall into three main categories:

I. Feed Your Mind: Develop Mind Power

II. Feed Your Soul: Develop Soul Power

III. Feed Your Heart: Develop Mood Power

Your inner strengths are defined by how well you feed your mind, feed your heart, and feed your soul. As you develop your mind power, mood power, and soul power, an amazing transformation takes place. You see, as you learn how to feed your mind, heart, and soul, you gain a new perspective on your appetite. Nurturing your mind, heart, and soul feeds your appetite for life. As you feed your appetite for life, your emotional hunger for food will lessen, and you will be less inclined to turn to food for fulfillment.

Your inner strengths endow you with purposefulness, happiness, conviction, self-control, inner peace, and inner joy. Furthermore, the greater your inner strengths, the less restlessness, the less EMT, the less attachment you will have to food and the better lifestyle choices you can make. You have already incorporated some of the major concepts of feed your mind, feed your heart, and feed your soul. They are the backbone and foundation to your pre-meal approach in the Golden Rules of Smart Eating. Now, it is time to understand the power of these tools in greater detail and to give you a more fulsome arsenal to further develop your inner strengths of permanent weight loss.

Your mind power, soul power, and mood power are your fundamental inner strengths. In time, these strengths turn into vital inner skills to the devotee of PWL. Be certain to refine and hone these skills over your lifetime. Get better at them every day. With repetition and practice, these skills turn into the habits that will keep you looking your best and feeling your best. Let's take a closer look at these vital skills.

I. Feed Your Mind—Develop Mind Power

a. Cultivate Dynamic Willpower and Won't Power

b. Develop the Three D's of Self-Control

c. Build Self-Confidence and Positive Belief Systems

II. Feed Your Soul—Develop Soul Power

a. How to Nourish Your Soul: The Art of Spiritual Nutrition

b. How to Create the Triangle of Divine Fire

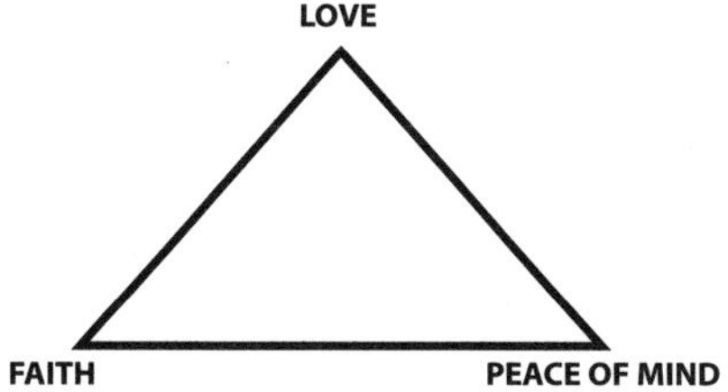

c. Define Your Purpose in Life

III. Feed Your Heart—Develop Mood Power

a. Develop Emotional Self-Awareness

b. Acquire the Habits of Happiness

c. Acquire the Mood Power to Sustain a Good Mood

22

Feed Your Mind—Develop Mind Power

YOUR mind has the power to influence your weight-loss program. The fact is, mind power can trigger the vision and ignite the necessary actions to win the battle of the bulge. Write this down. *Mind power is a must for permanent weight loss.* Let me tell you why.

Mind power is about developing a strong mind. It is about the strength of your thoughts and the power of your thinking. A strong mind is dominated by positive, clear, and calm thinking. The level of your mind power is determined by your ability to keep your thinking positive. These positive thoughts can breathe new life into your PWL plan.

A strong mind has the ability to manifest your thoughts and intentions. You think big, and then big happens! You get what you pray for. Your visions and your dreams turn into your lifestyle. This is the essence of mind power. It is something that everyone can attain. In fact, there is a science to achieving mind power.

The key is to make mind power a way of life, a lifetime habit just as success and winning are habits. Positive mind-powered thinking keeps your PWL program going well. Mind power gives you the tools to adhere to the Golden Rules of Smart Eating. In essence, mind power can be broken down into the following three LYF-Skills and inner strengths:

THE THREE STEPS TO ACHIEVING MIND POWER
• LYF-Skill #1—Cultivate Dynamic Willpower and Won't Power
• LYF-Skill #2—Develop the Three D's of Self-Control
• LYF-Skill #3—Build Self-Confidence and Positive Belief Systems

Mind power gives you the ability to focus on your weight-loss goals and develop the right belief systems to make them happen.

LYF-Skill #1—Cultivate Dynamic Willpower and Won't Power

Your willpower is the foundation to the strength of your mind. Your willpower and your eating habits have a hand-to-glove relationship. In fact, your willpower is the gatekeeper to your eating habits. As we've discussed, overeating and poor food selection will undermine your PWL plan. Your willpower can say yes to what's in and no to what's out. It takes a strong will and a clear mind to keep your eating habits in check. On the other hand, it is easy to check out and indulge your appetite, overeat to satisfy your palate, succumb to recreational eating, or take a break from your daily workout. A strong will follows through whereas a weak will is likely to give in when the going gets tough. Your willpower lays the foundation to mind power and PWL. And, *yes, yes, yes* you can *will* your way to wellness. A strong will empowers you to choose and control your everyday eating and living habits

Dynamic Willpower Is the Crucial Link

Your willpower is the intention of your thinking and the driving force behind your desires. Strengthening your willpower gives you the focus to carry out the highest intentions of your ambitions to achieve, sustain, and maintain PWL. In fact, you can measure your willpower by the degree of your intention. Let's take a look at the different levels of desire that underlie and define the strength of your will.

- **Wishes, Hopes, and Desires**—Wishes, hopes, and desires are mild intentions of thinking that are easily deterred and are backed by little or no attempt to manifest themselves.

- **An Intention**—An intention is a stronger desire or determination. Intentions have a higher yield. An intention is more likely to manifest itself.
- **Dynamic Willpower**—Dynamic willpower is a conviction. It is an expansion of your intentions. When you can exercise unyielding determination, around a specific intention, and manifest your desired result, you own dynamic willpower.

Dynamic willpower is a forceful and energetic willpower. Dynamic willpower abounds with kinetic energy; it makes things happen. Dynamic willpower has the ability to make what you most think about come to fruition. Your thinking tells you that it makes good sense to sport a fit and trim body. Your dynamic willpower is that very power that converts what you are thinking into reality.

Just how strong is your will? When you make up your mind to lose weight, does this mission get accomplished? Did you know that you can lose weight permanently when you use dynamic will to follow through? Dynamic will means that you keep on trying and trying no matter what the circumstances. Dynamic will is tenacious and penetrating and does not take no for an answer. When you continually exercise your dynamic willpower, you are in the most favorable posture to eat Smart Foods and master your eating habits.

Size Up Your Intentions

Dynamic willpower gives you the strength to manifest your vision of a toned, fit, and attractive body. Don't you want to look younger, sexier, and in shape? Just ask yourself how badly you want to achieve PWL. Don't make it a wish. Don't make it a hope. Don't make it a desire. Make it a dynamic volition, a dynamic willpower, that you can manifest the desired result.

I want you to take a short timeout. Be honest with yourself. Take a quiet moment and ask yourself:

- How much do you really want to lose your excess weight?

- Just how willing are you to make some changes?
- Do you have the will to have a trim and toned physique?
- Do you have the willpower to sustain a healthy metabolic rate that burns fat instead of storing it?
- Do you have the will to uphold your quest for the healthiest of eating habits?
- Do you make up your mind or tell loved ones that you are going to lose weight in the New Year, or after your birthday, only to fall back to old patterns and habits?
- Do you have the will to follow through on your LYF Program and achieve your ideal weight?

Before we move on, let me summarize the important features of willpower.

- Your willpower is the backbone to your mind power.
- Dynamic willpower is the vibratory power of your mind to purposefully control your behavior, your eating habits, your living habits, and your actions.
- Your willpower is a necessary link between your mind and your metabolic performance.
- Your willpower is the vehicle to manifest your intentions.

What is my goal for you here? I want you to use your willpower to develop the habit of successful weight control.

Your Willpower Can Make the Impossible Possible

I've seen it thousands of times. There comes a point, where anyone looking to lose weight has to put his or her foot down and say, "The time has come for my life to take a new direction." A clear-cut system and course of action are necessary to implement proper eating and living habits. With dynamic willpower, you can make choices, set goals, and take deliberate actions to achieve PWL in spite of opposition, difficulty, or adversity. Your willpower can guide you to maneuver through the thick and thin, the challenges, and the ups and downs of your everyday lifestyle. Your willpower can make something out of nothing, opportunity out of casual encounters.

Willpower Breeds Won't Power

Dynamic willpower can whip you into shape. When you fail to lose weight effectively, it usually suggests that your will needs to be stronger. When you find your willpower to be passive, tired, or insufficiently focused, it is common to:

- Make poor food selections
- Develop hazardous eating habits

The beauty about willpower is it fuels *won't power*. You see, a strong willpower and a strong won't power go hand in hand. If you have a dynamic willpower, sure enough, you will also have dynamic won't power. Your won't power is crucial to achieving and sustaining long-term weight control. It is a necessary link between your mind and the performance of your eating habits. You have to take a stand on what you won't eat anymore. You will have to say NO to what is self-defeating. You will have to say YES to what is self empowering. Take a look and practice affirming some of the wills and won'ts that characterize your willpower and won't power.

Willpower	Won't Power
• I will select Smart Foods. • I will follow the Golden Rules. • I will exercise my willpower through daily meditation. • I will exercise regularly.	• I won't indulge in overeating. • I won't develop self-defeating eating habits. • I won't eat the wrong foods. • I won't succumb to cravings and late-night indulgences.

Your Willpower Is a Spiritual and Mental Muscle

You can say that your willpower is a sign of your mental toughness. In fact, your willpower is a critical spiritual and mental muscle for your mind power.

I find it interesting that your mental and spiritual muscles respond like your physical muscles. When you do the bench press at the gym, you are exercising your chest muscles. The more you bench-press, the stronger your chest muscles become. Similarly, the more you utilize and exercise your willpower, the stronger your willpower becomes. When you exercise this spiritual and mental muscle regularly, you gain the know-how and the skills to put your mind power into action. Where there is a will, there is a way to get the job done well.

Take the Initiative: Exercise Your Will

You, and only you, can make the decision to have superior weight control. You can cultivate dynamic willpower. Your dynamic willpower can see to it that your desire for being at the right weight comes to fruition. Follow the action steps below to fortify your will. With the appropriate exercise, you can turn your will into the spiritual warrior called dynamic willpower.

Time for Action

Your action steps are going to be both tactical and technical in nature. Let's start with the tactical approach, and then we will incorporate the technical exercises to strengthen your will. The tactical approach will help you maneuver your thinking and facilitate the cultivation of dynamic willpower. In other words, the tactics below will sculpt the necessary mind-set you need to foster dynamic willpower.

Tactical Approach #1— Make the Commitment to Dynamic Willpower

Making the mental commitment is necessary to accomplish any goal. Make the pledge today to build dynamic willpower. In doing so, your commitment will enrich your dynamic will.

Tactical Approach #2— Believe in the Miracle of Your Willpower

You need to believe to achieve. Believing in your willpower is the same as emotionally feeding your willpower. It gives your willpower the energy it needs. Indeed, believing in the magical powers of dynamic willpower is sound emotional nutrition. It gives you heartfelt willpower—the most important kind. Your belief in your heartfelt willpower makes your willpower experiential and not just intellectual.

Believe in the magnetic vibration of sustained willpower. This will energize your will. When you energize your will and then learn to concentrate your will, your willpower is converted into dynamic willpower. When you embellish and amplify your thinking on losing weight, your will can become dynamic enough to manifest the desired result.

Tactical Approach #3—Perseverance Furthers: There Is No Such Thing as Defeat

Tell yourself that you will never give up. If tomorrow you binge on ice cream, do not let it get you down. Keep your resolve to move forward and lose weight. Perseverance, stick-to-it-ness, and enthusiasm refresh and recharge your willpower.

Dealing constructively with previous or present failures to lose weight and keep it off builds dynamic will. Learning from your past performances and actions can strengthen your resolve. Dynamic will means that you keep on striving and feel undefeated within, no matter what happens. In other words, do not lose heart and become discouraged by previous results. It is dynamic willpower that gives you the personal power to be rich in health and lose weight permanently. When you refuse to accept failure and when you don't let a dietary indiscretion get you down, your shedding of unwanted pounds is likely to take place.

Tactical Approach #4—Make PWL a Conviction

You want to make PWL a conviction, a principle of yours. Turning your desire to lose weight into a conviction helps your willpower. When you stand by your principles, you naturally and instinctively nourish your willpower. The magnetism of your conviction energizes your will. Developing conviction strengthens your will. So does standing up for your convictions. When you can hold your conviction against all odds and under the toughest and most adverse of circumstances, it will fortify your dynamic will.

Now that you have the right mental mind-set, let's give you some technical action tips for you to exercise your will.

Action Tip #1—Concentrate Your Mind: Concentration is Key to Dynamic Willpower

Concentrating your will creates favorable results. Your will has a vibration, a wave length, a frequency. Its intensity can crescendo and work for you to get your desired results. You may think to yourself that you intend to lose weight. But do you have the will to follow through? A lack of focus is a common root cause of failure to lose weight for the long term.

There is something you need to know. It's important to connect the dots. You need to know the relationship between your mind, your mind power, and the effects of concentration on your thinking. Your concentration skills act like a magnifying glass. On a sunny day, if you hold a magnifying glass above a newspaper, the newspaper catches fire. As you intensify your concentration skills, you amplify and increase your dynamic will. To successfully lose weight for the long term, it pays huge dividends to pause at regular intervals and take a few minutes to concentrate your thinking on fitness and your intention to lose weight. It works best, that is, you get the best results, when you follow your LYF Plan with superior concentration.

Pay Attention to What is Important to You

When you pay attention to your garden, your plants, flowers, and vegetables do well. When you pay attention to your family or spouse, your primary relationships improve. Pay attention to what it takes to lose weight permanently and you will. You need to concentrate on your courage and perseverance to achieve your weight-loss goals. You can enrich your concentration skills every day in your nutritional timeouts, your daily meditation, or silent prayer time. As your concentration skills improve, so will your willpower and mind power.

Concentrate Your Mind and Fortify Your Will through Meditation

There is a way to exercise your mind and get your willpower into shape. It's called meditation. In fact, in-depth concentration while meditating is one of the most efficient ways to cultivate dynamic willpower. It is of crucial importance to concentrate your will to increase the strength of your will. Ideally, daily focused meditation for fifteen to twenty minutes, preferably before breakfast and again before dinner, helps fortify your willpower. At a minimum, your three-minute drills during your nutritional timeouts are also designed to strengthen your willpower.

When you concentrate your will, it persists; it gives you the competitive edge to stick to your Smart Food plan. Make up your mind to develop dynamic willpower. Make sure to meditate every day in order to exercise, cultivate, concentrate, and magnify your willpower. Once you have read through the action steps on mind power, refer to pages 378-381 for our preferred technique for meditation.

Action Tip #2: Affirmations Strengthen Your Willpower

Affirmations are statements that reflect strong, positive convictions, beliefs, and feelings. Affirmations can be used to develop and strengthen your willpower. Positive declarations and assertions that you say to yourself quietly, over and over again, build dynamic willpower. You can affirm from your mind, or you can whisper your affirmations from your heart. You already have been introduced to affirmations in your three-minute drill during your nutritional timeout. Affirmations are also an integral part to meditation. Practice the following affirmations to strengthen your will. Start by incorporating these affirmations into your nutritional timeouts and daily meditations. Additionally, whenever you have a few moments, practice them throughout the day; for example, you can practice them while you wait in line at the store, while you wait for a friend to return a call, or while you wait at a stoplight.

SAMPLE AFFIRMATIONS
• I need to lose weight permanently. (3x) • I must lose weight permanently. (3x) • I will lose weight permanently. (3x) *** Note: Say the first affirmation three times. Then move on to the next affirmation and say it three times. Finally, say the last affirmation three times. This will complete one full cycle. Keep your concentration and try to say these affirmations in cycles of seven.

The ABE Technique Works!

Let me expand upon the affirmation drill I just provided. One of the most effective ways to incorporate affirmations is to turn to the ABE technique. ABE stands for Affirm, Believe, and Expect.

- **ABE = Affirm + Believe + Expect**

When you follow up on your affirmations with believing in them and expecting your assertions to come to fruition, you are implementing the ABE technique. This ABE technique will amplify your will like a magnifying glass amplifies the size of fine print. Apply the drill outlined below and become familiar with the ABE technique. You can use the ABE technique not only for PWL, but for any conviction that you own or want to manifest.

SAMPLE ABE TECHNIQUE
• I must lose weight permanently. (3x) • I believe I will lose weight permanently. (3x) • I expect to lose weight permanently. (3x) *** Note: Say the first affirmation three times. Then move to the next affirmation and say it three times. Finally, say the last affirmation three times. This will complete one full cycle. Keep your concentration and try to say these affirmations in cycles of seven.

I've noted that I would like you to attempt your affirmation and ABE drills in cycles of seven. The trick is to start slowly. If you can make it through one cycle with full concentration, you are beginning to develop significant mind power. Keep building up your concentration until you can do seven full cycles. When you are able to reach seven cycles, you will have improved your mind power and increased your conviction exponentially.

Action Tip #3: Your Imagination Has the Ability to Expand Your Will

Your imagination can favorably influence your willpower. The faculty of creating a new self-image at your ideal weight comes into play here. A positive self-image invites PWL. A negative self-image invites weight-loss failure. Achieving PWL calls for a new body image—one that is fit and trim. This can be achieved through visualization, or what I like to call picture power. Visualizing yourself at your desired weight is a powerful way of believing it will happen.

Picture Power: The AVE Technique

The AVE technique stands for Affirm, Visualize, and Expect.

AVE = Affirm + Visualize + Expect

Incorporate the AVE technique into your affirmation drills. Here is what makes your imagination so important. Use your imagination to visualize, detail-by-detail, exactly how you would like to look. In other words, form a mental image, a picture, of your ideal weight and shape. If you can't visualize yourself at your ideal weight, it suggests that you don't fully believe that you can get there. Remember. Seeing is believing.

AVE TECHNIQUE
• Step 1—Affirm – I must lose weight permanently. (3x) • Step 2—Visualize – Visualize, detail-by-detail, your ideal weight and shape. • Step 3—Expect – Intensify your visualization and expect it to take place. Try to experience what it will feel like when you achieve your ideal weight. Make this drill experiential and not just a mental exercise.

Additional Action Tips

Your willpower thrives on anything that builds your self-confidence and determination. Here are some additional action tips that will favorably influence your will.

Creative Self-Expression Counts	• Creativity in your self-expression can build dynamic willpower. When you creatively find solutions to your problems, it also builds dynamic willpower. Tap into your intuition and let your creativity flow. Your creativity will energize your willpower and give it more clout.
Accomplishment Builds Willpower	• Choose something that you want to accomplish and then try with all your might to achieve it. Once you are successful, move on to a more difficult task or achievement; keep building your will to succeed.
Keep to Your Word	• Whatever you say, have the will and integrity to follow through. This builds your will.

Be Decisive, Do Not Procrastinate	• Make a list of things to do that need to get done. Take the list and do something today that you have been putting off for a long time. It can be as simple as returning a phone call, sending an e-mail, or mailing a birthday card. Don't procrastinate. Do one every day and watch your willpower grow.

Now then, make dynamic willpower a way of life.

LYF-Skill #2—Develop the Three D's of Self-Control

Self-control is a vital, indispensable link to PWL. Self-control gives you the authority to take charge of your thinking, hold your impulses in check, and exercise control over your eating habits. In essence, self-control is the inner strength that takes command of your thinking patterns and, by extension, your eating and living patterns. In this manner, self-control gives you the power to effectively maintain and sustain smart eating habits.

Self-control is built on the foundation of a strong, dynamic willpower. It means saying no to detrimental impulses. I find it interesting that self-control recruits being calm and collected and enables you to be the master of making choices that are in your best interest. It has made me realize that nutritional self-control is born out of an inner calmness that governs your connection, attraction, or attachment to food.

You see, self control is the ability to govern the direction of your thoughts and thereby your actions. I have shared this secret of effective cognitive behavior therapy before. It is important for you to keep in mind that your thoughts precede your actions. In fact, your thoughts can modify or regulate your actions. You may be lured into the flavor of a grilled hamburger with cheese and bacon swarming over the sides, yet your self-control can step up and say no. You decide to pass. That is why mind power can take control of your eating patterns.

Self-Control Gives You the Power to Outfox Your Temptations

Temptations can be seductive and recruit the pleasures of your senses. Temptation is a sugar-coated distraction. It looks delicious, tastes great, and is mouth-watering to your palate. Keep in mind that your most delectable temptations may appear to offer amazing pleasures, but indulging in them often leads to fatigue, indigestion, or restlessness. When asked about his favorite foods, Oliver Wendell Holmes was noted for saying he could resist everything but temptation. Do not equate resisting temptation as a denial of all pleasures. It simply means that you recognize and realize that what pleases your taste buds may not be good for your metabolism, health, and weight management.

It might be harmful to your liver, pancreas, and nervous system. Your senses may try to entrap you. Temptations may be strong and appealing, but you are stronger than they are.

Through our senses, we learn to enjoy foods that are pleasing to our taste, smell, and touch. There are times that certain desserts or favorite dips or sauces look so good. The desire to reward ourselves with a particular feel good sensation can easily become a habit. The taste of alluring, forbidden foods may be sweet—but in the end, not so sweet at all. Once you have established an emotional bond or attachment to your favorite mood foods, the habit of self-indulgence can overpower you. You tell yourself that you are not going to binge on pasta and pizza this weekend; but by the end of the weekend, you do anyhow. Your ability to manage your temptations may very well tell the story of a success or failure with your LYF Program. It is common to be a victim of your pleasure-based, recreational eating habits. You can say that self-control is about pulling the strings and staying in command. Self-control can defend you against the hazards of indulgent eating habits.

Self-control will play a major role in helping you lose your excess weight and keep it off. Before we get into the technical action steps that develop self-control, there are two key tactical building blocks to establishing self-control that you need to be aware of:

THE TACTICAL BUILDING BLOCKS OF SELF-CONTROL
• Self-Awareness
• Self-Responsibility

Self-Awareness Leads to Self-Control

Keep the big picture in focus. Ultimately, what is in your best interest? Did you ever stop to wonder as to who might be in control of your eating habits? Is it your spouse, your family, your environment, a social event or work event? Let's make sure that we are on the same page on this subject. You, and only you, are in control of your eating habits. It is just a matter of choice. You can choose to be in control. You are in charge of what you think. You have a choice when it comes to what you eat. You can be the master or the slave. You can be the master and be in control of your eating habits, or you can be the slave and have your eating habits be in control of you. I find that knowing you have the choice to be in control of your life is very inspiring. It is a step in the right direction to develop the awareness that you, and only you, can take charge of your eating and living habits.

Self-awareness brings out the connection you have with yourself and gets you in touch with your thinking. The more in touch you are with your goals, ambitions, and intentions, the simpler it is to take command, exercise self-control, and make the appropriate choices.

Self-Responsibility Leads to Self-Control

Self-responsibility is the other tactical building block to your self-control. You see, *"response-ability"* means your ability to respond and your ability to make the appropriate choices and decisions. It is imperative that you take ownership and hold yourself accountable to your eating and living habits. The underlying theme is that, regardless of the temptation, *you* can respond by making the proper choices and necessary adjustments in your attitude and behavior. It is totally up to you. It is crucial to be responsible and take charge of your eating habits. It is necessary to be the hammer, not the nail.

Action Steps—The Three D's of Self-Control

Develop self-control and you will be feeding your mind, not your palate. Your mind power is enriched by your self-control. This protects you from the hazards of out-of-control overeating. Your LYF Plan teaches you that there are three D's to the mind power of self-control.

THREE D'S OF SELF-CONTROL
• Vitamin D1—Dynamic Willpower • Vitamin D2—Discrimination • Vitamin D3—Discipline…Self-Discipline, that is!

The three D's are complementary and synergistic. They empower you with skills to outsmart, outwit, and overcome temptations that can sabotage and ruin your PWL plan.

Self-Control is a Process

Achieving self-control is a process that calls upon the workmanship and integration of the three D's. Each component is autonomous and important in its own right, and yes, they are all interrelated. Self-control starts with dynamic willpower—the conviction and determination to make PWL a way of life. Dynamic willpower is an important beginning but requires the partnership of the subsequent two Ds to get results. Discrimination allows you to overcome your impulses and gives you the insight to know what's in and what's out. Finally, self-control calls for self-discipline—the ability to follow through on your intentions and your skillful discrimination. Self-discipline is the closer, the final ingredient needed to apply self-control. In summary, self-control is a three-pronged surgical process. You open and make the incision with dynamic willpower. You operate with vitamin D2, discrimination. You close with self-discipline. Let's take a closer look at how this all works.

Dynamic Willpower

Your self-control starts with your willpower. You need to have a strong, unyielding volition and determination that permeates your thoughts and penetrates your feelings. Your willpower is the engine that drives self-control. The stronger your willpower, the more horsepower behind your self-control. Never lose sight of your conviction and your commitment to lose weight.

Refer back to our discussion on willpower for action tips on developing dynamic willpower.

Discrimination

When your discrimination governs your thinking, you cannot be a prisoner of your temptations or bad habits. Discrimination is the ability to make the distinction between what is good for you and what's not so good for you.

Discrimination Feeds Won't Power

As I have said, your powers of discrimination can identify what is truly in your best interest. This feeds won't power. In a way, discrimination is the ultimate application of won't power. The better your discrimination skills, the stronger your won't power, and the less likely any intrusion of savory temptation can influence or affect you. You may fear that you will be giving up what you love to eat. When what you love to eat or how much you eat begins to take away from the quality of your life, you need to turn to your discrimination skills to get on track. Discrimination, then, gives you the edge to prevent sensory desires and peer pressures from controlling you.

Let's move on to your action steps that will help you build your discrimination skills.

Discrimination: Action Tip #1—Honor Your Nutritional Timeout

When the temptation or urge for your favorite snacks sets in, you must acknowledge the urge and then stop—think—reason—and ask yourself, "Am I hungry? Is this food good for me?" Anytime you feel that you're being overpowered by food desires or cravings, slow things down and take a nutritional timeout. Analyze what is happening and then take command of your thinking.

The beauty of the nutritional timeout is that it prevents you from acting on impulse and gives you a moment to get in touch with your conviction to lose weight and apply discrimination. Let your discriminatory powers take over. Your discrimination pays honor to your higher self. You know, intuitively, what is good for you and when your food choices are driven by impulses to eat. Whenever there is food available—whether it's at home, at the office, at the bank, or at a party—be sure to honor your nutritional timeout. This will help develop your discrimination skills.

Discrimination: Action Tip #2—Use the Benefit-to-Risk Ratio

When it comes to food selection, use the benefit-to-risk ratio to help you discriminate between foods. You can use intelligent guidelines to select Smart Foods. Refer back to LYF-Style Factor #2 for a review of smart nutritional guidelines. With this knowledge, you can discriminate against bad fuel. Learn to apply the benefit-to-risk ratio to sharpen your discrimination skills. This means selecting foods with the maximum benefits and minimum risks to your health. The benefit-to-risk ratio generates a profitable return on investment

(ROI) for your food selections. The idea is to invest in foods that will help you achieve and maintain your ideal weight.

Discrimination: Action Tip #3—Visualize Yourself in Control

Here are some drills to help you strengthen your powers of discrimination. When you have the time, take ten minutes and rehearse how you will handle food distractions or temptations at home, a party, or a social event. Try to envision a food that tantalizes your senses. Then visualize yourself taking a moment to restrain your impulse, going through the process of discrimination, and making the appropriate choice about what to eat (or not eat). The more you rehearse this, the better you will get!

You can also turn to the AVE technique to strengthen your discrimination skills.

- Affirm: I am in control of my eating habits.
- Visualize: Visualize yourself in a specific setting (at home, at work, at your favorite restaurant, etc.) and exercising your discrimination skills in your food selection.
- Expect: Expect and see yourself doing the right thing.

Again, the more you practice, the better you will get.

Recruit the Warriors of Self-Discipline to Master Your Self-Control

The process of self-control starts with dynamic willpower, passes through discrimination, and culminates with self-discipline. Self-discipline is rooted in the first two Ds. If you have dynamic willpower and discrimination, it becomes easier to follow through with self-discipline.

Self-discipline is key to self-control. In fact, self-discipline is the mental training to act in accordance with your preferred rules of conduct. When it comes to nutrition, self-discipline is the mental training to act in accordance with the Golden Rules of Smart Eating. Did you realize that self-discipline trains your thinking and your behavior? It brings order and obedience to your smart eating habits. What I need you to get is that self-discipline gives you the holding power to say no to temptation. You must say no to sensually appealing food temptations and mean no. Without self-discipline, you can very well become weak-willed and eat whatever may appeal to you at that moment. Self-discipline in following the Golden Rules gives you the willpower and won't power that you need to master your eating habits. It takes self-discipline to be a good student. It takes self-discipline to be a good doctor. It takes self-discipline to lose weight permanently.

You will need self-discipline to do the following:

• Eat Well	• Select Smart Food: say yes to the right carbs, proteins, and fats.
• Adhere to Your LYF Nutritional Program.	• Avoid Forbidden Foods: say no to the hazardous carbs, fats, and proteins.
• Apply the Golden Rules of Smart Eating.	• Avoid Indulgent Eating Habits.
• Exercise Regularly.	• Think Positively.

You have control over your actions. Let's take a look at how you can effectively discipline your mind.

Self-Discipline: Action Tip #1—Self-Discipline Is a Mental Muscle; Exercise It Frequently

The interesting thing about self-discipline is the more you use it, the stronger it becomes. If you can develop the self-discipline to exercise regularly, the easier it will be to acquire the discipline to eat Smart Foods and follow the Golden Rules. When you are confronted with a craving, apply the discipline to RIEXA the craving away. With practice, you will develop the self-discipline to overcome any distraction or temptation. Discipline yourself to earn your meals and exercise before breakfast and dinner. The discipline of exercising, eating well, and meditating every day feeds the warriors of self-discipline. In time, self-discipline becomes a way of life.

Self-Discipline: Action Tip #2— Learn How to Respond, Not React

Size up your impulses before acting. Impulsive behavior is reactive behavior. You walk by a doughnut shop and are allured by the sugary smell, or you're watching TV and get an impulse to eat or drink what is being advertised. You conjure up the feel-good impact of salty, crispy potato chips, crunchy crackers, and your favorite cheese. You have the option to react to your impulses and indulge in your senses. Alternatively, you can respond to the situation by stopping, taking some cleansing breaths, and relying on the RIEXA technique to defuse your impulse. Responding, as opposed to reacting, will enable you to take control and develop the self-discipline to follow through.

Self-Discipline: Action Tip #3—Meditate before Meals

Meditation is the preferred weapon against the lure of temptation. Meditating before breakfast (Sunrise Cleanse) and before dinner (Sunset Recharge), and taking your nutritional timeout before lunch, will give you the discipline to overcome unhealthy food temptations. The deeper you meditate, the stronger your self-discipline.

Self-Discipline: Action Tip #4— Anticipation Leads to Self-Discipline

Train yourself to think ahead and use the best ingredients when planning your meals. Make sure to plan out your meals, especially when traveling. Thinking through your plans ahead of time will make it easier and give you greater resolve to follow through appropriately. Know what healthy snacks you need to have on hand for challenging circumstances. Be sure you have access to liquid nutrition when there is nothing healthy available to eat. Anticipating your meal options will help you select Smart Foods under all circumstances.

LYF-Skill #3—
Build Self-Confidence and Positive Belief Systems

Your self-confidence is an integral part of your mind power. In this chapter, you will find out how self-confidence influences your mind power and why it is key to achieving PWL. You'll also learn how your self-confidence can work for you whereas self-doubt can work against you. When you have self-confidence working for you, you get results. Experience teaches us that self-confidence is a crucial link to healthy eating, as well as healthy thinking and exercise habits.

What does it mean to develop self-confidence? Simply put, self-confidence is about believing in yourself. It is fueled by trusting in yourself and having faith in yourself and your abilities. Self-confidence is an attitude; it's an attitude of self-reliance and self-respect. When your prevailing mind-set is self-confident, you find it second nature to love yourself, value yourself, believe in yourself, and expect the best for yourself. These types of feelings and powerful beliefs in yourself lead to a positive self-image and, in turn, self-enriching choices and behaviors. Furthermore, when you believe deeply in yourself and have a strong sense of self-worth, you strengthen your willpower and bolster your self-control. That's right—self-confidence strengthens all of the necessary components for developing mind power. In this way, self-confidence will help you navigate the PWL process and achieve the results you desire.

Self-doubt is the opposite of self-confidence. When your prevailing mind-set is that of self-doubt, it is common to experience low self-worth and feelings of inadequacy. This feeds anxiety, depression, and fear-based belief systems. Self-doubt has a way of undermining and subduing your willpower, weakening your self-control, and deteriorating your mind power. If left unchecked, chronic self-doubt develops into emotional stress and EMT that will further debilitate your PWL plan. The combination of compromised mind power and elevated EMT is a recipe for weight gain.

Let's take a closer look at the dynamics of self-confidence and the inner workings of self-doubt and what you can do to create a prevailing mind-set of self-confidence.

Believe in Yourself

Your self-confidence is shaped by your beliefs and expectations. In fact, you will need to believe deeply in yourself to sport a dynamic self-confidence. Let the truth be known, self-confidence is a belief system—the *believe-in-yourself* belief system. Self-confidence is rooted in a series of positive beliefs in yourself. For example, self-confidence is based on the belief in your ability to succeed. Self-confidence is also based on the belief that you deserve the best, otherwise known as your self-worth. Finally, self-confidence is founded on the belief that you expect the best to happen. In a nutshell, self-confidence is a state of mind where you believe that you deserve the best, you are capable of achieving the best, and furthermore, you expect the best to happen.

Self-confidence can go deep. You need to believe in yourself from the depths of your conscious mind, your subconscious mind, and your soul.

Release Your Inner Powers

Beliefs are magical. Believing in yourself is likewise magical. Your beliefs reverberate throughout your body and vibrate in the amphitheater of your conscious and subconscious mind. Your beliefs have an energy all to themselves. Believing in yourself is both inspirational and motivational. In other words, believing in yourself unleashes an inner power that lights the fire in your belly. These beliefs and deep convictions in yourself fuel dynamic, penetrating mind power. They release the kind of mind power that empowers you to accomplish whatever it is you put your mind to.

Your life is not only greatly influenced by what you believe in, but you are usually most successful at what you believe in the most. Believing in yourself feeds the highest levels of self-confidence. Remember, belief systems have infinite healing powers but work within the boundaries defined by the physical laws of the universe. You can believe that jumping off the Coronado Bridge is not going to hurt you, but this is obviously disrespecting the laws of gravity. You can stand in front of a moving car and believe that you will not get hurt, but you will find that this is not so.

Your Beliefs Shape Your Self-Image

Your self-image is very important when it comes to PWL. Your self-image is linked to the image you have of your body. In order to effectively change your outward bodily appearance, you need to start by changing your inward perception of yourself. Your self-image is how you see yourself, how you think about yourself, and how you look at yourself. It is an image that is imprinted on both your conscious and subconscious mind.

How do you see yourself when you walk into a party and a room full of people? Do you feel confident and attractive, or do you feel inadequate? I find it very interesting that your beliefs about yourself and your self-worth sculpt your self-image. In many ways, your self-image is a simple reflection of your self-worth and self-confidence. When you believe in yourself, value yourself, and have a deep sense of self-confidence and self-worth, you inevitably produce a positive self-image.

For most people it isn't an obvious connection, but your self-image plays a major role in your choices, actions, and behavioral patterns. In fact, your self-image can dominate your eating habits. A positive self-image invites healthy, disciplined eating habits whereas a negative self-image invites overeating and weight gain. Your self-image is one of the key factors that influences your food choices. Let's explore this relationship a little further.

Your Self-Image Governs Your Choices

As we've discussed, your beliefs shape and impact your behavior. You see, your beliefs frame your thoughts and your patterns of thinking. These very thoughts govern your choices, actions, and behavior. When you believe in something, you take action to support it. When you believe in your children, your spouse, or your best friend, it is easy to take positive action to support them. When you believe in yourself, the result is no different; you take positive action to support yourself! When you have a positive self-image—that is to say, when you have a strong belief in yourself—you tap into a powerful inner strength that governs your choices and behaviors. A positive self-image guides you to make self-enriching choices. Why? Because you will naturally want to support your healthy self-image with self-empowering decisions and actions.

Alternatively, a negative self-image will inevitably be supported by choices and behaviors that are self-defeating.

In this way, a positive self-image supports PWL, and a negative self-image is detrimental to your eating, living, and exercise habits. In summary, your self-image influences your choices; your actions; your behavior; and, therefore, the manifestation of your weight-loss goals—or lack thereof.

The Inner Workings of Self-Confidence

Positive Beliefs	➡	Positive Patterns of Thinking	➡	Self-Confidence	➡	Positive Self-Image	➡	Self-Enriching Choices
	➡	Self-Enriching Actions	➡	Positive: • Eating Habits • Exercise Habits • Self-Discipline	➡	Weight Control		

Negative Beliefs	➡	Negative Patterns of Thinking	➡	Self-Doubt	➡	Negative Self-Image	➡	Self-Defeating Choices
	➡	Self-Defeating Actions	➡	Negative: • Eating Habits • Exercise Habits	➡	Weight Gain		

Now you can see why a diet, in and of itself, cannot correct long-term weight issues. Without addressing self-image, it is unlikely that you can incorporate beneficial choices and actions for the long term.

You Are What You Believe

Let's take your belief systems one step further. Your belief systems have a way of becoming self-fulfilling prophecies. You believe you can lose weight permanently, and you knock on the door of success. When you sincerely believe that you deserve to be happy, healthy, and fit, it is only natural that you look good and are proportioned well. You are afraid that you won't lose the weight, and you wind up struggling with your weight. Yes, your beliefs are the sacred keys that shape your behavior. In fact, a lack of self-confidence is one of the most common pitfalls facing those trying to lose excess weight. Your self-confidence shapes the way you think and perform. I have observed over and over again, that, without the inner strength that self-confidence generates, it is improbable that you will accomplish your weight-loss goals. As a doctor of the behavioral sciences, let me assure you that your belief systems are going to be crucial to the PWL process.

Self-Confidence vs. Self-Doubt

When you lack self-confidence, you are plagued by poor self-worth. A lack of self-confidence becomes the story of having profound self-doubt. As you can see in the previous chart, this negativity derails your self-image and can sabotage your PWL program. A sense of inadequacy interferes with the thinking and eating habits necessary to achieve effective weight loss. Feelings of inadequacy and a lack of self-confidence feed anxiety, depression, and fear-based belief systems.

With self-confident, *take-charge* belief systems, you can stay in shape the rest of your life. However, when fear dominates the way you feel, believe, and think, self-doubt appears and your self-confidence becomes eroded. This gets in the way of your PWL plan. Your beliefs of fear, inadequacy, and insufficiency represent negative belief systems. These negative patterns of thinking create patterns of behavior that can sabotage your efforts to lose weight. Remember how your beliefs can become self-fulfilling prophecies? Your fear of failure causes failure. Fear of abandonment creates abandonment. Fear of intimacy causes relationships to break down. Fear of rejection breeds rejection. Fear of not being good enough creates emotional isolation. Similarly, your fear of not losing the weight causes weight gain. Fear of weight-loss failure breeds weight-loss failure. Now you see the pattern. It is only when love and self-worth are central to how you feel about yourself that you will not sabotage your weight-loss plan.

The Origin of Our Thinking Patterns

Let's trace the origins of our thinking patterns. The majority of folks suffer with an inferiority complex that begins in their childhood or early adolescence. It carries over into adult life, shows up as a nervous habit, and turns into a self-defeating behavior. People who suffer from being overweight are no exception. In fact, it is common that people who are overweight often are inwardly frightened, plagued by a deep sense of inadequacy or insecurity. They are known to use their eating habits to medicate, withdraw, or escape from these fears. A poor self-esteem, low self-worth, not believing in yourself, and a negative self-image are all cut from the same piece of cloth. In your mind, you are just plain not good enough, not smart enough, not attractive enough, or not worthy enough. People who are overweight are usually riddled with inner turmoil. Their self-worth is in doubt. They will need the inner strength of mighty self-confidence to overcome this turmoil. They often live in the shadow of defeat and ineffectiveness, waiting for something to go wrong or settling for less than they deserve. A lack of self-confidence is emotionally draining. Gaining self-confidence solves this dilemma.

Let me summarize these important issues. When you incarcerate your self-confidence, you feel different levels of inadequacy or worthlessness. This devalues your self-esteem and negatively impacts your food choices and nutritional decision making. You may feel unworthy of having a trim and toned physique. Maybe it will attract too much attention from the opposite sex. Maybe you like to insulate yourself from others so that you will not get hurt or rejected. Maybe you are addicted to suffering. In time, low self-worth invites self-defeat and weight-loss failure. A negative self-image will dampen and diminish your self-confidence. This becomes an obstacle to your intention to look good and be fit. A negative self-image is often the prevailing mind-set of those who suffer from obesity and being overweight.

Size Up Your Self-Confidence

As you have discovered, your self-confidence can either make or break your weight-loss plans. Take a moment and recognize whether you are self-confident or suffer from poor self-esteem. You and only you know whether you own a self-confident mind-set. Can you afford to have more confidence? Do you have the confidence that you can look your best, or do you sometimes find yourself doubting that you will ever get thinner? Do you really believe that you can lose your excess weight and keep it off? Do you have a bruised self-worth? Have you been programmed to suffer from self-doubt? Are you bottling up your self-confidence?

Take a few moments to fill out and answer the "Self-Confidence" quiz below. Score your answers from 1 to 10, with 10 being the highest score. After each question, ask yourself:

- What it would take to score a 10 on each question?
  - What would you need to do?
  - What would you need to think?
  - What would you need to believe?

This will help you size up your self-confidence and determine what it takes to own the self-confidence and positive belief systems you will need to go all the way.

	Score (1–10)	What you need to do, think, or believe to score a 10?
Do you believe in yourself?		
Do you believe that you can have the kind of body you want?		

Do you believe that you can lose all your excess weight?		
Can you see your physical body toned, trim, fit, and looking right?		
Do you believe that you are worthy of prosperity, success, and happiness?		
Do you respect yourself?		
Do you love yourself?		
Do you look up to yourself?		
Are you an inspiration to yourself?		
Do you have confidence in who you are?		
Total Score		

Score	
• **80–100**	• A score above 80 suggests high levels of self-confidence. Work on the following action steps to take your self-confidence to the next level. Self-confidence is something you can never have enough of.
• **60–80**	• Scores from 60–80 suggest you need to fortify your self-confidence.
• **50–60**	• Scores below 60 suggest too much self-doubt. Pay close attention to the action steps that follow and watch your self-confidence soar.

• **50 and below**	• Scores below 50 suggest a prevailing mind-set of self-doubt. Not to worry. The following action steps will help you establish a prevailing mind-set of self-confidence and eliminate negative thinking patterns and self-doubt.

Action Steps to Building Your Self-Confidence

Self-confidence comes from within. Yes, self-confidence breeds permanent weight loss. Self-doubt also comes from within. And yes, self-doubt leads to weight gain. You see, self-confidence gives you the peace of mind and the necessary decisiveness to effectively focus on your goals. When you suffer from weight gain, you are likely plagued with self-doubt. You are constantly second-guessing yourself and often immobilized by your sense of inadequacy.

It calls for a bold move to lose weight permanently. It takes a bold person to step up and lose this weight once and for all. A new way of life and new patterns of thinking are in order. Out with the old and in with the new. Here are the reliable steps to build your self-confidence. Begin today to take the following action steps. Be prepared to improve every day. Here is your LYF formula to building self-confidence.

TEN STEPS TO SELF-CONFIDENCE
1. Make the Commitment.
2. Be Proud of Who You Are.
3. Become an Optimist.
4. Believe in Yourself.
5. Reprogram Your Belief Systems into Winning Belief Systems.
6. Stand Up for What You Believe.
7. Expect the Best.
8. Respect Yourself.
9. Be Self-Reliant.
10.Have the Courage of Your Convictions.

Self-Confidence: Action Step #1— Make the Commitment

It is important to build up and fortify your self-confidence. It begins with a decision on your part. You, and only you, can generate your self-confidence. Make up your mind today that having self-confidence is important—very important. Self-confidence is essential to all components of life, not just for regulating your waistline. When you make something important to you, it gets your attention. Pay attention to your inner journey. Make the commitment to developing self-confidence. Make the commitment to achieve higher levels of self-confidence than you have ever experienced. Be tenacious and stay the course—no matter what, no matter what it takes. Your commitment to yourself will go a long way. Remember at all times that you are committed to self-improvement and expanding your self-confidence, regardless of the situation.

The Choice Is Yours

Taking charge of your thinking is the most direct path to acquiring self-confidence and enriching your self-esteem. Embrace the full responsibility for the way you see yourself. You are the custodian of your self-worth. Your thoughts dictate the pace. You can choose self-confidence, or you can select self-doubt. The choice is yours.

Self-Confidence: Action Step #2— Be Proud of Who You Are

Taking pride in yourself and your values is a key strategy in upholding a positive self-image and owning dynamic self-confidence. You are a unique individual. Honor your uniqueness. Be proud of yourself. Take a look at some of your accomplishments. Be proud of your values. Be proud of your knowledge, skills, expertise, and what you know about life. It is crucial that you revitalize and energize your self-worth.

The 10 A's to Self-Confidence

Take stock of your talents. Take a moment and write down your ten strongest attributes. Ask a loved one or close friend to write down what they see as your ten best traits and strengths. I like to call them the 10 A's. Refer to your 10

A's whenever you need to lift your spirits and take pride in who you are. Take pride in yourself. Find things to be proud of every day. What will it take to be proud of yourself? Have a sense of pride about your work, family, and integrity. Remember that there is only one of you. Be proud of it!

Self-Confidence: Action Step #3—Become an Optimist

A positive mental attitude is a must to sustain the growth of your self-confidence. You are what you think. Your attitude is a measure of your thinking. Your attitude can transform your self-esteem. Positive thoughts feed your self-esteem. Yes, positive thinking is a prerequisite for sustained levels of dynamic self-confidence. Optimism and enthusiasm are the attitudinal components that lead to increased self-confidence. Optimism empowers your mind and energizes your self-confidence. Enthusiasm revitalizes your self-confidence as well.

Taking charge of your attitude means taking charge of your optimism and enthusiasm. Individuals who are committed to excellent health and superior weight control own a positive mental attitude.

Become an Optimist

Learn to think positively, even in the face of adversity. Tell yourself, your friends, and your loved ones that you are going to enjoy the process of getting in shape and are really looking forward to gaining control over your eating habits. Generate enthusiasm for everything that matters. Enthusiasm and optimism go a long way in nurturing your mind and building your self-confidence. Stay cheerful and keep your spirits high.

Make a Point of Only Saying Positive Things about Yourself

Destroy any thoughts that tell you that you can't lose weight or you can't maintain an exercise program. Substitute positive thinking for negative thoughts immediately. You can't give up hot fudge sundaes? Tell yourself you can. You catch yourself thinking that you won't stay on your program when you visit your family next weekend? Change your thinking and remind yourself that you can and you will stay on track! Destroy the thought that you can't live without cheeseburgers, fries, mac and cheese, or whatever seems so indispensible.

Learn to master your thinking process. Catch yourself in self-doubt or self-condemnation. Rely upon your enthusiasm and positive nature to keep it light while you weed out any negative self-talk and unflattering inner chatter. Replace negativity with positivity. As you nourish your self-confidence and you purge your self-defeating thinking, your own style of self-confidence will emerge. Keep in mind that self-confidence is a powerful magnet. It attracts long-term results.

Self-Confidence: Action Step #4—Believe in Yourself

We have spent a lot of time talking about believing in yourself because it is of the utmost importance—perhaps the most important action step in creating long-term self-confidence. Believing in yourself lifts the spirits of your self-confidence. Your belief in yourself will release inner powers and give you the strength to go all the way, lose all your weight, and keep it off. Use affirmations to construct an unbridled belief in yourself and an undaunted self-confidence.

Use Affirmations to Build Your Belief Systems

Affirmations can help you develop and bolster the belief you have in yourself. Quiet your mind with some deep cleansing breaths. Look within. Whisper firmly from your heart, or affirm and write down:

- I believe in myself; I believe in the miracle of life. (3x)

Affirm this to yourself upon arising in the morning, before bedtime, and at least ten to fifteen times during the day or whenever you catch a nutritional timeout. You'll see amazing results in your self-confidence by just repeating this to yourself for three minutes. Once you have completed this three-minute drill, pause, remain silent, and experience the surge. Now, take a moment to complete this drill. Check out the depth of your belief systems. How deep is the well? Write down your answers to the following questions:

- What does it really mean to believe in myself?

- What might that look like?

Use the ABE Technique to Build Self-Confidence

We introduced the ABE technique in the action steps for strengthening your willpower. The ABE technique is versatile in its application and can be used to build positive belief systems and self-confidence as well. This simple, yet effective formula helps you take charge of your beliefs. The idea is to *think big!* Let's review the ABE technique as it applies to your self-confidence.

- "A" Stands for Affirmation
  - Make a bold stand. Say to yourself, "I believe in myself; I believe in love; I believe in happiness; I believe in fitness; I believe in success." or whatever you want to experience or manifest. It can be at the personal or professional level.
- "B" Stands for Belief
  - Believe in your above affirmation from the bottom of your heart.
- "E" Stands for Expectation
  - Look to see your affirmation take place.

Self-Confidence: Action Step#5— Reprogram Your Belief Systems into Winning Belief Systems

Reprogramming your belief systems takes believing in yourself to the next level. It is a must to think of yourself as a winner. Certainly, to achieve PWL, it is a must to see yourself as a winner. When you value yourself and believe in yourself, it is a simple matter to create positive, winning belief systems. It takes self-confidence to come out on top. The LYF Plan calls for a wholesome, healthy belief system. It reads—you can and will win the battle of the bulge!

Think Big, Really Big

You can be happy and healthy and look your best. A winning belief system embraces believing in yourself, believing in what you are doing, and nurturing the heartfelt belief that you deserve to be healthy, happy, and trim. When you love yourself and believe in yourself, you can fully believe that you can have it all. It is important to believe that you deserve a fulfilling life—physically, emotionally, socially, spiritually, and intellectually. Do you love yourself? Do you believe you deserve the best?

Three-Minute Power Drills

Precede all of these drills by taking a moment and looking at your 10 A's. Recognize that you have very specific talents and attributes that can command respect. Believe in yourself.

Drill #1—Resolve Any Disbelieving Thought Patterns

Get in touch with any negative beliefs about yourself or your life. Recognize the limitations and restrictions imposed by not believing. Do you believe that you can achieve prosperity? Do you believe that you can be happy? Do you believe that you can look good? Do you believe that you can be well off financially? Do you believe that you can find the optimal relationship? Do you believe you can find the optimal kind of work?

Bring to mind the most positive resolution to any disbelieving thought pattern that you recognize. For example, replace "I can't" with "I can." Remember, you can be anything that your determination and talent guide you to be. Put your life into focus with the uplifting mental telescope of winning belief systems. "I can't lose weight" becomes "I can and I will lose this weight forever!"

Drill #2—Turn to the AVE Technique

The AVE technique has already been introduced as an action step in building dynamic willpower. Like the ABE technique, the AVE technique can be used for multiple purposes. You can use your picture power to transform your belief systems. We'll use the AVE technique to open up your mind and then change and modify existing beliefs. The goal is to convert all of your important belief systems into winning belief systems that will serve you well. When you couple your affirmations with visualization and expectation, you impact not only your conscious thoughts but also your subconscious mind. This is particularly important because the core of any self-image issues resides in your subconscious. Therefore, reprogramming your belief systems requires reprogramming both your conscious and subconscious mind. Work on your AVEs and watch your self-confidence soar.

- "A" Stands for Affirmation
  - Affirm: "I am healthy, fit, and attractive." (3x)
- "V" Stands for Visualization
  - Visualize yourself, detail-by-detail, at your ideal weight and shape.
- "E" Stands for Expectation
  - Intensify your visualization and expect it to take place. Try to experience what it feels like.

Self-Confidence: Action Step #6—Stand Up for What You Believe

Standing up for what you believe is very important in fortifying your self-confidence. When you stand up for what you believe in, it makes your beliefs and convictions stronger and strengthens your sense of self-worth. Be ready to take a stand on what you believe in. Just what is your philosophy of life? What is it that you most profoundly believe? Wherein lie your strongest beliefs? Take a moment and write down what you strongly believe in:

- I strongly believe in ________________________________
- I strongly believe in ________________________________
- I strongly believe in ________________________________

Stand up for your cause. Stand up for your loved ones and friends. Stand up and defend your principles. Stand up for your beliefs. Take a stand on major issues in the following areas:

- Your Personal Life
- Your Home Life
- Your Work Life

Stand up for what you believe and watch your self-confidence grow!

Self-Confidence: Action Step #7—Expect the Best

The power of positive belief systems works to help your weight-loss journey. Keep in mind that there is a dominating principle in the mind-body connection as it relates to weight loss. This principle can be summarized as the following:

- Whatever the mind profoundly expects it seems to receive.

Building your self-confidence relies on the expectations of your thinking. When you expect things to go well, they have a tendency to go well. When you expect the worst, the worst often happens. Self-confidence is sculpted by expecting that your strongest beliefs will manifest. "All things are possible to he who believes."

Practice the art and science of positive expectations. Practice makes perfect. Be certain that your really want to lose weight. Be sure that your desires are coming from the bottom of your heart. What is the truth about your heart's desire? Expect the best results possible. You can do it! It is important to learn to expect and not to doubt. When you expect the best, everything falls into the realm of possibility. Expecting the best is expecting greater, bigger, and larger. You see, when you expect the best, you release an inner strength, an inner power. This magnetic force in your mind attracts the object of your desires. Sustained expectations trigger the mind power to make *the best* materialize.

Give It All You Got

Expectation requires dynamic action for your intention to manifest itself. Expecting the best means that you put your heart and soul into whatever you want to accomplish or see happen. Give of yourself and take the initiative. Take dynamic actions to implement your expectations. Become very clear about what it is you want and expect. Be willing to work hard to get your desired result. For example, follow the LYF Plan and achieve your weight-loss expectations. Be determined to lose all of your excess weight. Fire up your heart and soul. Become passionate about achieving your goals. Do not take no for an answer. Fire up your thinking this way.

Kindle Your Imagination

The gift of imagination is the mental genius, the untold power of your perception. Your imagination stands for the creative, constructive power of your thinking. You can use your imagination to create a new vision of yourself and your expectations. This gives you a new perspective on what you expect to accomplish. Expect to lose weight and keep it off. Let your expectations start working for you.

Kindling your imagination accelerates your weight-loss process and simultaneously blazes out self-doubt. Concentrate on your weight-loss goals and perform the following AVE technique.

- **A**ffirm—I expect to achieve my desired weight. (3x)
- **V**isualize—With your eyes closed and with a slight upward gaze, photograph your desired objective in your third eye—at the point between your eyebrows. Recruit your vivid imagination.
- **E**xpectation—Use your imagination and visualize your expectation turning into reality. Try to experience what it feels like to be at your desired weight. Believe, believe, believe. Recruit your picture power. The constructive, creative, imaginative faculties of your mind are a precious tool. Passionate imagination is transforming. Here is where your thinking really begins to catch fire.

Self-Confidence: Action Step #8—Respect Yourself

Self-respect is conducive to self-confidence. When you respect yourself, you own a strong level of esteem for the dignity of your character. In essence, you hold yourself in high regard. It makes good sense to look out for yourself, take good care of yourself, and look up to yourself. Self-respect is an interesting feature to the relationship you have with yourself. Why? Because self-respect can feed the depth of your self-confidence.

Here's the bottom line. Either you respect yourself, or you don't. When you respect yourself, you want to look and feel your best. You want to realize your full potential, make a big difference, and get the most out of life. To see the big picture, your self-respect is linked to your respect for life. When you respect being alive, when you respect creation, when you respect your creator—it is a simple matter to respect yourself.

I don't have to tell you that life is very precious. When you stop to think about it, you may very well realize what a privilege it is to be alive. You are born with the most incredible machine ever invented—the human body. The intelligence of its parts is beyond measurement.

Take Command of Your Thinking and Generate Self-Respect

Take a moment and ask yourself, "what does respect look like?"

- Do you really respect yourself?
- Do your habits and behavior indicate self-respect or disrespect?
- In one hundred words or less, write down what you need to do or say to win your own self-respect. Do it now! Make the commitment to respect yourself. You deserve it. You are a unique individual. Keep in mind that it will be difficult to respect others when you don't love, accept, or respect yourself. Your self-confidence is nourished and nurtured by your self-respect.

Respect Your Soul and Nourish Your Self-Esteem

Your mind has the ability to tune into the vibrations of your soul. Meditation and prayer help you dial into the presence of your soul. In becoming spiritually mindful, you learn to acknowledge the magnificence of your own pure essence. By dialing your mind into your spirit, you are reminded of your magnificence. Your appreciation for being alive is reflected in your self-respect. As you begin to respect yourself, you fire up your self-confidence. Your self-respect and your self-confidence are vital inner strengths that feed and nourish the necessary mind power to achieve PWL.

Self-Confidence: Action Step #9—Be Self-Reliant

Your self-respect is cultivated by your willingness to take responsibility for your life. In other words, self-sufficiency feeds self-confidence. When you are self-sufficient, you are the captain of your destiny. You make the decisions about your life. Learn to rely upon yourself for your health and your well-being.

Self-Confidence: Action Step #10—Have the Courage of Your Convictions: Do Not Believe in Defeat

Courage feeds self-confidence. Courage is the ability to face your difficulties with inner strength and without fear. The time is ripe for you to face up to your weight-gain dilemma. Losing weight permanently is simple, but not easy. In fact, letting go of old thought patterns and self-defeating behaviors can be very difficult. Courage will see you through. You can do this. Have the courage to stand up for yourself.

Make Your Intention to Achieve PWL a Conviction

Make your intention to lose weight permanently a strong conviction. Remember, you are what you choose to think and believe. Through these choices, you create wellness or illness, happiness or misery, success or failure, weight gain or weight loss. Have the courage to stand up for your conviction to achieve and maintain your ideal weight. In fact, standing up for anything that you believe in promotes courage and a healthier sense of self-worth.

Have the Courage to Work Out Your Conflicts

Your self-confidence gets lifted when you effectively square off against your main conflicts with losing weight and keeping it off. What is your main predicament? What keeps you from losing this weight forever? Solving problems boosts your self-confidence. When you tackle the hurdle of overcoming your excess weight, with courage, skill, and efficiency, you add invaluable depth to your self-confidence. Be determined to come to grips with whatever it takes to accomplish your weight-loss goals. Write it down now. What will it take for you to permanently lose those unwanted pounds? Have the courage to follow through.

Be Willing to Take the Risk

Be prepared to shift out of your comfort zone. You may find that your comfort foods are an important emotional support system. Your comfort foods may very well be your way to cope with emotional and financial stress. Be courageous, though. Be assertive and focused under the most challenging of circumstances. Go out to dinner with friends, go on vacation, and celebrate when it is appropriate. At the same time, be willing to face adversity and still be the master of your eating habits. When you travel or party, learn to have fun and celebrate without eating yourself into toxic overload. This pattern of behavior builds your self-confidence. Start with a friend at lunch and build up to bigger events. You can do this. Be confident of your ability to stand up for what you believe. Tenacity and decisiveness will promote a lasting sense of self-confidence.

23

Feed Your Soul—Develop Soul Power

THERE never has been—nor will there ever be—anything that can compete with or that is stronger than soul power. Soul power plays a huge role in permanent weight loss. You could say that soul power is a vibration; it's an energy—a magnetic force that grounds you, centers you, and keeps you calm and peaceful. In the simplest of terms, soul power is the source of all-encompassing inner fulfillment. How do you find soul power? Soul power is generated by establishing inner peace, inner joy, purposefulness, and fulfillment. It is the sanctuary of inner tranquility and peace of mind.

Let me take it a step further. Soul power is synonymous with the ultimate in inner strength and conviction. In the grand scheme of PWL, soul power gives you the crucial inner strength to stick to your LYF Program. It aligns you with your highest priorities. It empowers you to achieve your weight-loss goals. Soul power roots you. The strength of a tree is in its roots. The strength of your weight-loss plan is rooted in the depth of your soul power. You will need soul power to help you weather the storms and adversities that may come into your life.

Without inner peace, inner joy, and purposefulness—that is, without soul power—there is an inner void that is created. This void has a driving force. It is constantly looking to be filled. It is very common for people to look to food to fill this void. When you fill yourself with soul power, you won't need to look to food to fill an inner void. You won't need to use food as a crutch. The purpose of this chapter is to guide you to feed yourself with inner peace, inner joy, happiness, and purpose. In doing so, you won't be preoccupied with filling yourself with food.

The Villains of PWL

The true test of your ability to sustain weight loss is revealed by how well you fare in the face of the five villains of PWL. You may know what to do; you may have a plan to handle adversity; but your success will often come down to how well you can handle these five villains—restlessness, temptation, distraction, anxiety, and fatigue.

Time and time again I have seen people's weight-loss plans and convictions uprooted by these weight-loss offenders. So why do I make such a fuss over soul power? Soul power gives you the inner strength to fight off the restlessness, temptations, distractions, anxiety, and fatigue that undermine your PWL plan. Soul power will also help you overcome disappointments, indifference, cravings, and bad moods that are infamous for derailing your eating habits. Soul power gives you the authority to follow your LYF Program. It gives you the long-term self-control to defend you from being a victim of harmful eating habits. In essence, soul power gets the job done.

Soul Power is Necessary to Outwit Your Temptations

The bottom line is that soul power gives you the power to outwit—that is, to outfox—your temptations! As you know, temptation is nothing more than a sugar-coated distraction. Temptation appeals to your senses—the sight, the smell, and the taste of food. It may look good, smell good, and taste good, but much like cravings, temptations are short-lived and generally bad for you. You can learn to overcome temptations by tapping into your inner sanctuary and inner fulfillment that evolve with the acquisition of soul power. "Ever fed, never satisfied. Never fed, ever satisfied."

Soul power gives you the upper hand, so you can master your eating habits instead of becoming a slave to alluring, enticing food temptations. With soul power, you learn that there is a greater pleasure than the lure of the senses—and that is the joy of the soul. It seems like the soul is shackled to your body by the chains of worry, desires, obligations, troubles, and temptations. It makes better sense to yearn for something long-lasting—like inner joy, inner peace, and the bliss of the soul. In this chapter, you will learn that the most effective way to outsmart your temptations is to live in harmony with and experience the inner sanctuary of divine presence that accompanies the development of soul power.

Restlessness Works against You

You tell yourself you are going to fire up the will to overcome temptation and lose weight once and for all. However, "the best-laid plans of mice and men often go awry." Just ask folks about their weight-loss plans at the beginning of each New Year. Everybody is going to lose weight—few do. What is the predicament? I will tell you what it is. I see it show up in thousands of my patients. It is the same predicament in the United States as it is in South America and Europe. It is called restlessness. You can't stop your mind. You can't turn off your thinking. Restlessness is the predicament.

Restlessness feeds destructive eating habits. Restlessness leads to nervous, impulsive eating. When you are restless, you invariably find it difficult to concentrate or stay focused on one thing at a time. Before you know it, your jittery nature often spills over to your eating habits. Most people suffer from some form of restlessness. It often shows up as nervousness. Restlessness can also show up as anxiety, stress, depression, moodiness, mood swings, anger, fatigue, a wandering mind, or emotional tension. Being anxious, high-strung, tense, or apprehensive does not favor healthy eating. It favors succumbing to your temptations, cravings, food indulgences, and dietary distractions.

In other words, restlessness is an enemy to permanent weight-loss seekers. Restlessness is in epidemic form today. This feeling of uneasiness and inability to relax is commonly medicated with prescription tranquilizers, antidepressants, and sleeping pills. Doctors ink more than one hundred million prescriptions each year for these nervous disorders. Meanwhile, others choose to self-medicate with alcohol, caffeine, cigarettes, work, gambling, sex, or recreational drugs. And all too many others are tempted by food to appease their restlessness and uneasiness.

The bottom line is that restlessness undermines your eating habits. Restlessness can destroy your PWL plan. Why? Because restlessness commonly triggers hazardous overeating habits. Furthermore, restlessness invokes temptations and provokes emotional overeating. The truth is that restlessness, and its sister anxiety, are known to trigger food indulgences. Restlessness is often behind late-night eating, snacking, nibbling, raiding the refrigerator, or full-blown bingeing. In fact, many folks are accustomed to medicate their anxiety or restlessness with their favorite comfort foods. The remedy calls for the inner peace and the inner joy that emanate from soul power. Here is where soul power comes in handy.

Soul Power is Necessary to Overcome Restlessness

Soul power is necessary to prevent and overcome restlessness. When you have inner peace, restlessness cannot exist, just as darkness cannot exist where there is light. Soul power breeds the kind of serenity and calmness that heals whatever form of restlessness you currently own. Your soul power can take this debilitating nervous energy out of your lifestyle. It replaces disorder with orderliness. It replaces temptations with healthy preferences, distractions with self-control. How sweet it is!

From a practical point view, soul power takes the proverbial wind out of the sails of dietary temptations. Soul power gives you the muscle to overcome restlessness. It gives you the power to say no to the untimely ingestion of your favorite mood foods—foods that, at one time, may have had a hold on you. Soul power also gives you the strength to overcome purposelessness, apathy, depression, and anxiety that feed and invite your restlessness.

CAUSES OF RESTLESSNESS AND ANXIETY		
Mental Strain		
Emotional Stress		Restlessness
Financial Distress	➡	and
Emotional Bankruptcy		Anxiety
Soul Suffocation		

Take note of some of the causes of restlessness and anxiety listed above. You know what anxiety and restlessness do to your moods. They take them south of the border. You know what this does to your appetite; it takes it to the north pole. You know how this anxiety can get you to eat for comfort and deviate from your health plan. How well you manage restlessness, anxiety, and ongoing frustrations will tell the story of your success or failure in sustaining permanent weight loss. Feed your soul with inner peace, inner joy, and purpose, and you can say good-bye to the restlessness, nervousness, and anxiety that wreak havoc with your weight-loss goals.

Soul Suffocation: The Story of Restlessness

Soul power is the story of your inner essence. Sooner or later, you have to face the truth of your soul. Otherwise, soul suffocation can set in. How does soul suffocation present itself? It comes through the familiar adversaries that we've been talking so much about—restlessness, nervousness, and free-floating anxiety. It becomes a vicious cycle.

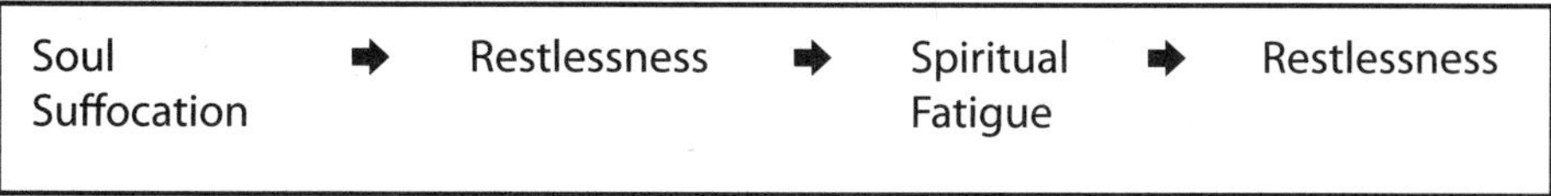

Let's take a minute to examine this cycle of soul suffocation, spiritual fatigue, and restlessness. Several factors can influence the onset of soul suffocation. Maybe it's that the time you spend every day is not allocated to the things that are most important to you. Maybe you spend too much time working and not enough time with your family and loved ones. Maybe you don't have the time—nor make the time you need—for your favorite hobbies or creative self-expression. In any case, you often feel that you are not doing what you want to be doing. You would rather be somewhere else, doing something different, or being with someone else. Your life feels like a stressful overload of duties, deadlines, demands, rules, responsibilities, and chores. Somewhere along the line, you have lost sight of your true sense of purpose. Somehow you find that you don't spend enough time doing the things that truly make you happy. These are all signs of soul suffocation. Over time, this suffocation develops into spiritual fatigue.

With spiritual fatigue, you usually lose the will to love, the will to improve, and the will to live your life to the fullest. Losing touch with your soul—and, as such, yourself—is a root cause of burnout, soul suffocation, and spiritual fatigue. In the presence of soul suffocation and spiritual fatigue, restlessness, much like an opportunistic invader, sets in.

Stay Focused

In way of summary, yes, yes, yes...soul power gives you the ability to stay focused and prevent the villains of restlessness and anxiety from undermining your PWL plan. Soul power gives you the moxie and the might to stick to the Golden Rules of Smart Eating. It gives you the swagger, the wherewithal, and the character to work through challenging nervousness and overcome temptation. As you study the techniques and strategies to cultivate dynamic soul power, you will develop new inner strengths. As you shift into the zone of soul power, you will gain the necessary edge to let go of your over-attachment to food. Soul power breeds a level of enlightenment that empowers you to have a healthy relationship with your diet. When you tap into the powers of the soul, it goes a long way in helping you let go of whatever dietary rituals and attachments that are more self-defeating than not.

Soul Power Is Inspirational

Yes, soul power, desire, and ambition are on the same page! When you are driven to improve yourself and fulfill your visions, you own the essence of soul power. When you are prepared to do whatever it takes to be well and stay in metabolic balance, the presence of soul power is shining through. Your soul power gives you your drive to experience the magnificence of spirit that is called life. Soul power is the strength of spirit swarming through your veins. Soul power feeds your appetite for life. It gives you the drive to seek fulfillment in your world. When you seek self-fulfillment through self-enriching, purposeful actions and behaviors, you will find that you can transcend food consciousness.

You know you have soul power when your prevailing mind-set is happy and peaceful. Yes, soul power is identified by the presence of an inner smile and substantial peace of mind. More often than not, you are serene and joyful. This empowers you to take charge of your life!

Your soul power inspires you as well as others. Soul power gives you the charm, influence, and inspiration to be the best at who you can be—for yourself and for others. It dials you into your gifted uniqueness and encourages its full expression. Soul power is an alliance with the true and real you. It is a fellowship with the convictions and secrets of your soul. Soul power inspires you to be the best at what you instinctively and intuitively know and do the best—being yourself.

Keep in mind that your soul is the spiritual part of your being. It is your spirit. In fact, it is spirit within your body. The seat of your soul is the center of your very essence. Your soul gives you the gift of life; and without a soul, there is no life as we know it. The light of your soul is the electricity that plugs you into life! Soul power keeps you connected to the light of your soul. It generates a lot of good energy.

How to Create Soul Power

A well-nourished soul generates soul power. Peacefulness, gentleness, blissfulness, and tranquility are the spiritual attributes of a well-nourished soul. The fruits of an empowered soul are love, joy, creative self-expression, and inner peace. Further, being lively, bold, forceful, and glowing speaks well for a vital spirit. A well-nourished soul has the ability to trump cravings, overcome bingeing, and regulate other kinds of impulsive eating.

Soul power works to keep your dreams alive. The purpose of this chapter is for you to find out how you can energize and activate your soul power. Just as there are white belts, brown belts and black belts in karate, there are multiple levels of soul power. Keep in mind that to achieve the highest levels of soul power, you must fully satisfy the longings of your soul and heal your emotional wounds. The truth is that you can develop and sculpt soul power into its most dynamic form. You can have soul power. Everyone can. It is something that lies quietly within us all. There are three ways to cultivate dynamic soul power and feed your soul. Use these strategies and techniques to overcome restlessness and the villains of PWL.

THE THREE STEPS TO ACHIEVING SOUL POWER

- LYF-Skill #1—How to Nourish your Soul: The Art of Spiritual Nutrition
- LYF-Skill #2—How to Create the Triangle of Divine Fire
- LYF-Skill #3—Define Your Purpose in Life

LYF-Skill #1—How to Nourish Your Soul: The Art of Spiritual Nutrition

Just as your physical body needs quality nutrition to thrive, your soul needs to be well nourished to grow and prosper. A healthy, well-nourished soul is the key to dynamic, invincible soul power. In other words, a well-nourished soul promotes the soul power that creates a playful, jubilant, cheerful, and animated lifestyle.

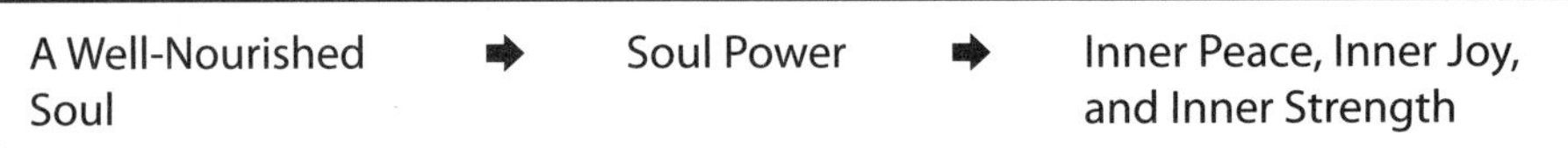

A Well-Nourished Soul
Soul Power
Inner Peace, Inner Joy, and Inner Strength

A well-nourished soul is absolutely a *must* for PWL. It supports good eating habits and Metabolic Fire.

Feed Your Soul What It Needs

Taking care of your soul goes beyond eating well and exercising every day. There are ten essential spiritual nutrients to a well-nourished soul. These life-giving principles keep your spirits high. Spiritual nutrition keeps your soul alive and well. Below are the ten nutrients that promote spiritual growth and, ultimately, soul power. Take a look at the importance of each one of these soul foods.

TOP TEN "SOUL FOODS" THAT NOURISH THE SOUL	
I. Standing Up for Your Beliefs	• Standing for the truth of your beliefs strengthens your integrity and your convictions and empowers the soul.
II . Purpose	• Purposeful living keeps you in harmony with your highest priorities and brings an inner fulfillment to your soul.
III. Creative Self-Expression	• Creative self-expression gets you in touch with your true uniqueness and invites you to express the depths of your soul.
IV. Spending Time with Nature	• Nature is very orderly and balanced. Nature is inspiring and soothing to the soul. Allow the spirit of nature to impregnate your soul.
V. Communicating and Spending Time with Loved Ones	• Heartfelt love is food for your soul.
VI. Satisfying Social and Cultural Activities	• Social health and interpersonal relationships feed your soul.
VII. Laughing	• Keeping it light is good for your soul. Laughter is your best medicine.
VIII. Eating Smart Foods	• Eating well protects your body, the temple that houses your soul. Smart Foods lighten up and purify your soul.
XI. Exercising	• Keep your feet moving. Exercise keeps your spirits high.
X. Meditation	• The key to your inner sanctuary of happiness, inner peace, and inner joy.

Size Up Your Soul Power

Take inventory, and see how well your soul is getting fed. Then, take a few quiet moments and reflect on what it would take for each soulful nutrient to become a more in-depth, regular, consistent support system in your life. Score each statement below based on the frequency and consistency in which you feed yourself with these important soul foods.

Do you...	Always (Daily)	Frequently (4x / week)	Sometimes (2x / week)	Rarely (monthly)	Never
Stand up for what you believe in?	5	4	3	2	1
Have a purposeful lifestyle?	5	4	3	2	1
Find creative self-expression regularly?	5	4	3	2	1
Spend time outdoors in nature being quiet, listening, and taking in your environment?	5	4	3	2	1
Communicate and spend time with loved ones?	5	4	3	2	1
Spend time in satisfying social and cultural activities?	5	4	3	2	1
Share laughter with kindred souls?	5	4	3	2	1
Eat Smart Foods?	5	4	3	2	1
Exercise vigorously?	5	4	3	2	1
Spend quality time in devotional prayer and/or meditation at least one time a day, if not two to three times a day?	5	4	3	2	1

Total Points	
40–50 points	• Suggests a well-nourished soul
30–39 points	• Suggests you are on the right track but need to nourish your soul more regularly.
29 points and below	• Suggests spiritual burnout. Pick out your favorite soul foods from the above list and start incorporating them into your daily activities.

Experience the Magic of Meditation

Among all of these ten soul foods, meditation is the Rolls Royce of spiritual nutrition. In fact, meditation is a spiritual super-nutrient. Meditation is as important to your soul as exercise is to your heart. I find that meditation gives you the opportunity to get in touch with the light in your life. You can also say that meditation enriches your state of self-awareness. It takes soulfulness to pay attention to the inner workings of your heart, mind, and soul. Meditation is that inner sanctuary, to be there for you whenever you need to make contact with yourself or spirit. Meditation feeds your soul power!

How Meditation Feeds Your Soul

Meditation is very soothing to your soul. Calming meditation quietly, but efficiently, feeds your soul. Meditation creates the inner sanctuary that empowers you to focus on your inner joy and inner feelings of bliss. Indeed, meditation is an inner journey. It shuts off outside distractions and tunes you into your divine presence of inner peace, love, and joy. Meditation is an opportunity to communicate with your own heartfelt vibrations that nourish your soul. It is a way to experience your higher loving self. Unless time is spent developing your inner life, it could easily be neglected.

What really is meditation? Although the word is often associated with yoga, relaxation, and stress management, I find it interesting to look at the original description given to the art of meditation by scholarly yogis. They would tell you that ***meditation is sustained concentration on and devotion to Spirit.*** This one pointed concentration on your heart and soul is the kind of harmony that we can all stand to enjoy. As you turn to your meditation to connect the dots in your life, it feeds your soul power.

Meditation ➡ Spiritual Super-Nutrition ➡ Soul Power

Meditation gets you in touch with your inner peace, love, and inner joy. The more you meditate, the deeper you will experience these feelings throughout the day and the less you will have to deal with restlessness, temptation, and anxiety. This bodes well for your eating habits and making self-enriching choices and behaviors that support your PWL plan.

Additional Benefits of Meditation

Meditation is a spiritual, mental, and emotional tonic. It cleanses your soul, uplifts your soul, and feeds your soul power. Meditation purifies your emotions and can be very emotionally supportive. Further, it soothes your mind and gives you the clarity to keep your eating habits on track. This tonic has incredible benefits for the body. It has been scientifically documented to lower blood pressure, increase blood circulation, and effectively help the body reduce stress. It revitalizes your nerves and rejuvenates your hormones.

Quiet Your Mind and Experience Your Inner Peace

You see, the idea in meditation is to calm your overactive mind. People tend to have wandering minds. Commonly, you can have too much on your mind and your thinking can become overactive. Even when you are relaxing, you may have a tendency to waffle from thought to thought. You might be thinking about a project at work, your financial situation, or a relationship issue. The point is, unless you can quiet your mind, you will miss out on the guiding voice of your inner silence. When you make the effort to meditate, you work to break the endless distractions of your thinking. It can be very difficult to get through this self-defeating mental static. When you put an end to the inner chatter, you gain eligibility to experience the love, peace, and wisdom within yourself.

With effective meditation, you begin to identify your true feelings, touch base with your real self, and gain emotional intelligence. This is why meditation is so important for everyone. It can decompress your stress and put a smile in your heart.

Make Meditation a Daily Habit

Like exercise and good nutrition, making meditation a daily habit is important. You could not exercise one day a week and consider yourself fit any more than you can meditate once in a while and bring yourself into spiritual harmony.

The overwhelming majority of people who practice meditation find that it supports them. The key is to inspire yourself to do it. It takes practice, regularity, and consistency to make progress with your meditation—your inner journey to the source of your life. When you begin to get somewhere with your meditation, it relaxes you, empties your mind, and empowers you to get rid of the chaos and disorder in your chain of thoughts. In time, you learn to get your mind out of the picture. When the clouds dissolve, you can experience the sun in its full form. Similarly, with your mind out of the picture, so to say, you can make the connection with the presence of your soul. Eventually, the feelings of inner peace and joy that you experience during your meditation will be the prevailing feelings you experience throughout the day. In this way, you can best nurture your soul.

Embrace the Discipline

It is very important to develop everyday meditation skills. It is interesting to note that the more sustained and concentrated your meditation, the higher the level of self-attunement and the more soul power you generate. This gives you the upper hand in dealing with the distractions of restlessness, anxiety, frustration, disappointments, depression, and difficult life challenges. I want to strongly recommend that you embrace the discipline to be consistent with your meditations. You need to know that you will be challenged by the cycles, changes, and inconsistencies known to influence our human behavior. Meditating every day will support a new level of consistency in your efforts to achieve and maintain your ideal weight.

Meditation Comes in Different Forms

Meditation brings together prayer, ritual, self-discipline, and celebration. That's a lot. It can be simplified. I find that, from a practical point of view, there are three main types of meditation. Each one of these holds the promise of fortifying your soul power.

THREE BASIC FORMS OF MEDITATION
• Mental Relaxation • Creative Imagination • Self-healing

We are going to focus on self-healing as the meditation of choice for acquiring the inner strength you need to achieve PWL. To give you a better frame of reference, however, let's quickly review the other forms of meditation as well.

Mental Relaxation, also Known as the Shangri-La Meditation

This kind of meditation gives you the opportunity to lighten up and retreat from your daily stresses, struggles, and strain. The following methodology details the steps you can take to practice mental relaxation.

- Step 1—Fix your mind on a peaceful, natural setting. For example, fix your attention on some green trees in the forest, a white sandy beach at sunset, or beautiful flowers in your favorite garden. Likewise, you can gaze at the waves or watch the setting sun. You can also sit and listen to the waves at sea or the birds in the forest.
- Step 2—Now then, shut off your thoughts, and let yourself go. Use deep cleansing breaths to slow down and calm your mind.
- Step 3—Try and become one in mind, body, and spirit with your natural element. For example, become emerged in the sound of the waves crashing at the beach. Let all tension drift away as you relax and feel yourself come alive. Stay with it for at least ten to fifteen minutes.

Creative Imagination

This kind of meditation relies on the picture power of guided visual imagery. Here, you use your imagination to create the kind of events you want to experience in your life. This is where you tap into your vivid imagination and use the mind power of expecting the best to trigger your dormant soul power.

- Step 1—Visualize the circumstances at work, home, and play as you desire. Do one at a time. Direct the movie of your own mind and see yourself as the main interesting character.
- Step 2—Be sure to not only see the experience but, more importantly, to become emotionally involved with your clearest visions. Feel the emotional surge while at the same time keeping your focus on your vision. Feel triumphant in whatever you are visualizing. It is your creation. Practice this for ten to fifteen minutes to feel the full benefits.
- *The One Best Thought Meditation Technique*—Another type of creative imagination is the "One Best Thought" meditation technique. Determine the single most positive thought that you can create in your mind. It can explore the full scope of happiness, fulfillment, and enlightenment. Visualize this thought manifesting itself. Get emotionally involved and try to experience it from the depths of your heart. Stay with this thought and vision for at least three minutes, and when you have the time, longer and longer.

Self-Healing Meditation

Concentrating on the healing powers of your soul is the foundation to self-healing meditations. Affirmations that invest and validate the power in your spirit are commonly used. Affirmations are statements of strong intent and belief repeated silently to yourself and then out loud. When repeated in a mantra-like fashion, affirmations open up and interface a great deal of internal communication with your inner powers. In fact, repetitive, silent chanting releases your soul power. For example, say any of the following affirmations to yourself three times:

- I am a pure channel of love and light.
- My heart is alive with pure love and joy.
- I have the power of spirit to achieve __________.
- I believe in myself.

In the process of meditation, your soul naturally unfolds into its ultimate manifestation as a pure channel of love. This generates enormous supplies of soul power. It takes practice, but it is worth it. By practicing self-healing meditation, the instrument of your soul comes alive. You can go deep, feel the love in your heart, listen to your inner voice, and you will discover the secrets of your soul power. Eventually, you can turn to your meditation to purge the darkness of spiritual blindness, spiritual indigestion, and spiritual restlessness out of your life. Keep in mind that self-healing meditation stabilizes and regulates your eating habits.

How to Meditate

As discussed, there are many different ways to meditate. Any inspirational technique or deep prayer that allows you to concentrate fully on your heartfelt love, your soul, or divine consciousness can be an effective meditation. Meditation is a mind-set. It is a zone. It allows you to focus your undivided attention on experiencing inner peace, love and joy, and healing from within.

With that in mind, let's discuss the specific steps I would like you to take to incorporate meditation into your daily routine. The ultimate meditation embraces a relaxed physical body, a pure loving heart, deep breathing, and a one-pointed, calm mind. Put a smile in your heart, your soul, and your eyes. This will recharge your spirit.

I have worked out a powerful ten-step technique to help you cultivate the skills of meditation. Please review and practice the following ten essential steps. In time, this will lead to effective, in-depth meditation. This LYF self-healing technique will teach you how to meditate and generate soul power.

- **Step 1: Relax**—Relax your physical body. (Precede meditation with exercise, yoga, or tai chi).

- **Step 2: Posture Counts**—Sit up straight; keep your spine straight and head upright; and steady your eyes. Get ready to look within, quiet the mind, and focus on your spirit.
- **Step 3: Find Your "Third Eye"**—With your eyes closed, gently gaze up and concentrate on your third eye—the central point between your eyebrows. Be sure to relax the eye muscles in the front and back of your eye. Find the light of your soul. Try to find the light in the darkness at the focal point of your gaze, just as you might see the light of a candle. Try not to move your concentration away from your third eye. When your focus shifts away from your third eye, your mind is typically wandering. Keep your eyes steady on your third eye throughout the meditation.
- **Step 4: Cleansing Breaths**—Cleansing breaths are next. Practice deep cleansing breaths using a rhythm of 2:4:4:2. (Inhale for two counts, hold for four, exhale for four, and then hold for two.) Work up to 4:8:8:4. Concentrate and listen to your breath. Breathe loud enough so that someone walking by would hear it.
- **Step 5: Heartfelt Love**—This step highlights the importance of heartfelt meditation. Return your breathing pattern to deep, natural breathes. With every breath, fill your heart with love. Allow your heart space to expand. Feel the bliss and the unconditional love for yourself, others, and Spirit. Open your heart and experience the light of your soul.
- **Step 6: The LYF "Cease-fire" Technique**—The purpose of this step is uniting heartfelt meditation with the light of your soul. I call this the cease-fire technique because it stops your mind from wandering while you meditate. Experience the love radiating from your heart while concentrating your gaze on your third eye. This quiets and empties the mind and puts a cease-fire on any inner mental chatter. Heartfelt meditation is the panacea for a wandering mind; it enables you to enter a higher level of awareness and consciousness. When you are in a state of bliss, there are no thoughts on your mind. You get the chance to experience your inner peace and inner joy.
- **Step 7: Healing Affirmations**—Focus on healing affirmations that are strong feelings of purpose, conviction, belief, and self-acceptance. Affirmations open your heart and heal your soul. Believe in the destiny

of these affirmations. Expect these affirmations to ring the bell of truth. Experience your soul power much like you experience the warmth of the sun when you are sunbathing. Practice the following affirmations or make up your own. To get the best results, repeat these affirmations for at least one minute. You get exceptional results when you can devote three minutes or more, as your time frame allows. Be certain to keep your upward gaze steady and focused on your third eye.

SELF-HEALING AFFIRMATIONS	
• I believe in myself.	• I expect to be happy.
• I love life.	• Heal my mind, heal my body, heal my heart, and heal my soul.
• My faith will make me whole.	• The power of creation loves me!

- **Step 8: Practice Your ABEs and AVEs**—In this step, you take your weight-loss affirmations to the next level. Three effective weight-loss affirmations are:

  – I need to lose weight permanently.
  – I must lose weight permanently.
  – I will lose weight permanently.

  Using these affirmations, this is where you can practice your ABE or AVE techniques introduced in mind power. Beliefs are self-fulfilling. Creative visualizations make all the difference in the world. When doing an ABE, focus on your belief in your affirmation. When doing an AVE, tap into the power of visualization. See your dreams come true before you. Guide your imagination to visualize an optimal situation, lifestyle, or circumstance. Picture power counts.

- **Step 9: Expect**—Finish your affirmation with a deep expectation that your affirmation will be achieved. Try to experience what it feels like to achieve the goal of your affirmation.

- **Step 10: Let Go and Flow**—Relax, let go, and flow with inner joy and peace. Transcend your busy mind, and bliss out! Concentrate on your feelings of heartfelt love, joy, and peace. Experience the inner peace of your soul power.

Practice makes perfect. Use this self-healing meditation technique to achieve your PWL goals. It won't let you down.

LYF-Skill #2—How to Create the Triangle of Divine Fire

Divine Fire is one of the keys to lasting soul power. Divine Fire is your strength of spirit. It is the penetrating flame of soul power.

It can be said that Divine Fire is the love of Spirit, the love of life, the love of being alive, the will to live, and the will to love—all wrapped up in one. It is an all-consuming heartfelt love. It goes deep and addresses the urgency of your heart. It heals the heartaches of your soul while it purges negative thoughts and feelings within. Divine Fire is your appetite for life—your appetite for fulfillment, happiness, prosperity, thrills, and excitement. It gives you a step in your walk and a sparkle to your eyes.

Divine Fire Is the Path of Self-Inspiration

In effect, Divine Fire is the life principle that sustains you. It blazes the path of self-empowerment, self-awareness, and self-realization. It is the path of self-inspiration. You will need all the self-inspiration you can get to maintain good health, wellness, and permanent weight loss. Your self-inspiration and your appetite for life will empower you to overcome the five villains of PWL and the everyday ups, downs, and disappointments that play havoc with your eating habits. Divine Fire is strong enough to reverse negativity and neutralize the hazardous impact of worry, doubt, fear of inadequacy, and emotional stress.

The Triangle of the Divine Fire

The foundation to your Divine Fire is a triangle of dynamic inner powers. Divine Fire is accurately symbolized by the following equilateral triangle. There are three main sides, three main corners, and three equal forces. Together they make for strength and stability. Yes, there are three spiritual muscles—love, faith, and peace of mind—that need daily exercise for you to develop the Divine Fire.

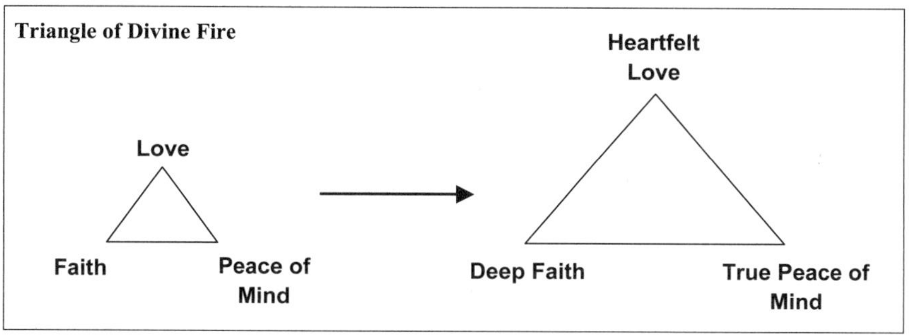

Faith in spirit, heartfelt love, and peace of mind come together to enrich your soul power. You see, with love in your heart, faith in your spirit, and peace in your mind, you create a sound and strong equilateral triangle of support that feeds your soul. Divine Fire replaces restlessness with inner peace, nervousness with inner joy, and anxiety with a strong belief in yourself. In this way, Divine Fire naturally suppresses your appetite for food, makes you less susceptible to temptations and distractions, and supports self-enriching choices and behaviors. Divine Fire works because of the synergy between your faith, heartfelt love, and peace of mind.

Divine Fire, Corner #1—Deep Faith

Vitamin F is one of the essential keys to building Divine Fire. Vitamin F, or faith, is having confidence in what you believe. Remember that you heard it from me first. You can never have enough faith, Divine Fire, or soul power.

With Vitamin F, your intentions and your beliefs work together, synergistically helping you to achieve superior weight control. Faith is the willingness to believe in the fulfillment of your dreams. As it might relate to your metabolism, faith is knowing in your gut that you will lose your excess weight and keep it off for good.

Faith is also knowing that you can grow in all circumstances. In other words, adversity has a silver lining. Vitamin F sees to it that regardless of the challenges, disappointments or setbacks you may incur, *you find the way to make the necessary adjustments in your mood, attitude, inner resolve, and circumstances* to stay on track with your LYF Program. When you own the faith, you have a total belief that you have the inner power to be whole, fit, trim, and happy. You really believe that you can go all the way. No matter what the predicament, the faith dictates that you will find the inner strength to see things to a favorable resolution and achieve your PWL goals.

Faith Feeds Divine Fire

Faith is a way of believing in your mind and heart that things will work out and that you are capable of working through any challenging situation. This may sound simple, but it will help resolve persistent anxiety or fear in your life. This simple belief is food for your soul. It puts you at ease and gives you the conviction to do whatever you need to do to achieve your goals.

You Need to Have the Faith

The faith is a spiritual muscle. It needs to flex to grow. You can do this. Day by day, develop the faith to overcome any dilemma by believing in the power of your faith. Develop the habit of having the faith. This will activate your faith to grow and grow. Start with the small predicaments that challenge your eating habits. Catch yourself when you get down on yourself and buy into negative inner chatter. Turn to Vitamin F to turn things around.

Think about this. How do you rebound from a dietary blunder? For example, you are at your best friend's birthday party and binge on birthday cake. Count on Vitamin F. What do you do to keep from getting depressed and self-critical when you have not lost all the weight you had intended to lose for your sister's wedding? Use Vitamin F to stay on track in the face of adversity or disappointment. See how faith has a powerful organizing influence on your mind.

Faith is the union of belief, trust, intention, and spiritual conviction. It grounds your soul to the possibility of miracles. Life is a miracle. Do you appreciate being alive, or do you take the gift of life for granted? It is high time to realize that life is miraculous and that you have the opportunity to achieve permanent weight loss. Faith steers you through the storms of your life and keeps you on track with your eating habits. Faith breathes oxygen to the spirit, without which the Divine Fire of the spirit has no flame. You can build the bridge of faith. Follow the action steps below and watch your faith take over your life.

FAITH: ACTION STEP #1— "HOW TO CULTIVATE FAITH" MEDITATION

- Find a Natural Setting—Find a natural setting to meditate. Skillfully relax your body and mind. Sit up straight, and listen to your breathing for a few moments. Relax fully. Breathe deeply and put your focus within. Feel your heart center. Steady your eyes. Now then, do the following:

- Reflect on Your 10 B's—Warm up to the faith by asking yourself what blessings in life you have to be thankful for? Now write your top ten blessings on a piece of paper. I like to call these blessings your 10 B's. Reflect on your 10 B's and it will help you get in touch with your faith. Once you have warmed up to your faith, relax and let go even further.

- Use Your Imagination—Imagine yourself in a room where you are surrounded by a warm bright halo of light—warm like sunlight. This warm light represents your faith. Inhale the warm sunlight; and as you bring the warmth and light into your body, feel the faith expanding within your body much like your breathing expands your lungs. As you inhale, ask yourself what in your weight-loss program needs to get better? Is it your focus, your attitude, your exercise, or maybe your late-night eating habits? Then listen! The key is to listen in silent prayer to yourself, and tune into the intuitive wisdom of your inner voice.

- Action Steps—Be patient, and await your answers. Now ask yourself, "What specific actions can I take to improve my weight-loss plan?" Then move forward with your strong and active faith in yourself to get the job done.

- Recruit the Faith—Keep the faith through thick and thin. Keep breathing into your expanding balloon until you feel swollen inside with the faith. Keep in mind that faith is food to your soul just as love is nutrition to your heart. Practice this exercise so you may recruit the faith to resolve conflicts and further strengthen your Divine Fire.

Faith: Action Step #2—Additional Faith Meditation

Another meditation technique for developing the faith is to repeat over and over the affirmation, "My faith will make me whole." Say this often in silent prayer.

Remember, with practice, discipline, repetition, and focus, you can learn to use your faith to heal your soul, contribute to Divine Fire, and keep your spirits high. Try to believe that no matter what the predicament, you can find the inner strength to see it through to a favorable conclusion. Now then, to apply it right now, answer the following question:

- What kind of things can you do, starting now, to build your faith?

Stand by Your Faith

With your faith guiding you, open your mind, expand your awareness, and believe in the infinite healing power of your Divine Fire. When you have the faith, you are comfortable in emotionally surrendering your deepest spiritual convictions to the higher order of the universe. "Let thy will be done," Paramahansa Yogananda teaches, is the single most effective prayer there is. Faith is born out of complete yielding to the will of the Spirit. Faith is one of the keys to opening the magic door of the Divine Fire. Do you have the faith in the healing powers of your own Divine Fire?

When you move forward in your life with a strong active belief in yourself and in your LYF program, you are on the path to having faith. Strong characters of faith know the more you experience faith, the more Divine Fire you will generate and unleash. Make the commitment to develop the faith and embellish your Divine Fire.

Divine Fire, Corner #2—Heartfelt Love

Heartfelt love is the foundation to Divine Fire. Heartfelt love is the next spiritual muscle to awaken as you follow down the path of Divine Fire. Love is the most powerful healing force in the universe. The deeper the love connection in your most valued love relationships, the greater the love in your life is—and the more meaning and fullness to your life. These deep feelings of love and fulfillment feed your soul.

Be Rich in Love

You have the option to experience love or experience fear as the dominant emotion in your life. You can choose your love for life over your fear of rejection or abandonment as your prevailing mind-set. Your level of heartfelt love is the catalyst to the awakening of Divine Fire. It is only through your ongoing expansion of heartfelt love that your soul can eventually ascend the different levels of consciousness and become spiritually awakened to healing your soul. Heartfelt love breeds positive belief systems, self-confidence, inner peace, inner joy, and fulfillment. I have observed that heartfelt love is a magnet that attracts positive energy, conviction, and success. Alternatively, fear breeds negative belief systems, self-doubt, inadequacy, restlessness, and anxiety. I've come to realize that fear can also act as a magnet and will inevitably attract failure.

Rich in love, rich in life. Rich in money and not rich in love? Not rich in life. How rich in love is your life? Do you usually feel loving and giving, or do you typically feel deprived? I believe that the quality of your life can be measured by the kinds and amounts of love in your life. Self-inspiration makes you love and appreciate life to the fullest. Indeed, Vitamin L, love, and Vitamin F, faith, open the gates to Divine Fire!

How to Be Rich in Love, Rich in Life

How do you become rich in love? Make a difference in other people's lives. Enrich others. Pour your love into those you believe in and trust. As John Lennon said, the more love you make, the more love you take. Indeed, the more love you radiate, the more you will get back in return.

Heartfelt Love: Action Step #1

At the end of each day, be sure to ask yourself the following questions:

- How much love did I generate today for the people who came into my life?
- How often do I tell the people in my life, "I love you?"
- What can I do to make those I care about feel more valued, loved, and appreciated?

Feel yourself pregnant with love. This is an important technique for developing love in your heart. Expand your love relationships. Become a channel of love. Carry this love with you everywhere you go.

Heartfelt Love: Action Step #2

To enhance your feelings of heartfelt love, go back and look at the most basic primary love relationships you have with the following:

• Yourself	• The Divine
• Loved Ones	• Nature

Now, one at a time, experience the energizing love you have for each one of these relationships.

- Turn your attention to your heart. Feel the soft, beautiful warmth within your chest. Take some cleansing breaths.
- Affirm softly with each inhalation, "My heart is alive."
- After a deep inhalation, pause, enjoy the breathless state, and focus your attention on the love you have for one of the four primary love relationships listed above.
- Then with expiration, say, "With pure love and joy."
- Therefore, "My heart is alive" (inhalation), pause, and focus on a primary love relationship, and then say, "with pure love and joy" (expiration).

This affirmation technique enables you to feel the expansion of love, Vitamin L, in your heart. Experience the love you have for each primary relationship and stay with it. Try to experience it from deep in your heart. For each primary relationship, repeat this affirmation for three to five minutes. The full cycle of affirmations should take you approximately fifteen to twenty minutes.

Heartfelt Love: Action Step #3

Acknowledge your love for life. To do this, follow the ATG's below.

- "A" stands for Appreciate: in your daily prayer/meditation time, spend some time reflecting on how much you appreciate being alive.
- "T" stands for Thankfulness: every day acknowledge your thankfulness for all the blessings in your life
- "G" stands for Gratefulness: life is meant to be loved. Be grateful and never take the miracle of your life for granted. Take a moment and write down your 10 G's, the ten things you are most grateful for.

Experience Heartfelt Love

From the inner reservoir of your love for self, loved ones, the divine, and nature, your love grows into strength and compassion. This inspires you to believe in yourself and feeds a very positive self-esteem. These are powerful allies in your quest for permanent weight loss.

Loving people are happy people, and those who feel the most love, feed their heart the right kind of soul food. Heartfelt love that feeds your soul takes your appetite for dietary food away. You know you are tending to your Divine Fire when you feel pure love and joy in your heart. This is enriched by a deep pride in being alive. When your thankfulness and gratefulness are exemplified by your inner powers of inner joy and heartfelt love, you are on your way to feeding the flames of Divine Fire. It is important to note that your love power is there for you to embrace at all times.

Divine Fire, Corner #3—True Peace of Mind

Vitamin P, peace of mind, is the third vital component in creating the triangle of Divine Fire. Inner peace is a cornerstone to your Divine Fire. It enriches your life and puts a smile in your heart. Inner peace, or Vitamin P, completes the corners of the equilateral triangle of Divine Fire.

The inner working of these three spiritual muscles is the essence of Divine Fire. Together, faith, heartfelt love, and peace of mind will help you sustain good eating habits and a strong Metabolic Fire. No one but you can bring inner peace to your life. It is up to you to tap into your source of inner peace. When you take the time to get in touch with yourself, you'll realize inner peace is the natural state of your inner being. All you have to do is dial into it. When you stop and quiet things down, tranquility is the natural feeling deep in your soul.

When you figure out what is important in your life, it is easy to find this inner peace. By making important things important to you, and paying attention to what is important, you can generate even greater levels of inner tranquility. By keeping your life in stride, you can slow down inside. Inner peace is the antidote to unresolved emotional stress or EMT.

Lasting, real peace of mind is the skill of heightened self-awareness. Get in touch with your love for life and experience the peace. This inner peace begets creativity, productivity, and sound decision making. Furthermore, peace of mind is a soothing tonic for your soul. Real peace of mind results from being at ease with who you are and at one with what you are doing with your life. Peace of mind is the kind of soul food that takes your appetite for cravings and overeating away. Vitamin P is a strong advocate of the Golden Rules of Smart Eating.

Peace of Mind: Action Step #1— Shangri-la Can Be Yours

Practice this simple Shangri-la exercise whenever you are restless, nervous, anxious, uptight, upset, or out of touch. It will help you find your inner calmness.

- Relax, take some cleansing breaths, and tune into the love in your heart. Center yourself. Close your eyes, and steady your eyes with a gentle upward gaze at your third eye.
- Now then, with your eyes closed, see yourself climbing a flight of story-book stairs to one of your favorite vacation retreats. Feel the exhilaration of being where you love to be.
- Turn your visualization into your Shangri-la, your heavenly dream setting. Create a Shangri-la environment with your imagination. Use your vivid mind to embellish your favorite retreat with all the circumstances

and details of how you would love to spend your time. Recruit birds singing, the wind whistling, and the sunshine and the sunsets that go along with a fabulous adventure and vacation. Consider the kind of people you would have there with you. Imagine having them to be the most fulfilling love relationships you have ever had. Long lost feelings are coming back. Hold this vision, and feel this experience. Enjoy.

- Now let yourself go. Become the happy star or starlet of your own movie. You are the hero or heroine in Shangri-la. Lights, camera, action! The scene is set. Spend fifteen minutes enjoying this movie. Take this peace and calmness of Shangri-la with you wherever you go.

Now then, think about your everyday lifestyle. Ask yourself:

- What action steps can I take to create more peace of mind at home, at work, and with my social life?

Peace of Mind: Action Step #2

Peace of mind comes from within. Whenever you meditate, make sure to take a few minutes to concentrate on feelings of heartfelt love, inner joy, and inner peace. These are the true feelings that exist within us all once we take the time to shut off our minds and outside distractions. Experience what this inner peace, love, and joy feels like. Capture these peaceful feelings and try to carry them with you throughout the day. Whenever you feel stressed, anxious, restless, or nervous, take a minute to get back in touch with those feelings. The more you meditate, the more inner peace will permeate your feelings throughout the day. Remember, it is important to dial in. Inner peace is always there no matter what the circumstance. It is just a matter of slowing things down, quieting things down, and getting in touch with it.

Focus Your Willpower to Synergize the Components of Divine Fire

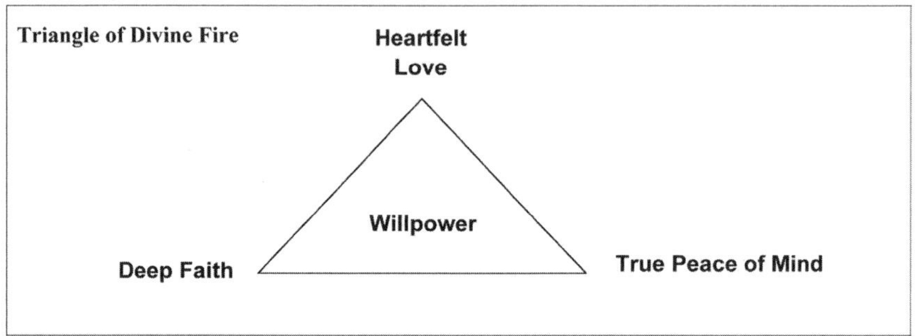

At the center of your healing triangle is your willpower. Sitting in the center of the vortex of this triangular energy, your willpower drives your spiritual muscles and whips them into shape. You need your willpower to keep your focus on your Divine Fire, your eating habits, and your Metabolic Fire. You need willpower to monitor your intention.

Your willpower aims to develop your soul power, as well as your faith, love, and peace of mind. Make it a deep conviction of yours to develop these necessary components of Divine Fire. Keep the faith, be peaceful, and, above all, experience the love and light in your soul. You know you are drinking the nectar of the Divine Fire when you experience more love, joy, and peace every day. This will show up as self-control and effective self-regulation of your eating habits. With a strong will, you can zoom in and stay focused on your love for Divine Fire. This transforms you into a new level of awareness that makes it a simple matter to eat Smart Foods and eat them well.

LYF-Skill #3—Define Your Purpose in Life

Your purpose in life is a very important part of your lifestyle. In fact, your purpose in life plays a pivotal role in sustaining your soul power. Your soul power thrives in the context of a meaningful, purposeful life. How so? Having purpose means spending time doing things that make you happy and bring you a sense of inner fulfillment. This motivates, inspires, and energizes you. This inner fulfillment resonates deep in your soul. Purposeful living is conducive to inner peace and joy. It enables you to live in harmony with your deepest beliefs and convictions. Living a soulful, soul-filled, purposeful life is Smart Food for your soul. Your purpose in life feeds your spiritual health and is a stepping-stone to long-lasting soul power.

I find it fascinating that, just as the mind needs to think positively, the heart needs to love, and the body needs exercise; the soul needs purpose! Everyone has his or her own unique purpose. In addition, we all share a similar purpose in our efforts to be healthy, happy, fit, and well. It takes some quiet time looking within to clearly define your purpose. Then it takes the rest of your life to follow it.

Let's get down to basics. Your purpose in life is your direction in life. It is your cause, your mission, your objective. The purpose in your life touches your heart and activates your soul to come alive. You see, your purpose shapes your identity. Simply said, your purpose is defined by what means the most to you and what has the greatest value to you. Your purpose is your endless determination to find your place in the sun. In time, it becomes the ceaseless commitment to your happiness and well-being and the prophecy of your soul. Have you spent some time determining whether you have found your purpose in life?

Your Soul Needs Purpose to Thrive

Living with purpose breeds inner fulfillment, inner peace, and inner joy. Purpose inspires and motivates. Yet just as purposeful living nourishes the soul, the opposite also rings true. A lack of purpose is very stressful and creates restlessness and self-defeating anxiety. This is more than disruptive to your eating habits. Purposelessness erodes soul power. It takes the wind out of your sails and is conducive to depression. It weakens the immune system and essentially increases your vulnerability to illness. When you lack purpose, you feel trapped. Your soul suffocates and begins to burn out. This is most clearly seen in successful executives who, within two years after retirement, are either dead, severely depressed, or suffering from cancer, heart disease, or other disabling, degenerative illnesses. What happened? These people had purpose with their work. Their work gave them a sense of usefulness and being needed. Once their work ended, they lost their purpose in life. They did not cultivate purpose outside the boundaries of their work, money, or career. This apparent lack of purpose becomes unsettling to the point where it actually affects people's health. It would be unfair to single out successful executives as the only people struggling with their purpose in life. Look at the common life crises of teenagers, college graduates, people turning thirty or forty, mid-lifers, menopausal women, divorcees, retirees, or career changers. These crises center on one common thread. People are reevaluating the direction or purpose in their life. They are saying to themselves, "There has to be more to life than this." Well, I am here to assure you that there is.

As long as you are breathing, you have a purpose in life. Lack of purpose in life is really a mirage. Purposelessness, in fact, is an escape. It is convenient to say you have no purpose because it often represents the path of least resistance. The fact is we all have a purpose in life. You are endowed with a unique purpose with special qualities and individual features to develop this purpose. You and I and every living soul on this planet have a special mission in this lifetime.

You Are the Captain of Your Soul

In looking for purpose, once again, it is totally up to you. You face the challenges of staying in harmony with your purpose in life. This is no simple matter since your purpose in life changes in accordance with how your values change. It is your responsibility to know yourself and get in touch with what turns on your heart and soul. Only you know what means the most to you. Everyone has the privilege to validate their mission and develop their unique qualities.

We Have More Than One Purpose

Our purpose in life is multidimensional. Your mind, body, spirit, and heart each have purpose. You also have purpose in your connection with loved ones, family, and friends. You can also have a purpose in relationship to your career. There are a number of different ways to look at your purpose in life. You can find purpose in life spiritually, emotionally, mentally, and physically. Purposeful living is defined as being the best at being yourself. You can find purpose in being needed, in being useful, and by enriching the lives of others.

In speaking to a spiritual master, one may say that your purpose in life is to become self-realized and to know the depths of your blissful and peaceful soul. It can be argued that your purpose in life is to be reborn every day, to be fresh and alive, and to be totally yourself. Others might reason that your purpose in life is to grow up in your first twenty-five years, raise your family and dedicate to your career from twenty-five to fifty, and thereafter, find enlightenment. Some others may argue that your purpose is to die well with a smile on your face. Whatever you discover, a conscious commitment to your purpose in life will lead you to the highest levels of soul power.

You can also say that the purpose in life is to be happy, healthy, and free. The key is that when you pursue whatever it takes to be happy, healthy, and free, you will naturally come to terms with your purpose in life. Why? Because your happiness, your health, and your freedom guide you to long-lasting fulfillment and purposeful living. Staying on purpose means you are addressing your most important needs, not just your transitory wants and desires. This feeds your happiness and feeds your soul.

Purpose Feeds PWL

Let's take a look at all of the ways that purpose, or a lack thereof, can impact your PWL plan.

Purpose	➡	• Fulfillment • Happiness • Harmony with Beliefs and Convictions	➡	Soul Power	➡	• Smart Eating Habits • Weight Loss
Lack of Purpose	➡	• Restlessness • Anxiety	➡	Spiritual Fatigue	➡	• Self-Defeating Behaviors • Poor Eating Habits • Weight Gain

Without purpose, you cannot sustain wholesome, smart eating habits. When you lack purpose, restlessness can dominate your lifestyle, leaving you vulnerable to self-destructive eating and living habits. The time has come to take action and live in harmony with your purpose.

Purpose: Action Step #1—How to Find Your Purpose in Life

The following questions will help you become comfortable with finding your purpose in life. Find an inspiring, tranquil setting, and with pencil and paper in hand, answer these questions:

- What is missing in your life?
- What means more to you than anything else in your life?
- In what area of life do you want to make a difference more than any other?
- What kind of contribution do you want to make to your fellow man and woman?

- What, more than anything else, do you want to do with your precious life?
- What is it in life that you long to experience?
- How would you prefer to spend the majority of your time?
- Do you wake up each morning with love in your heart, enthusiastic and excited about a new day? If not, what will it take to feel this way!

Find Your Purpose

When you have purpose, you are excited and ready to be alive and live a fulfilling lifestyle. Sometimes, you have to get past thinking about duties, obligations, and responsibilities to get to know your purpose. For example, use the following questions to gain insight that can be supportive in your search.

- If you were a millionaire and money was no object, how would you spend your time?
- How would you spend the next six to nine months if you were told you only had that much longer to live?
- What do you live for?
- What is your cause?
- What are you trying to get people to understand?

Purpose: Action Step #2—Soulful Introspection

Finding your purpose in life is facilitated by getting to know your higher loving self. Through a regular, consistent, in-depth meditation program, you can become tuned into your inner wisdom and find your purpose. Creative, soulful introspection is the guiding light and strategy that will give you your answers. Run your purpose by the kingdom of God-consciousness within you.

Use the following formula to find your purpose in life.

- Spend time alone in a quiet, tranquil, natural, outdoor setting. For example, listen to the crashing waves, the birds in the morning sun, or the penetrating rhythm of a mountain stream.

- Feel the bliss in your heart, quiet your mind, steady your eyes, and find the secrets of your soul. Ten deep cleansing breaths will enable you to let your mental barriers down and let go.
- Focus on what you are feeling; turn off your mind and your thinking. Listen to your breathing. Feel and experience inner silence.
- Let the silence lead you to recognize your inner essence, and acknowledge the uniqueness of your very own self. Fully accept who you are; appreciate and love yourself.
- Look within and see yourself meeting up with a wise sage in your natural setting. Ask him or her, "What is my cause? What do I most strongly believe in? What is my purpose in life?" This is just a way to enable you to communicate with your inner self. The wise sage you are speaking to is your soul!
- Wait for the answer. Keep repeating this exercise daily until the answer is revealed.

How to Chart Your Purpose

Now then, make three separate columns for each different purpose you discover. In the first column, list your purpose. In the second column, note any obstacles to this purpose. In the third column, determine the action steps necessary to make this purpose a reality. Follow the examples in the columns below for this exercise.

Purpose	Obstacles	Action Steps
1. Find true love.	• Negative thinking.	• Take charge of my attitude and beliefs.
2. Teach English to learning-disabled.	• Trapped at present job.	• Get new credentials.
3. Heal my body.	• Digestive troubles.	• Change my diet; reduce my stress.

Purpose: Action Step #3—Passion Leads to Purpose

Another major technique for determining your purpose in life is to find out what really turns you on. In other words, be true to the passions in your life. Think back to what truly turns you on. Make a list of the top three things that you are most passionate about and love the most. How often do you spend time doing these things? Taking time engaging in the activities that you love the most will rekindle your passion for life. In pursuing your passions in life, you will bring your purpose into clear focus. Do not allow anything to stop you from being happy, joyful, and purposeful.

Now, take some time to answer the questions in this look-within quiz. This will help you find out what turns you on. After you get impregnated with your passions, go for it! Honoring and pursuing the passions in your life will bring purpose to your life.

LYF "Look Within" Quiz

1. My joys in life are ____________________.
2. I love to ____________________.
3. ____________________ turns me on.
4. I find ____________________ to be the most exciting thing in my life.
5. The thrill of my life is ____________________.
6. I enjoy being alone and doing ____________________.
7. The secret, untold fantasies in my life are ____________________.

8. I find ____________________ more interesting than anything in my life.
9. My greatest fascination in life is ____________________.
10. The most fun things in my life are ____________________.
11. The kinds of things I want to do with my life and have not yet done are ____________________.
12. ____________________ will give me more freedom in my life.
13. To be happy, I need ____________________ in my life.
14. More than anything else, I care about ____________________.
15. I have the strongest belief in ____________________ in my life.
16. I find joy in my heart when ____________________.
17. I want to take an adventure to ____________________.
18. ____________________ makes me feel really good inside.
19. ____________________ takes me to the limit.
20. My emotions are aroused by ____________________.
21. ____________________ inspires me to live each day to the fullest.
22. I would like to do ____________________ that nobody else has ever done.
23. The inconsistencies I am perplexed by are____________________.
24. I cannot stand ____________________.
25. In my free time, I like to ____________________.

Turning on to the passion, joy, and love in your life transforms the mystery of your life into the miracle of your life. These simple revelations of what turns you on triggers creative self-expression. This enriches your soul power. This gives you the strength of character you have been looking for. What a great feeling! Pursue your passions, and it will give you purpose. This natural process opens the door to keeping your Divine Fire and Metabolic Fire fully alive.

Purpose Leads to Soul Power

Use the guidelines in this chapter to find the mission and passion in your life. You will find your purpose. Honor yourself and your true feelings. Take your purpose to the next level. What will it take to get you inspired? When you are prepared to pay any price, bear any burden, and are willing to meet any hardship to be true to your purpose, you are playing the game of life true to your soul powers. Remember, point yourself in the direction of what turns you on and what feels right for you. Stand up for what you believe. Find the passion in your life and kindle its fire in the seat of your soul. Creatively express yourself and your spirituality, and you will be in stride and on target.

With purpose, you will experience emotional infinity in your spiritual timelessness. This will overcome any restlessness, worries, or anxieties that could disrupt your eating habits and sabotage your LYF Plan.

With these points in mind, what is your purpose in life?

____

____

____

____

____

____

____

____

24

Feed Your Heart—Develop Mood Power

DID you ever stop to realize that your emotional life is always present? Typically, your mood tells the story of your emotional life. You may have noticed that your mood is one of the more colorful aspects of your personality. Your mood refers to your humor, temperament, or disposition at any particular time. In the simplest of terms, your mood is your emotional frame of mind. Your mood is the prevailing feeling that determines your outlook on life. You will often hear folks speak about being in a good or bad mood. When you are in a good mood, you are present to life and tuned into all its wonders and opportunities. A good mood gives you a sense of happiness and well-being.

Have you noticed that your mood is the lens through which you see life? Looking at life through the lens of a good mood highlights all of the great things that are happening around you. Alternatively, when you look at life through the lens of a bad mood, it restricts your vision and dampens your thinking. A bad mood invites negativity. A bad mood lends itself to irritability, anxiety, grumpiness, and uneasiness. When you are in a bad mood, you lose touch with your sense of happiness and are typically consumed by stress and emotional tension. Yes, moods have either a positive or negative charge to them. At the end of the day, there are just two types of moods—those that are self-enriching and those that are self-defeating.

Your Moods and Your Eating Habits

So why are moods so important when it comes to PWL? We have learned that moods have an enormous influence over our behavior, actions, and habits; especially our eating habits. In fact, it is imperative that you realize that it is very common for people to turn to food to regulate their moods. It is true, good moods invite wholesome eating habits. But equally or more important, bad moods often threaten and sabotage your eating habits and PWL plan.

Mood Power Is the Ability to Self-Regulate Your Mood

When you come to terms with what it takes to lose weight permanently, it becomes time to answer to your moods. My thousands of weight-loss consultations have made this very clear to me; when your prevailing mood is positive, it is a simple matter to follow the Golden Rules of Smart Eating. You will need mood power to do this.

This chapter is about developing mood power. Mood power fortifies your LYF Program and helps you achieve your permanent weight-loss goals. How so? In its most basic form, mood power is the ability to self-regulate your mood. So what does it mean when you can self-regulate your mood? Self-regulating your mood comes down to your ability to be positive and stay positive. It is up to you to keep yourself in a good mood. When you can self-regulate your mood, you know how to secure a good mood in friendly, supportive, as well as trying circumstances.

The purpose of self-regulating your mood is to keep yourself upbeat and to keep your spirits high; in other words, to keep yourself in a good mood. The stability and durability of your mood power is seen in your ability to withstand stress, disappointments, emotional tension, emotional upheaval, or financial pressure. It takes a strong person to stay emotionally grounded and anchored to weather the storms that may come in and out of your life. This means that, except for tragedy or significant loss, it is up to you to keep your prevailing mood positive. Life has many ups, downs, and disappointments. It is a simple matter to let things get under your skin and cause bad moods or mood swings. The predicament is that to master your eating habits you need your prevailing mood to be positive. When you lack mood power, moodiness and mood volatility can take over. When your prevailing mood is more negative than positive, it triggers off an incredible vulnerability to overeating and food indulgences. Yes, it takes inner strength to raise your spirits and bring your prevailing mood back into the light and away from the darkness.

The Three Muscles of Mood Power

There are three important muscles that build the necessary horsepower you will need to self-regulate your mood and generate mood power.

THE THREE MUSCLES OF MOOD POWER
Learn how to: 1. Create a Positive Mood. 2. Sustain a Positive Mood. 3. Quickly Recover from a Bad Mood.

Exercising these three muscles is the essence of mood power. You will learn how to do this by following the guidelines and action steps outlined in this chapter. When you have mastered these skills, you will have acquired the habits of happiness that will keep you in a good mood.

Your Moods Can Change

No one is in a good mood all of the time. Furthermore, I do not believe it is humanly possible to stay in the same mood permanently. The best of moods get challenged by life's ups and downs. We all experience disappointment from time to time, whether at home, with the family, or at work. The sun does not shine every hour of every day, nor is it cloudy all the time. Even the worst mood will eventually swing back in the other direction at some point in time. When you can't shake a bad mood, you often find a negative, self-defeating mood has taken hold. Along with a bad mood, it is common to find yourself in the midst of food cravings. You may want to turn to food to comfort you and boost your mood. When you take charge of your emotional life, however, you can get back on track. This is what I like to call emotional self-responsibility.

Emotional Self-Response-Ability: It Is Up to You

It is up to you to keep yourself in a good mood. It is up to you to tune into how you are feeling. Unless you tune into your radio, you are not present or aware of what at that moment is on the airways. After all, who really knows what you are feeling and how it is affecting you except for yourself? Your mood certainly is not anyone else's responsibility. What does it look like to be responsible for your moods and emotions? It looks good. It looks like emotional self-responsibility.

Emotional self-response-*ability* is the ability to respond to circumstances constructively and sustain a favorable mood. In essence, emotional self-responsibility describes your ability to be accountable to your emotional life. The kind of emotional self-responsibility that leads to PWL is the responsibility to keep your prevailing mood upbeat. It is the emotional equivalent of owning a positive mental attitude. Emotional self-responsibility is a cornerstone to mood power.

In way of summary, everyone knows what it is like to be in a good mood. Your prevailing mood tells the story of your emotional life. When you have mood power, you are typically in a very good mood and know how to keep it that way. When your prevailing mood is lighthearted, chipper, bright, and happy, you are in the throws of being in good spirits, better known as a good mood. A good mood is conducive to self-control. Alternatively, when you lack mood power, you are vulnerable to mood swings; shifts in your mood tend to be more dramatic, volatile, and unpredictable. An unfavorable mood favors impulsive, compulsive behavior. Furthermore, mood swings commonly trigger hazardous food swings.

The Four Cycles of a Bad Mood

You can be proactive or inactive in dealing with your moods. The predicament is as follows: when you are inactive, self-defeating moods can dominate and self-defeating behavior is the rule. Self-defeating moods are the enemy—the stick in the mud—to those looking to achieve PWL. The good news is that there is a solution. You can learn how to purge self-defeating moods. First, let's take a brief journey and see what happens to a bad mood. There are four possibilities.

A bad mood can:

1. Be self-regulated back to a good mood.
2. Eventually revert to a better mood.
3. Persist as is.
4. Escalate into a more negative mind-set.

Let's take a closer look at these scenarios.

1. A Bad Mood Can Be Self-Regulated Back to a Good Mood.

Getting your emotions back on track is a tricky business. It takes know-how. Sometimes, you can quickly shake off a sour mood. Sometimes, the bad mood can drag on. Happy, well-adjusted people still get tested by the stress and strain of modern-day living; and minor, short-lived mood swings are common. Depending on the situation, they may even be normal, natural reactions to troublesome events, disappointment, or upsetting news. But when it comes to those everyday bad moods, the quicker you bounce back, the better your physical and mental health will be. Mood power is your ability to be resourceful and resilient and gracefully bounce back into a good mood.

2. A Bad Mood Can Eventually Revert to a Better Mood.

Were you to wait long enough, something usually happens within hours, days, or weeks to bring you back into a better mood. It is like the way the body repairs itself after you have had a cold. Eventually, the body catches up, and the cold or flu goes away. The longer the bad mood lasts, however, the more you are susceptible to self-defeating behavior. It is up to you whether you want to be proactive or inactive to the onset of an unpleasant mood.

3. ***A Bad Mood Can Persist As Is.***

   Low-level depression, pervasive malaise, impatience, brooding, grumpiness, irritability, apathy, or an indefinable sadness can linger for hours, sometimes days. Typically, your eating habits are in jeopardy. More so, the longer the moodiness persists, the more likely a dysfunctional eating habit is on the horizon.

4. ***A Bad Mood Can Escalate into a More Negative Mind-Set.***

   Bad moods may extend into deeper depression, heightened anxiety, and extreme irritability. Sometimes, these escalations occur suddenly. You may be in the middle of a normal conversation; but within minutes, your temper flares, and you lose all composure. Other times, bad moods spread slowly, insidiously taking root until you're trapped, and you can't remember when you last felt happy.

The Five Factors That Influence Your Mood

By now it should be clear that your PWL plan will benefit from being proactive in self-regulating your mood. So how do you go about doing this? By regulating the key components that impact your mood. Your mood is a result of the interaction between your nerves, your hormones, and your emotional profile. There are five important factors that influence your mood. When you can favorably influence these factors to create a good mood, sustain a good mood, and quickly recover from a bad mood, you will have achieved a level of mood power that will feed your heart and keep you light in mind and body. Take a look at the "Mood Pie" that follows, which details these five dimensions.

The Mood Pie

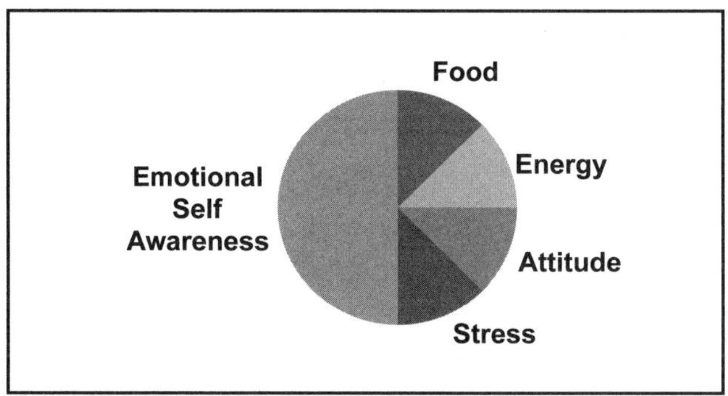

As an example, let's take a look at two of these key factors, your energy and stress levels, and see how they might influence your mood. When you are energetic and calm, you tend to be in a better mood. Alternatively, when you are tired and tense, you are more prone to a bad mood. As we walk through each dimension of the mood pie, you will be given the tools to work these factors to your favor. This will support a healthy emotional life and outlook. Before we move on, take note of how each factor can either support mood power or moodiness.

Mood Power	Moodiness
• Emotional Self-Awareness	• Faulty Emotional Self-Awareness
• High Energy	• Fatigue
• Positive Mental Attitude	• Negative Mental Attitude
• Calmness and Peace of Mind	• High Stress
• Smart Foods	• Unhealthy Foods

I believe that now is the time to take a closer look at how these factors impact you. This will help you to develop your mood power, take charge of your moods, and safeguard your eating habits.

Mood Factor #1— Emotional Self-Awareness

Emotional self-awareness is defined by knowing how you feel and standing up for yourself and what you need to be happy. When you are emotionally self-aware, you know:

- What you are feeling;
- How to experience the scope of your feelings, good and bad;
- How to size up your feelings and put them in perspective;
- How to express your feelings constructively to others; and
- How to shift into a better mood and stay there.

It is common for people to go through mood changes each day depending on their circumstances. It is going to take emotional strength and emotional know-how to embrace the dynamic process of emotional self-awareness. Yes, emotional self-awareness calls for emotional know-how. The know how to do what? The know how to do the following:

- Create a good mood.
- Sustain a good mood.
- Recover from a bad mood.

That is, you'll need emotional know-how to work, apply, and use the three muscles of mood power.

As illustrated in the following table, emotional self-awareness is a three-step process. The first step, emotional self-discovery, will teach you how to create a good mood. The second step, emotional attunement, details how to sustain a good mood. The third step, emotional self-discipline, will be necessary to quickly recover from a bad mood. Take a closer look at each stage below and the emotional tools required in each step.

Stages of Emotional Self-Awareness		
I.	**II.**	**III.**
Emotional Self-Discovery: How to Achieve a Good Mood	**Emotional Attunement: How to Sustain a Good Mood**	**Emotional Self-Discipline: How to Recover from a Bad Mood**
• Emotionally Proactive • Emotional Preparedness	• Emotionally Active • Emotional Resourcefulness	• Emotionally Responsive • Emotional Adaptability

Let's start by looking at the process of emotional self-discovery and how it will help you achieve a good mood. We will then move on and review the emotional skills you can develop to sustain a good mood and recover from and outfox a bad mood.

I. Emotional Self-Discovery: How to Create a Good Mood

To achieve a good mood, you must create an environment that supports a good mood. When you are at peace with yourself and in harmony with your environment, your setting, and your relationships, it is a simple matter to create a good mood. When you are out of sync with yourself and your environment, your mood structure begins to falter. You need to know what works for you. Emotional self-discovery gives you the know-how to make your life and your moods work for you. You see, emotional self-discovery is an inner journey.

Emotional self-discovery is about finding out what makes you tick. It is about *identifying* and *satisfying* your most basic needs. Simply said, when your needs are met and you are doing what turns you on, you are naturally going to be in a more friendly and agreeable mood. Mood power comes to light when you see to it that you actively satisfy your most fundamental needs. Emotional self-discovery guides you to being true to yourself and sets the stage and is the foundation for a good mood.

While this may sound simple, it is not easy. Most people suffer from unnecessary stress and demoralizing friction in their lives because they are not satisfying their most fundamental needs. When you don't take the time to address your basic needs, it is difficult to achieve and sustain a good mood. Instead, you may find yourself constantly feeling uneasy, stressed, or perturbed, and putting out the fires of a bad mood. Trust me—it is easier to start from the foundation of a good mood and work to sustain it than to continually try to recover from a misguided lifestyle and the underpinnings of a bad mood.

Your Needs and Your Happiness

So what do you think you need to be happy? When you take the time to reflect on it, you'll discover that you need to love and be loved. You need to be needed and feel useful. You'll also find out that you need to be appreciated and acknowledged. Other needs include the need to be yourself. You have a driving need to belong. You have an intuitive need for fulfilling relationships with the people who mean the most to you. You have a need for job satisfaction and making a difference in others' lives. As you advance on your spiritual path, you'll come to realize that you need to feel the love for life and for spirit within. Mood power gives you the greatest gift in your life—emotional fulfillment. You can achieve emotional fulfillment when you actively satisfy your most fundamental emotional needs.

As usual, it is all up to you. Pursuing your needs, working toward your goals and your dreams, and actively paying attention to what makes you happy will keep your mood up. When you neglect yourself and your needs, it dampens your mood. By failing to deal with your goals, dreams, or personal desires, you can slip into a state of apathy, moodiness, indifference, or depression.

You Are the Captain of Your Destiny

Keep in mind that you are the world's authority when it comes to yourself and what is in your best interest. You know more than anyone what feels right to you. You are in the driver's seat when it comes to achieving happiness for yourself. The more you know and discover about yourself, the more responsibly you can choose your actions. It is best to go through the growing pains of emotional self-discovery and learn how to keep yourself and your moods upbeat.

Simplify Your Life: The Key to Emotional Self-Discovery

Emotional self-discovery starts and ends with simplifying your life. Simplifying your life is a matter of recognizing and paying attention to the things in your life that have the greatest value. In other words, pay attention to IT! What is IT? IT is you! When you dial in to what really matters, your life can thrive. Simplifying your life gives you the code to the vault. It empowers you to live your life in harmony with your values, your principles, and your personality. There is no sense trying to put a square peg in a round hole and getting stressed out by its misfit.

Unnecessary stress rains on the parade of your mood power and is known to drain your mood. In order to maximize your mood structure, it makes good sense to minimize the drama and chaos that can show up. Drama and chaos have a way of wearing down your mood and turning it south. The fact is that you can avoid a large source of disruptive mood swings through prudent emotional self-discovery.

Emotional self-discovery teaches us that you need to be proactive in creating a fulfilling lifestyle and prepared to meet your needs. This is called being emotionally proactive and emotionally prepared. Emotional self-discovery breeds emotional wellness and will help you set the stage for a good mood. It is also your best form of emotional preventive medicine. By simplifying your life, you will prevent unwanted, unnecessary, and unneeded moodiness.

There are necessary strategies to help you find out what matters to you most, so you can set the climate for a good mood and prevent unnecessary mood distortion. Let's take a look at the strategies to help you simplify your life.

Simplify Your Life: Time for Action

Simplifying your life feeds your mood power and prevents unnecessary mood stress and moodiness. It can be done. To simplify your life it starts with knowing how to recognize what in your life has the greatest value. Again, it pays to know who you are. Simplifying your life embraces what it takes to acquire, preserve, fortify, sustain, and protect what is most valuable. For example, your body and your health have priceless value. Your love relationships, your family, your work relationships, your interests, your passions, and how you spend your time are all important. In other words, figure out what really matters to you. Be prepared to take full responsibility to know:

- Yourself,
- Your needs, and
- Your priorities.

Furthermore, to simplify your life, you will need to get the clutter and confusion out of your emotional life. Clutter and confusion typically deflate your moods. Let's take a look within. We all have the ability to dial in and come up with important "ahas" and realizations.

Honor your Priorities: How to Simplify Your Life

Simplifying your life is finding out:

- What makes you happy
- What makes you tick
- What makes you sick
- What turns you on
- What clutter in your life you must get rid of

To simplify your life, your lifestyle must be tailored to satisfy your most fundamental needs and your most basic priorities. When your needs are met and your priorities are in order, your life is simplified. When your needs are not met and you spend time neglecting your priorities, your life turns to mood stress, moodiness, chaos, clutter, confusion, and disorder. When your needs and priorities are in balance, you have discovered one of the secrets to creating and sustaining a good mood. Be certain that your foremost priorities get the most attention or, at the very least, enough attention.

Follow Your Priorities

Take a moment. Breathe in some fresh air. Take a few deep cleansing breaths. Grab a pen and paper. Now, fill out the table below by listing the priorities in your life from highest to lowest. When you are done, turn your attention to the column next to it and fill out the top seven things that take up your time, from highest to lowest.

What Are Your Top Priorities?	How Do You Spend Your Time?
1.	1.
2.	2.
3.	3.
4.	4.
5.	5.
6.	6.
7.	7.

Take a moment to answer these questions:

- Is there any one area that weighs so heavily on you that you neglect your highest priorities?
- What can you do to change this?

How do the two columns match up? When your priorities don't correspond to the way you delegate your time, you need to reevaluate. Make sure to do the following:

Tune In	➡	Know Thyself	➡	Find out what Matters	➡	Take Action

Follow-Through on Your Priorities

What percentage of your life are you willing to commit to find happiness, fulfillment, and well-being? If you want to devote more attention to your spiritual growth, do you really need the distraction of hours upon hours of TV shows? Is that higher salary worth the extra two hours you'll spend in transit every day? Ask yourself the tough questions. Do you have enough fun every day? Do you have enough time with your loved ones? Do you get to do what you love to do? Ask yourself what can go. Then get rid of it. Ask yourself what has to change. Neglecting your priorities works away at a good mood. Mixed priorities are conducive to mood stress, chaos, confusion, and mood swings. Misaligned priorities feed moodiness that trigger compulsive, indulgent food patterns and eating habits. Aligning your priorities feeds your heart.

Not simplifying your life is conducive to mood disorder and emotional confusion. When your relationships at home or at work are stressful, this often leads to a lifestyle of mood strain and emotional overeating. When you do not answer to the task of simplifying your life, you are out of sync with your highest priorities. This sets the stage for stressful upheaval and unnecessary complications. Life is an ongoing challenge. There is enough pain and suffering in the normal growth cycles that lead to happiness. Why hassle and burden yourself with unnecessary pain and suffering? This will keep you from experiencing the full passion and beauty in being alive! Living a topsy-turvy, helter-skelter, jumbled life is like shooting yourself in the foot—you cannot feel great, look great, and keep yourself in the right mood.

In summary, simplifying your life is the manifestation of emotional self-discovery. Allow yourself to get in touch with what really inspires you, and you will find out what really makes you happy. Get your basics covered. Everyone needs to love and be loved. Everyone needs a positive self-image. Everyone needs to be valued and appreciated. Everyone needs to be needed. Take care of these needs. Pay attention to them. Everyone needs to work their physical body, and everyone needs to have a purpose in life. Meet your needs, simplify your life, and achieve mood power.

Now that we've gone through the process of emotional self-discovery, let's revisit the questions that we posed earlier in the chapter. Take a minute to reflect on and answer these questions:

- What makes you happy?
- What makes you tick?
- What makes you sick?
- What turns you on?
- What clutter in your life must you get rid of?

II. Emotional Attunement: How to Sustain a Good Mood

The second step in the process of emotional self-awareness is emotional attunement. Whereas emotional self-discovery gives you the framework to *create* a good mood, emotional attunement gives you the nuts and bolts to *support* and *sustain* a good mood. Emotional self-discovery calls for being emotionally proactive whereas emotional attunement relies on being emotionally active. Active in what? Active in being in touch with how you feel.

Being tuned in to the world inside you is the first step in establishing self-attunement. Self-attunement is about being in touch with your feelings. When you know how you are feeling, you can be emotionally active and act in your own best interest. When you are in touch with your feelings, it's a natural process to self-regulate your mood. When you are not dialed into how you feel, it is more than difficult to self-regulate. When you are disconnected from your feelings, it is not possible to self-regulate what you don't have a feeling for. Unless you know how you are feeling, how can you keep your spirits high? This is why emotional attunement is a crucial step in developing emotional self-awareness.

When you deny, suppress, or lose touch with your primary feelings of love, fear, pain, frustration, hurt, and disappointment, secondary feelings of anger, resentment, and worry start to accumulate. Repressed emotions disrupt your mood, build up mood stress, and throw you out of balance. Emotionally repressed individuals have lost touch with their feelings. As a result, their internal signals are mixed. Therefore, they find it exceedingly difficult to sustain a good mood because they're so accustomed to burying everything. At some point, repressed feelings will inevitably erupt and disrupt your mood. When you are not actively in tune with your real feelings, it is common to become fixated on work or obsessed with alcohol, drugs, money, sex, gambling, TV, or codependent relationships. What's the solution? Tune into how you feel!

Emotional Self-Assessment: Tune into How You Feel

Tuning into how you feel empowers you to sustain a healthy, positive mood. It is imperative to know your true feelings and not run away from them. Are you so busy with what is going on around you that you are unaware of emotional experiences you feel each day? Are you in touch with your own level of happiness? How often do you take the time to appreciate being alive and love your life? Is there room for more happiness in your life?

Emotional self-attunement calls for an honest declaration of underlying feelings. By taking inventory of how you feel during the course of the day, you can find out whether you are operating from a position of loving strength or stressful mood fluctuations.

To help you get acquainted with the spectrum of what you feel, consider what percentage of a typical day you spend feeling the following emotions:

EMOTIONAL SELF-ASSESSMENT		
Happy ________%	**Sad** ________%	**Mad** ________%
glad	lonely	angry
excited	heavy	aggravated
hopeful	troubled	exasperated
joyful	helpless	irritated
satisfied	gloomy	agitated
delighted	grief	furious
encouraged	overwhelmed	enraged
grateful	distant	infuriated
confident	despondent	hostile
inspired	discouraged	bitter
cheerful	distressed	pessimistic
content	dismayed	resentful
proud	disheartened	disgusted
Tired ________%	**Scared** ________%	**Confused** ________%
exhausted	afraid	frustrated
fatigued	fearful	perplexed
inert	terrified	hesitant
lethargic	startled	troubled
indifferent	nervous	uncomfortable
listless	panicky	torn
weary	jittery	withdrawn
overwhelmed	horrified	apathetic
fidgety	anxious	embarrassed
helpless	worried	hurt
heavy	anguished	uneasy
sleepy	lonely	irritated
Peaceful ________%	**Loving** ________%	**Playful** ________%
tranquil	warm	energetic
calm	affectionate	effervescent
content	tender	invigorated
engrossed	appreciative	zestful
absorbed	friendly	refreshed
expansive	sensitive	stimulated
serene	compassionate	enthusiastic
loving	grateful	alive
blissful	nurtured	exuberant
satisfied	amorous	vibrant
relaxed	trusting	adventurous

Now that you have an idea of the range of emotions you feel in a typical day, let's take your self-attunement a step further. Over the course of the day, take the time to catalog your feelings. Take inventory in the morning, midday, at sunset, and before you go to bed. Take particular note of the times of the day when you are stressed or rushed and not likely to be in the best of moods. Take some deep breaths, give yourself a few moments to get in touch, and then ask yourself what you really feel (not what you think). Do you feel right or not? Be patient until you break through and get to your real feelings.

Time of Day	Prevailing Feelings
Morning	
Midday	
Sunset	
Before Bed	

In this way, you can become an expert with what you are feeling. Within a few days you will get good at it. Otherwise, you can get so wrapped up with survival, chores, and details that you become a victim of your own emotionally constipated lifestyle. Remember, feelings are not what we think about how we feel. For example, "I think I'm happy; I seem to be excited; or I believe I'm angry." Feelings are felt from the heart, such as "I feel happy; I feel excited; or I feel embarrassed."

Take note of the fact that when your needs are being met, your predominant feelings can usually be found in the Emotional Self-Assessment table, under the categories of Happy, Peaceful, Loving, and Playful. Alternatively, when your needs are not being met, you'll find that your most prevalent feelings will be found in the categories titled Sad, Mad, Tired, Scared, and Confused.

The Habits of Happiness: How to Sustain a Good Mood

Self-attunement invites happiness. In fact, self-attunement is the steppingstone to longstanding happiness. Anywhere you travel, any place you choose to go, all cultures have one language in common. People everywhere want to be happy and in a good mood. A happy face, a happy smile, and a happy laugh are the ever-present signs of a good mood. Making happiness a habit can become a way of life. It is going to call for and recruit your emotional resourcefulness. Acquiring the habits of happiness will give you the mood power to sustain a good mood. When you acquire the habits of happiness, it teaches you to come to your own emotional rescue and become your own hero or heroine. Thomas Jefferson, one of the founding fathers of this great country, had it straight when he wanted every American to have the right to life, liberty, and the pursuit of happiness. Indeed, the habits of happiness are the nuts and bolts of sustaining a good mood.

The Habits of Happiness Feed Mood Power

Happiness invigorates, inspires, and energizes your mood. Happiness is the emotional key to wellness. When you are happy inside, it feeds your heart and your heart comes alive. Happiness is heartfelt inner joy. In the simplest of terms, making happiness your prevailing mood makes your life worth living.

Good moods keep you in touch with the lighter side of life. When you are happy, you feel special and excited to be alive. True happiness is a bright, shining candle that brightens up your life. In fact, one of the reasons you are in a good mood is that you have things to look forward to all day long—from work, to passion and romance, to your hobbies, friends, and family. Happiness is the manifestation of your love relationship with life. It takes your breath away. It empowers you to fill up each day with loving and healing energy to enrich the lives of others and yourself.

On the other hand, depression, anxiety, and unhappiness drain your life and shift your mood into a downward spiral. Emotional self-abuse, emotional mediocrity, boredom, and loneliness drain your lifestyle and de-energize, deaden, muffle, smother, and subdue you mood. Negative feelings can interfere with how you function, think, and make decisions. In fact, when bad feelings arise, they trigger an internal radar telling you that something is not right. This is called anxiety. It is telling you that one of your emotional needs is being threatened or that something is missing in your life. These are the times to be emotionally resourceful. Instead, people commonly turn to food to comfort themselves through this. The habits of happiness will give you the emotional resourcefulness and the know-how to jump these challenging hurdles on the path to long-lasting mood power.

Rich in Mood, Rich in Life

You see, this mood-powered habit of happiness teaches you to make the best of your life and to make light of your troubles. It guides you to create a favorable emotional response to the changes in your life. It encourages you to find the good in any and all circumstances. The habits of happiness also teach you to turn your conflicts into opportunities and triumphs and, in so doing, create your own emotional fulfillment. Furthermore, the habits of happiness teach you how to stay in touch with your feelings, both good and bad. Disappointments, emotional disturbances, and emotional upheavals are a very real part of life. Few of us have had any skilled emotional guidance or emotional mentors, so we are usually not prepared for emotional upheaval.

Emotional Consistency Is the Key

Keep in mind, the habit of happiness feeds mood power. The bottom line in making happiness a habit is about being able to maintain a spirited good mood throughout most of the day. Day in and day out, day after day, do you consistently see life as a gift? Are you so ecstatic to be alive and feel so privileged to live on this planet that your mood reflects your gusto and appreciation? Mood power is one of the main benefits that emerges from consistently owning the habit of happiness. Having the courage to live up to, and be in harmony with, your deepest heartfelt emotional convictions on a daily basis breeds this kind of emotional consistency.

You can measure your mood power by your level of ongoing happiness. Do you usually find yourself upbeat and happy? Or do you find that you have only episodic moments of happiness mixed in with a prevailing heavier emotional outlook?

Mood power is an acquired skill, as are the habits of happiness. Being a great person requires the same level of skill as being a great surgeon! Imagine learning surgery without a mentor, a teacher, or a professor. Cutting out healthy tissue or making improper incisions would eventually teach you by trial and error, but why pay the price?

Mood power skills and happiness skills are one and the same. Happiness skills teach you to create a positive inner lifestyle, no matter what is happening in your life on the outside. The habits of happiness train you to take emotional positivity into consideration. Happy people retain their sense of humor and have a natural way of being lighthearted and fun-loving. Happy people act with the greatest of ease to reach the goals or objectives they have in mind. Why? Because happy people know how to stay in a good mood. They have mood power; they have a love for life, a love for their loved ones, a love for spirit, a love for the universe, a love for God, and a love for themselves! The good news is that the habits of happiness can be learned. Emotional consistency is within your reach. All you have to do is practice the following exercises and action steps.

Action Steps: The Seven Emotional Tools to Build the Habits of Happiness

Emotional consistency stems from your daily commitment to yourself to be healthy and happy. Do you make the effort? Have you made the commitment to be consistently happy and healthy? You need emotional consistency to sustain the habits of happiness. Emotional consistency is a bridge builder. It builds the bridge to the habits of happiness. To be sure you have emotional consistency, you will need seven emotional tools. You can learn to build on these seven emotional tools that feed the habits of happiness.

The Seven Emotional Tools that Build the Habits of Happiness	
1. Emotional Rebound	• One step back means two steps forward.
2. Emotional Pursuit	• Go for it!
3. Emotional Perseverance	• Stick with it!
4. Emotional Magnetism	• Happiness attracts.
5. Emotional Self-Reliance	• Count on yourself.
6. Emotional Support	• Create a rich network of social support.
7. Emotional Balance	• Life is a question of balance.

Emotional Tool #1: Emotional Rebound

Emotional rebound is a crucial skill to sustaining a good mood. The idea is to spring right back from a disappointment. A disappointment doesn't need to put you in a bad mood. What did you learn from the disappointment? What did you learn from your setback? For example, if the job you want doesn't come through, determine what it will take to secure such a position. Make the necessary adjustments and be optimistic. *When disappointment comes, one step back can be followed by two steps forward.*

You can convert your emotional setbacks into opportunities for personal growth and development. They say that opportunity stares you in the face everyday—the difficulty is that you just plain don't see it! Don't get bent out of shape when things don't go your way. Adversity often shows up. We all grow and get tougher with adversity. Regardless of what happens, use the momentum from what you have learned in your disappointments to spring you forward to improve your quality of life, your business, and your relationships with family and loved ones. This is what emotional rebounding is all about. It's all about your resourcefulness and your thirst for happiness. Life is happening and so are you.

Emotional Tool #2: Emotional Pursuit

Emotional pursuit is the driving force behind sustained happiness. Reach out and pursue the things that turn you on. When fervor and passion move you, take a stand and go after it. When you feel and experience the ring of truth, follow it! Pursue and fulfill what matters to you; this will help you maintain the appropriate mood chemistry that goes along with healthy, prosperous living.

Happiness is everywhere, but you have to look for it. You can only find what you are looking for. If you are not looking for it, you will not find it! When you are not looking to stay in a good mood, it may slip away. I remember from medical school, when you do not look for an enlarged heart, you will not find it. Similarly, when you do not look for a new job, it usually does not come knocking on your door. It is not common to meet new people in your backyard. Make the effort. Pursue what makes you happy.

Earlier in this chapter, in learning about emotional self-discovery, you were prompted to reflect on your most fundamental needs and interests. Emotional pursuit is about following through and pursuing whatever it is that is most important to you. When you pursue your natural interests, you become happier. Spending your time emotionally involved and doing what you love to do keep you in the best of moods. Emotional pursuit gives your emotional life a chance to thrive. Go forward. Go for it!

Emotional Tool #3: Emotional Perseverance

Emotional perseverance calls for the kind of endurance that turns all endeavors into positive, favorable emotional experiences. Stick with it! You get good at what you practice. When you practice becoming a good tennis player, parent, pianist, or husband, eventually you will get better at it. Practice adjusting your mood when you do not feel right. There will always be difficulties and setbacks in life. These are not opportunities to succumb to temptation and forego healthy eating habits. Utilize these tougher moments to fortify your resolve. Make sure being happy and establishing your mood power is one of the main goals in your life. Be patient with yourself. Emotional perseverance will breed the habits of happiness.

Remember, perseverance furthers. Be persistent. Emotional perseverance teaches staying power. This means you keep the faith and build mood power into all circumstances to maintain and sustain your happiness.

Emotional Tool #4: Emotional Magnetism

Mood power works like a vibrant, strong emotional magnet. Mood power attracts value, joy, excitement, and happiness into your life. An enthusiastic, good mood is a magnet to positive energy. You can tell you have the habit of happiness when there is an abundance of love and joy around you and within you. You know you can improve your habits of happiness when you can have more love and joy in your life.

When your mood carries a happy, vibrant, and enthusiastic charge, good things will come to you. Focus on your heart, and radiate pure love and joy. This will lift your mood. Allow nothing to interfere with your most positive loving vibrations. Send your healing, loving vibrations to all your loved ones, and feel the love for your loved ones every day. This expands the depths of your magnetism.

Remember to feel love for life on a consistent, daily basis, especially in the morning when you awake and at night before you go to bed. To become an effective emotional magnet, practice this meditation for five to ten minutes whenever possible.

Emotional Magnetism Meditation

Send love and joy to your loved ones for at least five minutes, and then spend another five minutes receiving love and joy back into your heart. In other words, radiate love and joy; then magnetize love and joy. Radiating and magnetizing love and joy feeds your heart, fortifies your mood power, and strengthens your emotional magnet. In turn, your mood power will attract more love and joy. In time, your emotional magnet will carve out a lifestyle of favorable, expansive, heartfelt experiences. Alternatively, if you are negative and unhappy, your negative emotional magnet will attract more and more negative things in your life. Radiate happiness, and happiness will come back to you.

Emotional Tool #5: Emotional Self-Reliance

Put your hands on the wheel and take charge of your emotional life. It is your full responsibility to see to it that your emotional needs are met. Emotional self-reliance means you are the only one who can create happiness for yourself. Other people can support and inspire you, but they cannot provide the happiness for you. Happiness does not come from "when-itis" or "if only" scenarios. You cannot rely on outside circumstances to fulfill you—for example, the following conditions won't lead to your happiness: "if only I made a little more money, I would be happy" or "when I meet the man of my dreams, I will be happy." It is important to realize that happiness comes from within!

Emotional self-reliance leads to emotional self-control and feeds emotional consistency. When you are emotionally self-reliant, you can rely on yourself to self-regulate your moods and keep yourself on the up-and-up. Emotional self-reliance is fueled by your own personal, insatiable appetite for life. Your love for life shines through. Life is always happening … are you?

Be strong, warm, sensitive, and vulnerable. Be compassionate and understanding. Forgive yourself for being perfectly imperfect. Your inner voice wants you to be happy. Learn to trust your own feelings.

In summary, becoming emotionally self-reliant breeds emotional consistency and sound emotional judgment. In time, emotional self-reliance makes you emotionally independent and feeds the courage it takes to sustain a good mood.

Emotional Tool #6: Emotional Support

Emotional support means you create resourceful intrapersonal and stimulating interpersonal emotional support systems. Take a stand. Stand by the people you love and believe in. Be emotionally supportive to loved ones and people in your life. Create lasting friendships. Learn to listen and be a good friend. Give and share with others. Create a diversified emotional support system among friends, loved ones, hobbies, and interests. This will feed the depths of your mood power and lead to lasting happiness.

Also, recruit your intrapersonal support systems. Specialize in being your own best friend. Nurture and understand yourself. Stand by your convictions, and stand up for what you believe. Be true to yourself. Get in touch with who you are and what you love to do. Not only share it, but make it happen and recruit the proper support. When you have fallen in love with love itself and have a wide variety of friends and recreational activities, you will know what it means to have emotional support in your life.

To further your emotional consistency, practice the following "Midas Touch" meditation for five to ten minutes when you have the chance. Close your eyes, breathe deeply, and picture everything you touch become richer in happiness and love. See everyone with whom you come in contact become healthier and happier.

Emotional Tool #7: Emotional Balance

Mood power invites you to become an emotionally balanced person. By keeping in touch with the love in your heart and appreciating the positive things and blessings in your life—no matter what you are going through—you will be able to stay centered and grounded in the bedrock of mood power. Staying young at heart will keep you youthful and balanced. Search for personal freedom and commit to lasting happiness. Stay present to the moment, look after your affairs, and keep to your agreements. By keeping yourself in a good mood, it feeds mood equilibrium and emotional balance.

When you are emotionally balanced, you live each moment in life to its fullest. You can appreciate yourself, as well as the magnificence of life, and see the beauty in others. When you are in balance, you can keep in touch with the love in your heart, no matter what you are going through. Acknowledge the beauty around you, and appreciate the love within you. Why not have a positive emotional reaction to whatever comes up or goes down around you? This leads to emotional equilibrium, which feeds your mood power. This will balance your emotions and help you sustain a good mood.

Size Up Your Habits of Happiness

Please review and score from 1–5, 5 being the strongest, how well you fare with these seven emotional skills.

	Strong		Average		Weak
1. Emotional Rebound	5	4	3	2	1
2. Emotional Pursuit	5	4	3	2	1
3. Emotional Perseverance	5	4	3	2	1
4. Emotional Magnetism	5	4	3	2	1
5. Emotional Self-Reliance	5	4	3	2	1
6. Emotional Support	5	4	3	2	1
7. Emotional Balance	5	4	3	2	1

Total Points	
28–35	• Strong sense of happiness. You've got the mood power habit!
21–27	• Happiness is incomplete and can escape you. Identify the emotional tools that you can improve on. Be consistent. Concentrate on making a little more effort at finding happiness, regardless of your situation.
7–20	• Suggests a weakened sense of inner happiness. Focus more on getting in touch with your feelings and having more fun. Keep it lighter at all levels!

Develop the habits of happiness and take your mood power to the limit. Just commit to being happy, and discover what makes you happy. Have fun every day, and remember your sense of humor. Create lasting friendships, share, and be close to your loved ones. Keep it simple, keep it light, keep it balanced, and enrich other people's lives. Your mood power has game and endurance. It will not let you down.

Now, in one hundred words or less, describe in detail:

- What it is that really makes you happy; and
- What it will take for you to really stay in a good mood.

Then determine what action steps you can take to feed your heart, heal your heart, and own the habit of mood-powered happiness.

III. Emotional Self-Discipline: How to Recover from a Bad Mood

Emotional self-discipline is the third stage on the path to emotional self-awareness. We've been through the process of emotional self-discovery, then on to emotional attunement and, its tactical sister, the habits of happiness. As you develop these skills, it will lay the foundation for achieving and sustaining a good mood. However, sooner or later, we all have to work our way out of a bad mood. Emotional self-discipline empowers you to bounce back and quickly recover from a bad mood. It is a lot simpler to turn a bad mood around when it first appears than after it lingers. This is why you take a proactive approach to a down mood, work it out, and then come back to ready position—feeling great about being alive.

It takes emotional self-discipline to keep your prevailing mood favorable. It takes even more self-discipline to convert a bad mood to a good mood. Emotional self-discipline is essentially emotional self-control. You need emotional self-discipline to prepare yourself to handle emotional unpredictability, upheaval, or troubles. Emotional self-discipline empowers you to stay with your feelings, work out what it will take to make you feel better, and make the heaviness go away. Each time you handle emotional tension with positive action, you practice emotional self-discipline. By dealing with your true feelings, good and bad, you are taking responsibility for your emotional life and honoring your emotional needs. When you feel good, you follow through on your feelings. When you don't feel good, you need the emotional self-discipline to take a timeout, determine what you are feeling, and figure out what it will take to make you feel better. Emotional self-discipline trains you to keep in touch with your primary feelings and avoid being moody or emotional when it is unnecessary.

Emotional self-discipline requires that we open up and truly experience our feelings instead of stifling them with food or other addictions. As humans, we hate to feel vulnerable, and we will do almost anything to avoid it. Nancy overeats. Jack depends on alcohol or drugs. James turns to compulsive gambling. Anything to numb the fear and discomfort. Because we are accustomed to bottling up and blocking out pain, frustration, disappointment, and anxiety, these emotions often trigger negative food choices. We deny our feelings, turn instead to food for a quick-fix mood change, and snack our upsetting emotions into submission.

Although negative emotions disturb our comfort zone and interfere with our sense of security, they are a part of everyday life. Keep in mind that emotional self-discipline keeps your emotional life up to date. It prevents you from accumulating emotional tension, which can go on to cause emotional burnout. Emotional burnout is a state of mind where you have lost full connection to your feelings or moods. Essentially, emotional burnout numbs out your feelings. Regrettably, most of us have been brought up to regard bad moods not as currents to ride out but tidal waves that might drown us. Instead of dealing with disappointment and frustration, we medicate ourselves with our most comforting mood foods, Mommy-Daddy foods, or other addictions.

Emotional Self-Discipline Empowers You to Say No

As we've discussed, people often turn to food to medicate and soothe their mood. To change this dysfunctional coping mechanism, we have to summon the courage to face our every feeling. Emotional self-discipline gives you the discipline to not indulge in eating while you are transitioning from a negative, heavier mood into a lighter, better mood. Yes, emotional self-discipline teaches you not to eat when you are emotional or in a bad mood. As soon as you recognize that you're feeling upset—but before you reach for the plate of brownies—emotional self-discipline guides you to take alternative action and not be victim to stress-related eating.

Emotional Self-Discipline Leads to Emotional Adaptability

In order to stay in emotional balance, you will need emotional adaptability. That means that you can adjust to life's negatives and positives, ups and downs, and quickly recover from a bad mood. To do this you are going to need to be emotionally vulnerable and be willing to face your fears, worries, and underlying anxieties. When you have the emotional self-discipline to experience and stand up to your feelings, and the emotional self-discipline to be response-*able* and respond with positive action to reestablish a good mood, you will have achieved emotional adaptability. In this manner, emotional response-*ability* and emotional adaptability go hand in hand with emotional self-discipline.

RIEXPA to the Rescue

You may think you've seen a similar acronym to RIEXPA in "Master Your Eating Habits." Well, you are right! RIEXPA is a "mood-ified" version of the RIEXA technique. Whereas RIEXA was used to deal with and overcome the onset of a dysfunctional eating habit, RIEXPA is the technique of choice to deal with your moods before a craving or food indulgence appears. The RIEXPA technique that follows gives you the tactics to bounce back from a bad mood and convert a bad mood into a good one.

Why does RIEXPA work? Well, RIEXPA teaches you to deal with the emotions that drive you to eat, so you can reprogram your response to mood stress. Therefore, instead of *reacting* to a bad mood and indulging in self-defeating behavior, you can constructively *respond* and put yourself in a better mood. Without a clear mind and an open heart, it's easy to react and use food to relieve tension. Practice the following steps when you feel like you are in a bad mood, so you can respond and take positive action to offset a bad mood. When you are exercising your emotional self-discipline, you are exercising emotional response-*ability*.

The RIEXPA Technique Gets Results!

- **R: RECOGNIZE** that you're in a bad mood. Recognize the need to take charge and reprogram your mood.
- **I: IDENTIFY** the specifics of your mood. Identify what you are truly feeling. Please do not edit or censor your primary feelings. For example, if you are feeling angry and resentful, your primary feelings may reveal that you are actually hurt or wounded. Tune in. Your feelings count.
- **EXP:** Honestly **EXPRESS** how you feel about your situation and allow yourself to **EXPERIENCE** the full scope of feelings that underlie your mood. This is the time to experience any sensitive feelings of worry, anxiety, or fear that are bringing down your mood. Allow yourself to experience your emotions. Then, after the initial discomfort has passed, start to put the emotions into perspective. This calls for action.
- A: Take **ACTION**. Nurture yourself to enrich your mood. This does not involve a food reward. The prescription of choice to overcome a bad mood is the strategy that follows. I like to call it the EH-MN strategy.
  - **E: EXERCISE.** Keep your feet moving. Get your heart pumping and your lungs working. This will relieve mental and physical stress and prompt the natural release of your body's "feel good" endorphins. In this way, exercise has a way of counteracting even the worst of moods.
  - **H: HYDROTHERAPY.** Hop in the shower and alternate hot and cold water (15 seconds hot, 5 seconds cold) for three to four cycles. Alternatively, if you are near a fresh body of water—such as an ocean, a river, or a lake—submerge your head and body a few times for a complete hydrotherapy recharge. Hydrotherapy recharges your nerves and revitalizes the mind and body.
  - **M: MEDITATION**. Find your inner sanctuary. Get in touch with your inner joy and inner peace. Realize that the attunement to the love in your heart will help regulate your mood.
  - **N: NURTURE.** Finally, nurture yourself in a way that does not involve a food reward. Put on a favorite CD. Light a scented candle. Take a Jacuzzi. Phone a close friend. Wrap yourself up in a blanket and read a good book. Make yourself a cup of warm

herbal tea, or take a short walk to appreciate the season, whatever it may be. Whatever you choose to do, make sure to engage in something you enjoy that will constructively uplift your spirits. If you are looking for a nutritional pick-me-up, turn to your super-nutrients for a boost in energy.

- The EH-MN technique is designed to be sequential, so follow the steps in order for best results. A lot of times, exercise—or exercise and hydrotherapy—is all you need to get your mood back on track. If that is the case, it is up to you whether you would like to complete the remaining steps.

Mood Factor #2—Your Energy Level and Your Mood

Your energy level has a huge influence on your mood. Have you ever noticed that, when you are energized and feel great physically, you have an extra strut in your step and your mood naturally elevates? Did you realize that, when you are listless, tired, or lethargic, your mood can dampen?

The relationship I'm trying to highlight is simple. High-energy lifestyles breed mood power. Low energy, fatigue and burnout in your lifestyle inevitably invite mood instability, moodiness, and mood swings. The key is to learn and adhere to the wellness plan we have outlined, and you will have a massive amount of energy. Regular exercise, Smart Foods, a positive mental attitude, and your share of love and laughter are conducive to high energy and healthy, cheerful, light, and positive moods.

Fatigue can sabotage your mood structure. Everyone knows that you are more vulnerable to stress when you are worn out and tired. When you are tired, it is common to be more irritable. I have seen it in one patient after another; mental and physical burnout have a negative impact on your mood structure. When you are tired and fatigued, it is common to indulge and medicate yourself with your favorite foods to alter your mood. When Debbie feels tired and moody in the afternoon, she snacks on a couple of cookies to give herself a short-term boost. Jeff, on the other hand, reaches for his favorite candy bar. In any case, it is common to react to fatigue and moodiness by turning to food. This can be more than hazardous to your weight-loss program.

Let me solve the fatigue problem for you. Follow your LYF Plan. As you lose weight, your energy level will increase. Take the boulders out of a hot air balloon and the balloon rises. The LYF Nutritional Plan is guaranteed to increase your energy level. When you find fatigue setting in and affecting your mood, take action. Turn to the EH-MN technique to reenergize your mind and body.

Mood Factor #3—Your Attitude and Your Mood

Your attitude has a major influence on your mood. In fact, there is a direct connection between how you think and how you feel. When you are optimistic and enthusiastic, it becomes a simple matter to keep your mood elevated. Positive thinking triggers positive feelings. Positive expectations and constructive beliefs lend themselves to a good mood. When you are excited about being alive and are looking forward to the different and interesting parts of your day, you can maintain an energetic, vibrant, zestful, and exuberant mood. All in all, the best attitudes yield the best moods.

Alternatively, pessimism and negative mind chatter bring your mood down. When you expect things to go wrong, expect your mood to falter. Negative thinking drains your emotional life and makes you more prone to moodiness, depression, and mood swings. Resentment, irritability, and endless frustration contribute to mood volatility. You know the movie. You have seen it before. Downtrodden moods are attracted to food indulgence.

The best-case scenario, then, is to be energized; sport a positive mental attitude and outlook; and be tuned in emotionally. This supports mood power and mood stabilization. Fatigue, negativity, and emotional lethargy breed mood lowering and instability. It is important to acquire the mood power to self-regulate your eating habits. Sustaining a positive mental attitude goes a long way to feed your mood power.

There are a few rapid-fire ways to take advantage of your positive thinking to generate mood power. When you feel your mood slipping, do the following:

1. Write out the ten things and the ten people you are most grateful for having in your life. Give some thought to each one. When you are grateful for being alive and are thankful for the blessings in your life, your attitude and mood naturally lift.

2. Sit down, close your eyes, and think of the single most positive thought you can imagine. Embellish it in your mind and watch your mood go up.

3. When you need to boost your attitude, you can rely on your EH-MN technique. Exercise, coupled with hydrotherapy, goes a long way in

establishing a positive mental attitude. In addition, meditation is the single most powerful instrument to maintain a positive mental attitude and shift your mood upward. Your meditation time is the time you need to tune the musical instrument of your mind and set your thinking to a positive note. Finally, when you take some time to constructively nurture yourself, your attitude has a way of turning to the positive.

Mood Factor #4—Your Stress Levels and Your Mood

High stress levels feed moodiness. Calmness and peace of mind feed mood stability. You see, high stress levels can be unnerving. They often lead to anxiety and irritability. When you are stressed, rushed, or worried, it has a negative impact on your moods. The art of living is to keep your spirits high and mood upbeat in spite of potentially stressful life challenges. It is vitally important to know how to prevent unnecessary stress. It is also necessary to know how to effectively manage stress.

Keep in mind that high stress produces high levels of emotional tension. When you are tense, you are not going to feel your best. The heaviness of the stress weighs on your mind and deflates your mood. Eventually, the accumulation of emotional tension and the heaviness of prolonged stress weigh on your body as well.

Lighten Up Your Life

The bottom line is that mood power is about keeping it light. When you are light, it is a simple matter to maintain a high-spirited lifestyle. The goal is to lighten up your life and keep your moods light. Lightening up your life centers your personality around being lighthearted, fun-loving, and easygoing. This calms your mind and lightens up your thinking. This feeds a good mood. Lightening up involves unloading the heaviness of unresolved emotional stress. It also calls for letting go of stored-up bodily tensions and bottled-up emotional tension.

The opposite of keeping it light is to wear the heaviness of emotional stress. When you are heavy, it is likely that your mood can succumb to disappointment and everyday blunders. This heaviness burdens the heart, weighs down the spirit, strains the mind, and dulls the senses. Emotional distress leads to burnout and fatigue. This dampens your mood. Wearing this kind of heavy armor often leads to hazardous eating habits. In addition, this kind of stress is destructive to your immune system, can make you sick, and erodes your health.

Hopefully, it is becoming clear that the emotional sensitivity of mood power is fortified and preserved by high energy levels and a sense of optimism.

A light heart, easygoing nature, and the absence of stress and tension are also important in maintaining a good mood. You can do this. When order replaces disorder and serenity replaces chaos, you know that you have mastered the skill of lightening up your life.

Relaxation is the Key

Relaxation in mind and body is the prescription of choice to lighten up your life and stabilize a good mood. Relaxation is a way of life. It is a state of mind. It is the joyful feeling of being completely free. The art of relaxation is the art of being calm in mind and body. Keep in mind that real relaxation is effortless. When you feel good about yourself without feeling any strain or stress, you can enjoy being relaxed. This is very conducive to keeping a good mood. Relaxation is that breakthrough feeling of having no expectations and yet enjoying the moment in its total depth and dimension.

When you can feel at home wherever you are and with whatever you are doing, you've discovered the key to relaxation. Use these questions to help you determine whether you are relaxed in whatever you are doing. Remember, the more relaxed you are, the better your mood and your ability to prevent stress. Take a moment out of a busy day and answer these questions.

- Are you feeling lighthearted?
- Do you feel calm and peaceful?
- Do you feel a sense of inner joy in your heart?
- Do you feel like you are being yourself?
- Are you going at your own pace?
- Do you feel at home and good about yourself?

When you can answer yes to the majority of these questions, you are relaxed. When you answer no, you are not relaxed. The habit of relaxation is learned from being at one with yourself. The habits of relaxation lead to the habits of happiness. Do you take pride in the following:

- Knowing who you are?
- Knowing what you love to do?

Once you know who you are and what you love to do, it is easy to learn how to relax. Then you can just follow your heart. When you are relaxed, you can comfortably and successfully deal with any stress or surprise in your life. Relaxation leads to mood power. When you relax, you are centered, peaceful, and able to cope with whatever is happening in your life. Relaxation leads to light thinking. Light thinking leads to a light mood. Light thinking and light moods lead to healthy, lighter eating habits.

In order to utilize the most effective relaxation techniques to manage and prevent stress, there are three types of relaxation that you should be aware of.

THREE KINDS OF RELAXATION
• Passive relaxation • Creative relaxation • Active relaxation

Passive Relaxation

Going to the movies, watching TV, getting a massage, taking a nap, and going to a ballgame are all examples of passive forms of relaxation. They take you away from your hectic daily routine. These modes of getting unwound usually do not involve any effort whatsoever. On these grounds alone, passive relaxation can be valuable. Passive relaxation, however, can be limited in its benefits and effects. Creative and active forms of relaxation are much more effective in managing and preventing stress.

Creative Relaxation

Creative self-expression is important. The total mental and emotional involvement in writing, painting, composing, dancing, meditation, or playing a musical instrument, rechannels your energy into relaxed productivity. This is healing therapy for your mind, your nerves, and your mood. Creative relaxation gives you a heightened sense of well-being.

Active Relaxation

In addition to passive and creative relaxation, other forms of more active relaxation come into play. Active relaxation is meditation in movement. Active relaxation has a way of soothing both the mind and the body. It is involved participation in life, as opposed to being a passive spectator. In activities that are both mental and physical—such as jogging, yoga, swimming, dancing, exercising, lovemaking, or those physically adventurous times with your friends and loved ones—you can get the greatest benefits of relaxation. Meditation is also an effective active relaxation technique that coordinates the concentration of your mind with deep breaths and heartfelt love.

It is only through active relaxation that you can become powerful and grounded in regulating your mood. It keeps you balanced. Take a look at some of the different active, creative, and passive relaxation techniques listed below. Make a point to include more active and creative relaxation activities than passive ones.

Active Relaxation	Creative Relaxation	Passive Relaxation
• Meditation	• Playing a Musical Instrument	• Watching TV
• Exercise	• Painting	• Going to a Movie
• Yoga	• Writing	• Taking a Nap
• Tai Chi	• Dancing	• Going to a Ballgame

Begin Today and Be Consistent

Incorporating the right relaxation techniques will take you a long way in lightening up your life. Now, let's take it one step further. To master the habit of relaxation, make sure to come to terms with the following questions:

- What situations make you tense and make you feel uptight?
- What strategy can you take to prevent this?
- What are the main ways you know how to fully relax and have fun?

- How much time every day do you spend fully relaxing and having fun?
- Do you have a relaxation deficiency?
- Do you have enough fun and laughter in your life?
- If not, what can you do about it today?

Now, let's get at the root of any emotional burdens that may have a grip on your heart. It's important to face them, express them, grieve, and then let go. The following questions will help you figure out how you can go about lightening up your life.

- What about your thinking needs to lighten up (e.g., chronic worry, anxiety, insecurities, guilt, etc.)?
- What about your feelings needs to lighten up (e.g., unresolved stress, anger, fear)?
- What about your prevailing mood needs to lighten up?
- What about your body needs to lighten up (e.g., your weight, tension in your neck)?

Acquire the Habits of Active Relaxation

Regular exercise will teach you how to relax physically. Daily meditation will show you how to relax mentally. Deep breathing exercises will help you unwind and let go. Learn to do one thing at a time with full concentration, and this will lead you to an automatic state of relaxation. Learn to live in the moment—"Be here and now"—and this will relax your soul! Avoid borrowing problems from the past or worrying about the future. Learn to find your center, and stay in touch with your true feelings.

The habits of relaxation empower you to let go of the anxiety and restlessness that undermine and sabotage your eating habits. In this way, relaxation supports mood power. Count on it! Relaxation is conducive to a good mood. When you find yourself stressed and are having a difficult time relaxing, use the following seven-point formula to get you back on track.

The LYF Seven-Point Yield-and-Empty Relaxation Formula

The next time you find yourself uptight, call a timeout and practice this three-minute drill:

1. Find a natural setting; for example, a garden, a park, or the beach. Sit with your back straight and relax your physical body.
2. Quiet your mind. Experience the silence, and look within.
3. Identify with what you love the most. Inhale and expand with these feelings of inner joy.
4. As you exhale, yield and empty any tensions or anxiety in your mind or body. This will empty your mind. Continue to inhale and exhale in this fashion for at least three minutes.
5. Fully experience yourself in the moment. Be 100 percent involved in breathing in love and exhaling stress.
6. Continue to let go of all bodily tensions until you feel centered.
7. Relax and creatively enjoy your divine bliss!

Make Sure to Keep It Light!

Keeping it light empowers you to unload the emotional stress in your life. Most Americans suffer from a serious overload of seriousness. Our culture doesn't value relaxation. But imagine for a moment if you could replace all the stress in your life with relaxation. What a wonderful world it would be! Relaxation requires letting go and lightening up. Don't worry; it won't impede your professional progress. After all, it's common knowledge that people perform better when they feel calm, secure, and confident, as opposed to irritable, afraid, and impatient. So value downtime in your life. Make it a point to have fun. Encourage your sense of humor. Indeed, keep it light.

Mood Factor #5—Your Food and Your Mood

I think it is most valuable to take a closer look at the relationship between food and mood. I want you to understand the intimate connection between your foods, your moods, and your eating habits. This will help strengthen your mood power. Interestingly, there are entire new fields of nutrition emerging, with research delving into how nutritional chemistry influences your moods and your emotions. The art and science of emoto-nutrition has evolved over the last thirty years and analyzes the dynamic interplay between your diet and your emotions. These studies have revealed two fundamental principles that govern the food-to-mood relationship.

THE TWO FUNDAMENTAL PRINCIPLES OF EMOTO-NUTRITION
1. Your Moods Influence Your Eating Habits.
2. Your Food Selection and Eating Habits Influence Your Moods.

The first principle of emoto-nutrition, the art and science of the mood-food connection, is very simple. You are already familiar with it. This is a must-know. I know that you know this. It's essential to understanding what motivates you to eat.

Principle #1—Your Moods Influence Your Eating Habits

We've already established that moods have everything to do with appetite and eating habits. Perhaps most important, we have discovered that chronic, dysfunctional, compulsive, and impulsive eating habits are driven by unresolved emotional tension and can mask mood disorders.

The first principle of emoto-nutrition takes these ideas a step further. You see, mood stability and a sense of well-being groove your eating habits to fit your long-term intentions. When you are in a good mood, you are more likely to eat from hunger as opposed to appetite. You are typically absorbed in enjoying whatever you are doing; when the hunger pangs come around, you are usually ready for a meal. In other words, you feel good, and it feels right to honor smart eating habits.

Principle 2: Your Food Selection and Eating Habits Influence Your Moods

This is the flip side of the equation. Not only does mood influence food selection, but food influences mood. Not only is there a mood behind each food, but there is a food behind each mood. The Smart Food choices you make nurture and feed mood empowerment. Your mood benefits and so does your nutritional health.

How exactly do your food choices influence your mood? Smart eating habits do an excellent job of balancing your body chemistry. In addition, smart eating habits also balance your brain, or emotional, chemistry. Smart Foods have a steadying, stabilizing, neuro-chemical effect on your emotions. I have seen this a million times. Food plays a dominant role in determining mood. Smart eating empowers you to regulate your own neuro-chemical and neuro-glandular systems: your hormones, master glands, neurotransmitters, and nervous system. Smart Food promotes superior function of the liver, pancreas, adrenals, pituitary, thyroid, hypothalamus, limbic system, and immune system. In other words, you benefit from a strong set of nerves and a stockpile of emotional strength. When your nerves and glands are strong, you are in position to take charge of your emotional life and deal strategically with day-to-day ups and downs. Furthermore, Smart Foods are "pro-generative"—your body becomes healthier and healthier over time, enabling you to quickly adjust to setbacks. This ability to maintain your physiological and neuro-chemical balance is a key benefit of the Smart Food-mood connection. As a result, the Smart Food choices you make nurture and feed mood empowerment. Everybody wins! Your mood benefits and so does your nutritional health.

Feed your brain and nervous system Smart Food, and you'll achieve mood power. This is the purpose of understanding and adhering to principle #2 of emoto-nutrition.

Smart Foods
Mood Power
Smart Eating Habits
Mood Power
Permanent Weight Loss

Unhealthy Foods
Moodiness
Poor Eating Habits
Moodiness
Weight Gain

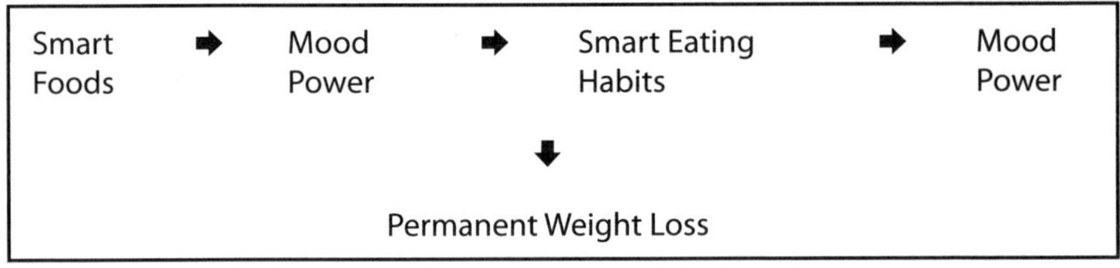

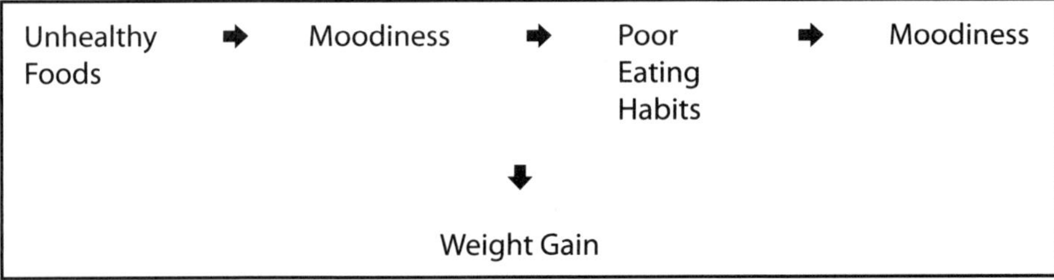

Know What Not to Eat: Avoid the Top Ten High-Stress Foods

We've discussed how Smart Foods can bolster your mood power. We've also reviewed how the wrong food choices increase stress and can exacerbate anxiety, trigger moodiness, and deepen depression. When you do not eat Smart Foods and own erratic eating habits, you are subject to moodiness and mood swings. When it comes to eating the wrong foods, some are worse than others. Check out the foods to avoid below. These foods play havoc with your metabolism, your nerves, your hormones, and your blood chemistry. They stress vital organs, such as the liver and the kidneys, and lead to moodiness and long-term fatigue. At this point, you're quite familiar with the culprits. They're many of the same foods that are hazardous to your long-term health and vitality.

TOP TEN STRESS FOODS
1. Candy, cookies, and other sugary sweets
2. Refined carbohydrates, such as pretzels, white crackers, white rice, white bread, and refined breakfast cereals
3. Soda and other sugary soft drinks
4. Ice cream and rich desserts
5. Alcohol
6. Caffeine
7. Bacon, hamburgers, and other beef and pork products
8. High-fat dairy products and cheeses
9. Junk food
10. Salted chips, pretzels, and party foods

About the Authors

Barnet Meltzer, M.D., is the founder and Director of the Meltzer Wellness Institute in Del Mar, California. He has been a board certified physician and surgeon for 40 years. Dr. Meltzer graduated Phi Beta Kappa from an Ivy League medical school, did his internship at UCLA, and then served two years of surgical residency at the University of California Medical Center in San Diego (UCSD). Dr. Meltzer is a pioneer and nationally recognized expert in the field of Preventive Medicine, Integrative Medicine, and Clinical Nutrition. He has authored six books and has an international following, having brought his teachings to South America, Mexico, Central America, and the South Pacific. Dr. Meltzer owns the distinction of being the first medical doctor to enter the clinical practice of Preventive Medicine and Alternative Medicine in Southern California, and retains a thriving private practice in Del Mar, California.

Jordan Meltzer is the President of the Meltzer Wellness Institute, and is integrally involved in the development and expansion of the institute's wellness programs. He is currently pursuing his PhD in Integrated Health Sciences. Prior to joining his father at the Meltzer Wellness Institute, Jordan spent 6 years working in finance; he spent 3 years investment banking for Goldman Sachs and 3 years working for the private equity investment firm, Friedman, Fleischer & Lowe. Jordan graduated with honors from the University of California, Berkeley.

INDEX